your pregnancy
week by week

parenting

your pregnancy
week by week

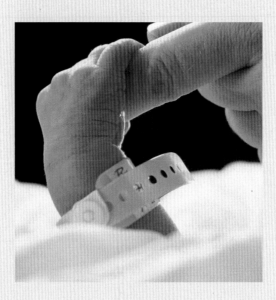

hamlyn

An Hachette UK Company
www.hachette.co.uk

First published in Great Britain in 2005 by
Hamlyn, a division of Octopus Publishing Group Ltd
Endeavour House, 189 Shaftesbury Avenue,
London WC2H 8JY
www.octopusbooks.co.uk

ISBN 978-0-600-61034-2

A CIP catalogue record for this book is available from the British Library

Printed and bound in China

15 14 13 12 11 10

Your pregnancy week by week has been produced in association with *Practical Parenting* magazine

Practical Parenting® is a registered trademark © IPC Media Ltd 2005

To subscribe to **Practical Parenting** call 0845 6767778 or click on www.ipcmedia.com

contents

foreword

Pregnancy is a special time in a woman's life, a unique journey to a new and exciting future. Pregnancy is also a time of great physical, emotional and social change, a time to look to new responsibilities, to explore, to learn new things about ourselves, and for the vast majority of women, it is a time of celebration and happiness.

Facing great and lasting change, however beautiful that change is, can be daunting. Having been a midwife for many years, I know the value of the support, advice and care that midwives give to women every step of the way, throughout pregnancy, labour and after the birth, and nothing can surpass the care of a professional. But, I also know that today's women seek to learn for themselves, to research, to question and to explore. Information is available everywhere, from friends and family, in magazines, in the media and on the Internet, and advice from so many sources, though good, can be overwhelming. With so much information, in so many different places, it's sometimes difficult to find what is needed.

This book will help to answer some of your questions about pregnancy. It will guide you through the physical and emotional changes that you will experience, and give you some tips on taking good care of yourself and involving your partner, family and friends in this journey. It will complement the support and care you will receive from your midwife and help you to ask her any questions you might have.

Enjoy this exciting time and enjoy the future to come. I commend this book to you, and I wish you all the very best on your own unique journey.

Dame Karlene Davis DBE
General Secretary
The Royal College of Midwives

introduction

Firstly, congratulations on having a reason to buy this book.

Whether you are thinking about starting a family or are already on the way to becoming one, you will no doubt be as anxious as you are excited. The amazing physical journey from getting pregnant to giving birth can seem completely overwhelming when it is happening to you, despite the very obvious (and also rather comforting) fact that many other women have done the exact same thing, often several times over!

You wouldn't be human if you didn't have weird and wonderful thoughts, hopes, fears and feelings, not to mention hundreds of questions that change and develop as your body changes and develops too. Whatever your questions, fears or anxieties, you won't find a more useful guide than the one in your hands right now. Created by a down-to-earth team of experts, many of whom are also parents, this book mixes practical advice, useful information and personal anecdotes to help deliver peace of mind to you as you wait to deliver your very own creation.

Dip in as every new question or symptom surfaces, or enjoy reading the book from cover to cover, but rest assured that the answers and inspiration you need are all here.

Enjoy this amazing time, and give your baby (or babies!) a welcome to the world hug from the team at *Practical Parenting*.

Best wishes for a happy and healthy pregnancy.

Mara Lee

Mara Lee
Editor
Practical Parenting

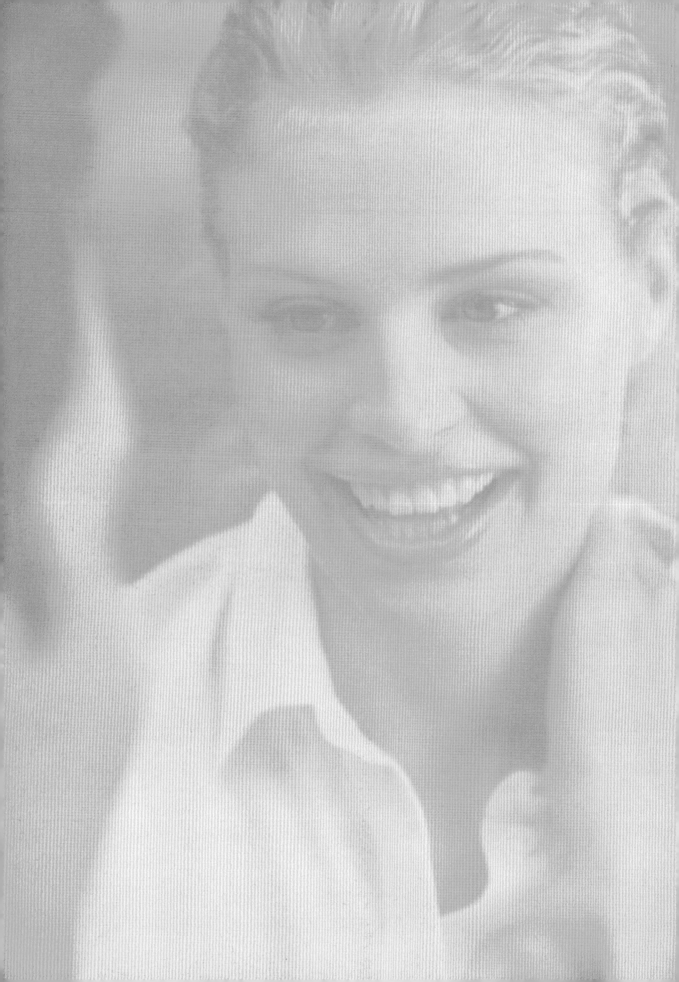

preparing for
pregnancy

Deciding to have a family is one of the most momentous decisions you are likely to make in your life, and the idea of becoming a parent can take some getting used to. Your mind may be brimming over with questions: When is the best time to try to get pregnant? Can I guarantee the sex of my baby? And, the dreaded one, what if I find out I cannot get pregnant? This section answers all these questions and more.

changing your lifestyle

Not everyone can plan their pregnancy well in advance, and many women have a perfectly healthy pregnancy with no special preparations at all. However, if you and your partner have the luxury of time to get in the peak of health and fitness before you conceive, you will improve your chances of conception and also have a greater chance of a healthy pregnancy and a healthy baby.

You should start preparing yourself for pregnancy at least 3 months ahead of trying for a baby, but ideally aim for 6 months or more. This will give you sufficient time to build up good nutritional reserves and eliminate all traces of the ill effects of alcohol and smoking from your system. Your partner doesn't get off scot-free either, because the quality of his sperm depends on his diet and lifestyle.

nutrition

One of the most important aspects of pre-conceptual preparation is optimizing your nutrition. The early weeks of your baby's gestation are crucial and, at this stage, before you even realize that you are pregnant, your baby will be taking all the nutrition he needs from your body's reserves. There are some nutrients in particular that you need to be well stocked up on before conception, the most important being folic acid. If you start taking a supplement of 0.4 mg (400 micrograms) a day at least 3 months before you conceive, and continue to take it for the first 12 weeks of your pregnancy, you will reduce your chance of having a baby with a neural tube defect (such as spina bifida) by 50–70 per cent.

other supplements

To ensure that you are getting all the vitamins and minerals necessary for you and your baby before you conceive, it is best to eat a balanced healthy diet. You may like to take a multivitamin supplement that has been specifically formulated for pregnancy, particularly if you follow a restricted diet, for example if you are a vegetarian or a vegan.

changing bad habits

Smoking in the 3 months before you try for a baby can reduce your chances of conception by a third. Caffeine may also affect fertility. The first month of pregnancy is when your baby is most at risk of alcohol-related abnormalities, so cut down or give it up altogether.

weight

If you are trying to conceive, it is best if your weight is in the healthy range (see the Body Mass Index chart opposite). Being either overweight or underweight can affect your fertility, and crash dieting, yo-yo dieting or excessive exercise can affect ovulation and your chances of conception. If you need to lose weight, do so sensibly and gradually well before you start trying to conceive. If you are underweight, aim to eat at least three nutritious, balanced meals a day – do not binge or fill up on fatty, sugary snacks because this will not help you to lay down the nutritional reserves needed to keep you and your baby healthy through pregnancy.

health checks

If you have specific health worries, or any conditions that you think might affect your pregnancy, discuss these with your midwife before stopping contraception. Mention any long-term medication you are on, as well as herbal supplements or homeopathic remedies, as some of these can affect your ability to conceive or harm the fetus. At the same time, arrange to have your immunity to rubella (German measles) checked.

If you have recently had a baby, your body may not be ready for another pregnancy. Generally, it is best to allow at least a year between full-term pregnancies.

If you are within the normal weight range for your height, you are less likely to suffer problems such as high blood pressure or diabetes during pregnancy. A BMI of 20–25 is ideal for optimum health.

Orange band (BMI under 17)
You may have difficulty conceiving. If you are poorly nourished when you become pregnant, your baby may lack nutrients before the placenta is fully developed and able to supply him from your blood.

Yellow band (BMI 17–19)
You are a little underweight, but if you gain at a reasonable rate your baby should be fine. You may need extra food to make enough milk in order to breast-feed.

Pink band (BMI 20–25)
This is the weight range associated with fewest problems.

Lilac band (BMI 26–30)
You are a little heavy, so are more likely to suffer discomforts such as heartburn, varicose veins, tiredness, breathlessness or skin irritation caused by friction and perspiration.

Purple band (BMI over 30)
Women in this band tend to suffer from health problems that can complicate pregnancy, such as high blood pressure and diabetes. Medical procedures such as fetal heart monitoring and epidurals can be more difficult, and the baby may be slightly heavier than average.

body mass index

The Body Mass Index (BMI) provides a guide to the best weight range for good health when you are not pregnant, regardless of your age or body type. You usually start to gain weight after about 12 weeks of pregnancy, so your midwife will record your BMI at your booking visit, to help her to assess risk.

body mass index chart

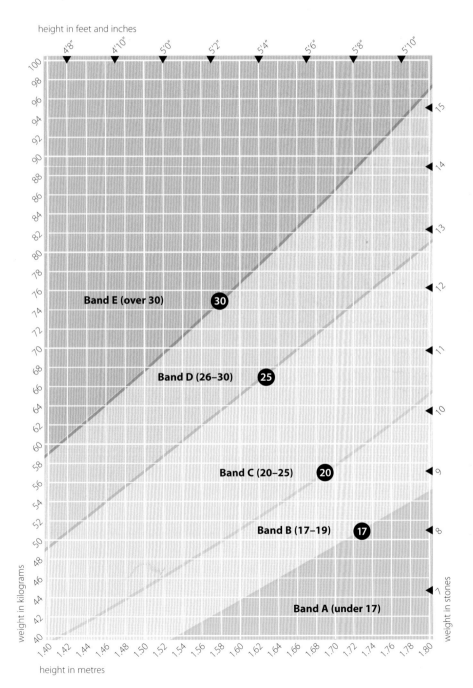

the female
body

If you think of everything that a woman has to do to bring a baby into the world, you realize what a feat of engineering the female body is. Your body has to produce an egg, ready to be fertilized by a sperm, and provide the right environment for that egg to grow and develop until it becomes a fully developed baby. Then you have to give birth, bringing that baby into the world, ready to lead an independent life.

female internal anatomy

Before you get pregnant, the uterus is roughly the size and shape of a pear and weighs about 60 g. The ovaries lie between the fimbriae at the end of the Fallopian tubes, through which a fertilized egg will travel to the uterus.

the female reproductive system

Before you start trying to conceive, it is a good idea to familiarize yourself with the workings of your reproductive system. You will soon be coming across words such as 'ovulation' and 'cervix' more often than you imagine, from the moment you attempt to get pregnant, throughout all your antenatal tests and check-ups, to the birth itself. The more you know about your reproductive body parts and what they do, the more in control and confident you are likely to feel when talking to your doctor or midwife. So the sooner you learn what all the different terms mean, the better!

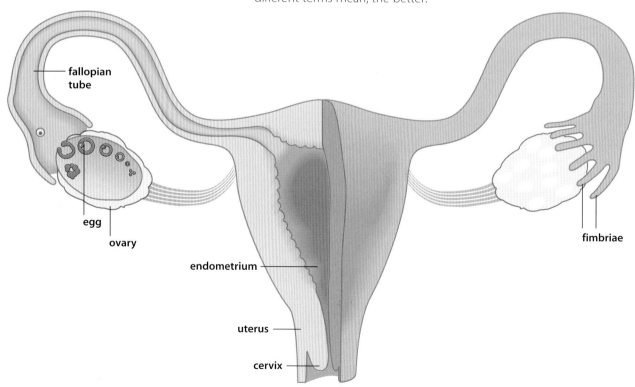

fallopian
tube

egg

ovary

fimbriae

endometrium

uterus

cervix

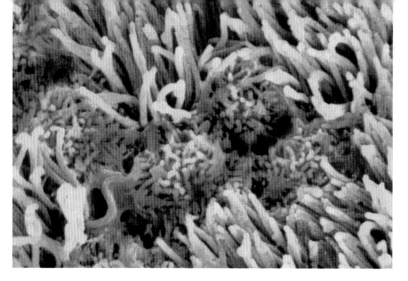

This magnified picture shows the cilia, the sea-anemone-like fronds that help stroke the egg down the length of the Fallopian tube.

ovaries

All the eggs you will ever produce are stored in your ovaries before you are born. When you begin menstruating, your body is finally mature enough to reproduce and one egg is released approximately every 28 days until you reach the menopause. The release of the egg is called ovulation, and usually each of your two ovaries produces an egg on alternate months. The ovaries also produce oestrogen which thickens the lining of the womb ready to receive the fertilized egg.

eggs

One egg is referred to as an ovum, while several eggs are ova. Each month, about 20 eggs begin to ripen inside the follicles in your ovaries. One egg will ripen before the others and be released from the follicle.

fallopian tubes

You have two Fallopian tubes (oviducts), one running from each ovary down to the uterus. When an egg is released from an ovary, it is drawn into the Fallopian tube. Slight contractions of the Fallopian tube help to move the egg towards the uterus. This takes a couple of days, during which time the egg may be fertilized by a sperm.

uterus

The egg moves into the uterus (womb), which is like a bag with a thick muscular wall and, if it is fertilized, it implants in the endometrium.

endometrium

This is the spongy lining of the uterus that has been prepared ready to receive the fertilized egg. If the egg is not fertilized, this lining is shed – this is your period. If a fertilized egg implants in the lining, it starts to develop, and a placenta will begin to form.

cervix

This is the neck of the uterus, through which the baby passes at birth. It is normally closed, with a tiny opening through which blood seeps during a period. In the early stage of labour, it dilates (opens) gradually – you are said to be in established labour when it is 2–3 cm dilated.

know your body

Understanding what is where in your external anatomy can be a help.
Labia majora (large lips). Folds of tissue enclosing the genital organs.
Labia minora (small lips) Just inside the labia majora, surrounding the openings to your vagina and urethra.
Perineum The area between the vagina and anus.
Urethra This opening carries urine from the bladder to the outside.
Clitoris This is the small protrusion between the labia minora.
Vagina Where your baby emerges.
Anus The opening at the far end of the digestive tract through which faeces leave the body.

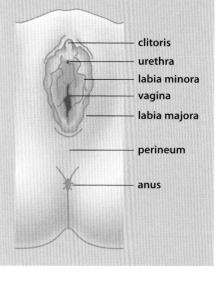

clitoris
urethra
labia minora
vagina
labia majora

perineum

anus

the male body

The body of a man is less focused on the business of reproduction than that of a woman. Once he has produced his sperm, his part in the process of starting a new life is finished, and the woman takes over as she spends the next 38 weeks with the baby growing and developing inside her. However, it is just as important for him to live healthily in the months before conception as it is for her.

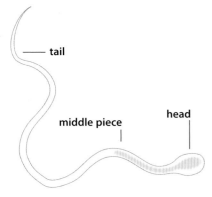

tail

middle piece

head

sperm

Healthy sperm can swim towards an egg at speeds of 2–3 mm a minute. Only a few hundred will reach the egg and only one of those will penetrate the outer layers of the egg to fertilize it.

the male reproductive system

This system is by no means simple and it is brilliantly designed to maximize the chances of impregnating a woman. Unlike a woman and her eggs, a man does not have a store of sperm when he is born.

scrotal sac

This is the bag of skin that contains and protects the testes. It holds them outside the body where temperatures are slightly cooler.

testes

Sperm are made in the testes (singular: testis), or testicles, and are constantly being replenished. Sperm production begins at puberty and continues until very late in life, although it starts to slow down in late middle age. It takes about 70–80 days to produce a mature sperm, ready for ejaculation. Of the hundreds of million sperm in any one ejaculation, only a couple of thousand survive the journey into the uterus and on to the Fallopian tube.

male reproductive organs

The scrotum is held outside the body in order to maximize sperm production, which is at its highest when the testes are about 1°C cooler than the core body temperature.

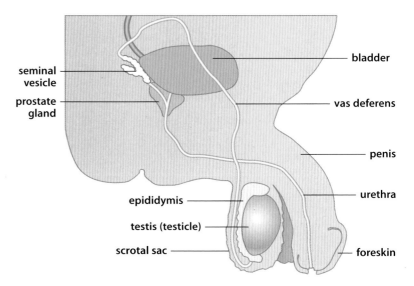

seminal vesicle

prostate gland

bladder

vas deferens

penis

urethra

epididymis

testis (testicle)

scrotal sac

foreskin

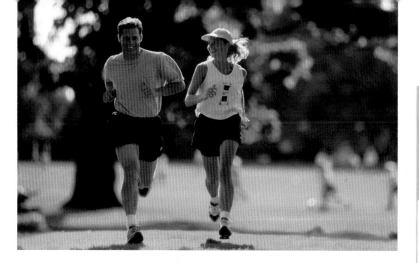

It's not just about you – your partner needs to be fit and healthy, too, for the best chance of conceiving a healthy baby.

sperm
Each sperm is about 0.05 mm long and consists of three parts: a head, which contains all the genetic information; a middle piece, which provides the energy for the sperm to propel itself along, and a tail, which swishes from side to side as the sperm swims towards the egg.

epididymis
The sperm mature in this part of the testis.

vas deferens
When the sperm are mature, they pass along the vas deferens (sperm ducts) from the epididymis to the seminal vesicles.

seminal vesicles
Sperm are stored here until a man ejaculates. The sperm mix with fluid made in the seminal vesicle, and other fluids from the prostate gland, to form semen, which is projected along the urethra.

urethra
During ejaculation, contractions at the base of the penis force semen along this tube, which runs all the way from the bladder, through the prostate gland and along the penis to its tip.

ejaculation
When a man ejaculates, semen containing sperm is projected from the seminal vesicle, along the urethra and out of the penis. In each ejaculation, between 2 and 6 ml of semen are released, each millilitre of which contains between 35 million and 200 million sperm. Not all of these are normal, healthy sperm – about a quarter of them cannot swim and have no chance of making it to the egg.

Q **I am getting fit and healthy, ready for pregnancy, but my partner is drinking and smoking as normal. Is it important for him to be healthy too?**

A   It takes about 70–80 days to make a sperm so it is important that your partner stays fit and healthy in the run-up to conception. An unhealthy lifestyle can increase the risk of abnormal sperm, which can compromise your chances of conceiving. Your partner should:

Cut down on alcohol Drinking more than 3½ units a day can reduce sperm count, so he should cut down at least 3 months before you try to conceive.

Stop smoking Cigarettes can damage sperm and increase the likelihood of birth defects.

Eat a healthier diet

Avoid stress This lowers a man's sperm count.

Keep fit – but not too fit! Excessive exercise or being underweight can lower the sperm count – but being overweight can raise body temperature, lowering sperm count. Your partner should aim to be in the normal range on a Body Mass Index chart and do moderate, sensible exercise.

Avoid wearing tight-fitting underwear and trousers These can raise the temperature of the testicles, which can lower the sperm count.

trying to
conceive

Once you are fit and ready for pregnancy, it is time to start trying to conceive. The decision to abandon contraception may produce a mixture of emotions: excitement, anxiety, happiness or apprehension. Do not get too anxious about counting days and time-tabling intercourse – studies show that you are more likely to conceive if you are relaxed and happy!

your ovulation time

There are a number of ways of working out the exact time of ovulation.

keep a calendar

Note the day your period starts and how many days it lasts. If you have a straightforward 28-day cycle, you probably ovulate on day 14. Otherwise, it is a little more complicated because ovulation generally occurs 14 days before the start of your next period, and this can be difficult to predict if your cycle is irregular.

keep a temperature chart

Just after ovulation, your body temperature increases very slightly and stays at this level until after your period. By taking your temperature at the same time every morning and plotting the readings on a chart, you can pinpoint when ovulation occurs (just before the temperature rise). You will need to take readings for a few months in order to work out an average pattern for your cycle.

monitor your cervical mucus

The mucus that your cervix produces to help sperm swim up to the uterus is often discharged from your vagina. By noting any changes in its texture, you can spot when you are ovulating. When you are fertile, the mucus looks like egg white and is stretchy.

ovulation kits

Most pharmacies sell ovulation-predictor kits. These are quite easy to use: you simply urinate onto a test-stick each day around the middle of your menstrual cycle.

The test, which is 99 per cent accurate, detects the increase in luteinizing hormone (LH) that predicts when you are about to ovulate.

remember to have sex

The key to getting pregnant is to have sex at least every 48 hours during your fertile period. This ensures that there are plenty of sperm available whenever there is an egg ready to be fertilized. It may help to stay in bed a while after having sex. Although sperm are designed to swim towards your cervix, you can help them on their way by lying down – or even sticking your legs in the air!

timing your pregnancy

Timing your pregnancy is tricky because it is impossible to predict how long it will take you to conceive. Every couple is different, and all sorts of things, such as age, general health and the type of contraception you have been using, affect conception. Generally, you should allow at least a year: 3 months for trying to conceive and 9 months for the pregnancy. If you want to improve your health and fitness (see page 10) beforehand, you should allow a further 6 months.

stopping contraception

Barrier methods of contraception, such as condoms or a diaphragm, allow you to conceive as soon as you stop using them. Once you stop taking the contraceptive pill or using an intra-uterine device (IUD, or coil), you should aim to have at least one 'normal' period before trying to conceive. Some women have a burst of fertility as soon as they stop taking the pill, while others find their

Your estimated date of delivery (see 'your due date' below for how to use this table)

		1	2	3	4	5	6	7	8	9	10	11	12	13	14	15	16	17	18	19	20	21	22	23	24	25	26	27	28	29	30	31
LMP	January	1	2	3	4	5	6	7	8	9	10	11	12	13	14	15	16	17	18	19	20	21	22	23	24	25	26	27	28	29	30	31
EDD	Oct/Nov	8	9	10	11	12	13	14	15	16	17	18	19	20	21	22	23	24	25	26	27	28	29	30	31	1	2	3	4	5	6	7
LMP	February	1	2	3	4	5	6	7	8	9	10	11	12	13	14	15	16	17	18	19	20	21	22	23	24	25	26	27	28			
EDD	Nov/Dec	8	9	10	11	12	13	14	15	16	17	18	19	20	21	22	23	24	25	26	27	28	29	30	1	2	3	4	5			
LMP	March	1	2	3	4	5	6	7	8	9	10	11	12	13	14	15	16	17	18	19	20	21	22	23	24	25	26	27	28	29	30	31
EDD	Dec/Jan	6	7	8	9	10	11	12	13	14	15	16	17	18	19	20	21	22	23	24	25	26	27	28	29	30	31	1	2	3	4	5
LMP	April	1	2	3	4	5	6	7	8	9	10	11	12	13	14	15	16	17	18	19	20	21	22	23	24	25	26	27	28	29	30	
EDD	Jan/Feb	6	7	8	9	10	11	12	13	14	15	16	17	18	19	20	21	22	23	24	25	26	27	28	29	30	31	1	2	3	4	
LMP	May	1	2	3	4	5	6	7	8	9	10	11	12	13	14	15	16	17	18	19	20	21	22	23	24	25	26	27	28	29	30	31
EDD	Feb/Mar	5	6	7	8	9	10	11	12	13	14	15	16	17	18	19	20	21	22	23	24	25	26	27	28	1	2	3	4	5	6	7
LMP	June	1	2	3	4	5	6	7	8	9	10	11	12	13	14	15	16	17	18	19	20	21	22	23	24	25	26	27	28	29	30	
EDD	Mar/Apr	8	9	10	11	12	13	14	15	16	17	18	19	20	21	22	23	24	25	26	27	28	29	30	31	1	2	3	4	5	6	
LMP	July	1	2	3	4	5	6	7	8	9	10	11	12	13	14	15	16	17	18	19	20	21	22	23	24	25	26	27	28	29	30	31
EDD	Apr/May	7	8	9	10	11	12	13	14	15	16	17	18	19	20	21	22	23	24	25	26	27	28	29	30	1	2	3	4	5	6	7
LMP	August	1	2	3	4	5	6	7	8	9	10	11	12	13	14	15	16	17	18	19	20	21	22	23	24	25	26	27	28	29	30	31
EDD	May/Jun	8	9	10	11	12	13	14	15	16	17	18	19	20	21	22	23	24	25	26	27	28	29	30	31	1	2	3	4	5	6	7
LMP	September	1	2	3	4	5	6	7	8	9	10	11	12	13	14	15	16	17	18	19	20	21	22	23	24	25	26	27	28	29	30	
EDD	Jun/Jul	8	9	10	11	12	13	14	15	16	17	18	19	20	21	22	23	24	25	26	27	28	29	30	1	2	3	4	5	6	7	
LMP	October	1	2	3	4	5	6	7	8	9	10	11	12	13	14	15	16	17	18	19	20	21	22	23	24	25	26	27	28	29	30	31
EDD	Jul/Aug	8	9	10	11	12	13	14	15	16	17	18	19	20	21	22	23	24	25	26	27	28	29	30	31	1	2	3	4	5	6	7
LMP	November	1	2	3	4	5	6	7	8	9	10	11	12	13	14	15	16	17	18	19	20	21	22	23	24	25	26	27	28	29	30	
EDD	Aug/Sep	8	9	10	11	12	13	14	15	16	17	18	19	20	21	22	23	24	25	26	27	28	29	30	31	1	2	3	4	5	6	
LMP	December	1	2	3	4	5	6	7	8	9	10	11	12	13	14	15	16	17	18	19	20	21	22	23	24	25	26	27	28	29	30	31
EDD	Sep/Oct	7	8	9	10	11	12	13	14	15	16	17	18	19	20	21	22	23	24	25	26	27	28	29	30	1	2	3	4	5	6	7

menstrual cycle takes a few months to settle down. If you want to wait until you are completely fit and healthy, you could stop taking the pill or have your coil removed and use a barrier method until the time you want to get pregnant.

your due date

Your midwife will use a chart similar to the one shown above to give you an estimated date of delivery (EDD). This date will be used to check your baby's growth and development.

Your EDD will be 40 weeks from the first day of your last menstrual period (LMP), not from the day you think you conceived. This is more accurate because not all women ovulate at the same stage of their cycle. However, because the date is based on an average 28-day cycle, only 5 per cent of women actually give birth on their EDD.

To work out when your baby is likely to be born, look up the day and month of the first day of your last period, then look at the line below to find your EDD.

fascinating facts

- Each month, you have a 20 per cent chance of conception.
- Your fertility begins to decrease (if you are a woman) from the age of 25.
- 75 per cent of couples trying for a baby conceive within 9 months of trying and 90 per cent do so within 18 months.
- In the United Kingdom, the United States, Belgium and Germany, more babies are conceived in November than in any other month. This is probably because of the winter nights drawing in. January is the most popular month in Switzerland and Holland, while August is the most popular month in Sweden.
- Sperm swim at 2–3 mm per minute.

boy or girl?

You may have a clear idea of what sex you would like your baby to be. Perhaps you want a baby of the opposite sex to your first child – or you may have medical reasons. In some countries, such as the United Kingdom, scientific methods of sex selection are legal only in cases of genetically inherited diseases so, if your reasons are a matter of preference, try some of the natural methods described here.

X or Y?

The sperm and egg are the only cells that contain 23 chromosomes rather than 23 pairs. The sex of a baby is determined by whether the sperm that fertilizes the egg carries the X or Y version of chromosome 23.

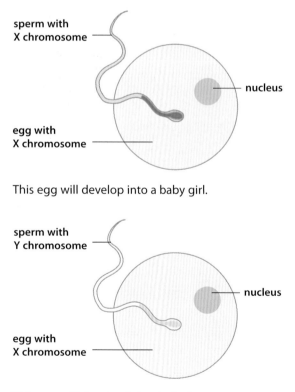

This egg will develop into a baby girl.

This egg will develop into a baby boy.

what are little boys and girls made of?

Every egg and sperm contains 23 chromosomes. Of these, one chromosome is a sex chromosome. Each egg contains one X chromosome, while every sperm contains either one X or one Y chromosome. If the sperm which fertilizes the egg contains a Y chromosome, the baby will be a boy; if it contains an X chromosome, the baby will be a girl.

Left to nature, there is a good balance of the sexes: about 103 boys are born for every 100 girls. However, there is a real danger that the scientific methods of sex selection currently being developed will upset this natural balance.

scientific sex selection

There are currently two main scientific methods of sex selection:

Pre-implantation genetic diagnosis (PGD) This procedure involves removing a cell from the developing embryo conceived through IVF (see page 30) for genetic testing to identify whether it has X or Y chromosomes.

Sperm sorting This involves separating male and female sperm either by spinning live sperm in a device called a centrifuge or by using a fluorescent dye to detect the X and Y chromosomes in the semen sample.

In some countries, such as the United Kingdom, PGD is illegal except where there is a high risk of a serious genetic disease being passed on (for example, haemophilia affects only boys, so if a couple is at risk of passing on a gene for this condition, a doctor could recommend sex selection methods to ensure they conceive a girl, see right). Fertility procedures involving frozen sperm or live embryos are regulated by the Human Fertilization and Embryology Authority (HFEA). Fresh sperm do not come under its jurisdiction and can currently be sorted for sex selection, although not at any clinic licensed by the HFEA.

natural sex selection

There are various natural methods that you can use to try to influence the sex of your baby. You can choose one that suits you or try a combination of them. However, even if you get the result you want, you will never know whether the method worked or if it was just chance.

timing intercourse

One of the most popular methods is timing when you have sex, which is based on the theory that male sperm swim faster than female sperm but die sooner.

For a boy Abstain from sex for 2–3 days before you ovulate, then have intercourse as soon after as possible so the speedier male sperm will reach the egg first.

For a girl Have sex 2–3 days before ovulation, so that the male sperm will have died by the time the egg is released, and the longer-living female sperm will have a greater chance of reaching the egg.

acid or alkaline?

Male sperm are said to prefer an alkaline environment while female sperm prefer an acidic environment. It should therefore be possible to influence the sex of your baby by making your vagina more acid or more alkaline. You should do this about half an hour before you have intercourse.

For a boy Flush your vagina with a solution of bicarbonate of soda (alkaline).

For a girl Flush your vagina with diluted lemon juice or vinegar (acid).

diet

Some women swear by dietary methods.

For a boy Eat foods rich in sodium and potassium, for example, meat, dried and salted fish, rice, pasta, potatoes and beans, and certain fruits and vegetables such as bananas, apricots and celery.

For a girl Eat foods rich in magnesium as well as calcium, for example, dairy products, eggs, nuts, soya beans, leafy green vegetables and fresh fruit juice.

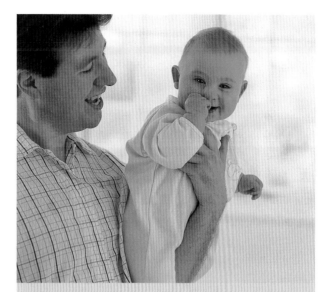

should you try to influence the sex of your baby?

As well as the danger of upsetting the natural balance of the sexes, there are other considerations. If you are keen enough to take measures to influence the sex of your baby, you may be very disappointed if they fail. This could lead to problems bonding with your baby and even cause post-natal depression. If this is a possibility, it might be better not to try for another baby, or to adopt a more laid-back approach, letting nature take its course and resolving to accept whatever sex of baby you have.

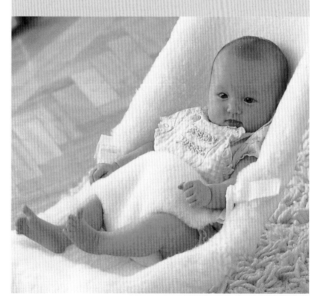

fertilization of the egg

When your partner's sperm meets your egg and the two fuse together at the moment of fertilization, a miraculous event occurs: the beginning of a brand-new life. From this point onwards, the fertilized egg assumes a life of its own, growing and developing at an amazing rate until, some 9 months later, a fully formed, unique, complex human being emerges into the world.

the first few days

the journey of the egg

Once the egg has been released from one of your ovaries (ovulation), it is drawn into the Fallopian tube. Slight contractions of the tube help to move the egg towards the uterus, helped by tiny hairs, called cilia, which wave and shift the egg along. The egg can survive in the Fallopian tube for 24 hours and, if it is not fertilized, it will be reabsorbed by your body.

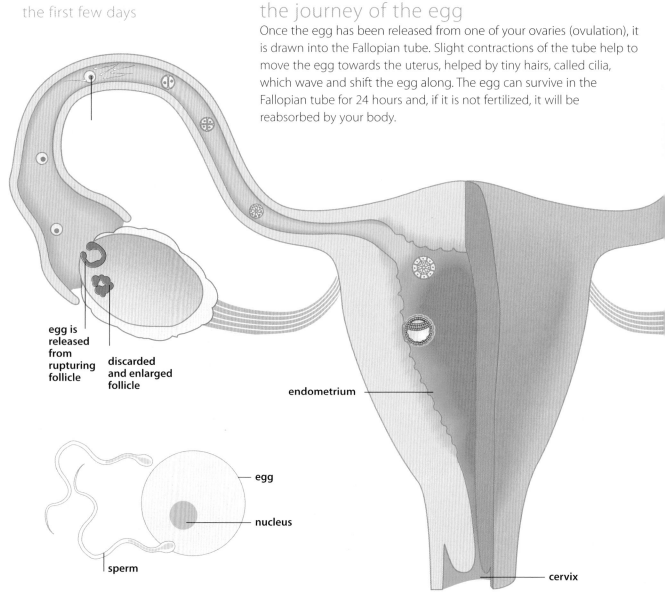

egg is released from rupturing follicle

discarded and enlarged follicle

endometrium

egg

nucleus

sperm

cervix

As the egg is released, your body begins to prepare for the possibility that it may be fertilized: the lining of your uterus, the endometrium, becomes thick and spongy, ready for a fertilized egg to implant. If fertilization does not take place, the endometrium will come away and you will start to bleed as another menstrual cycle begins.

the journey of the sperm

After ejaculation, the sperm swim very quickly from the vagina into the cervix (the neck of the uterus), through the uterus and into the Fallopian tube towards the waiting egg. The egg releases chemicals that tell the sperm where it is and attracts them towards it. The sperm race to penetrate the egg, but only one sperm will succeed: once penetrated, the egg releases chemicals that 'seal' it so that no other sperm can break through. Once the sperm has broken through the surface of the egg, its tail breaks off.

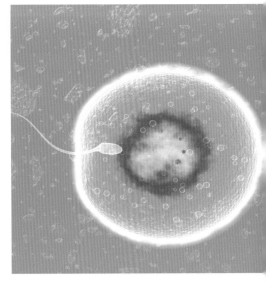

Only one of the millions of sperm released during ejaculation will fertilize the single egg.

after fertilization

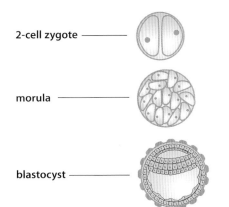

Once the egg and the sperm have fused, they become a new type of cell, called a zygote. The sperm and egg each contained 23 chromosomes, so the zygote contains 46 chromosomes. The zygote then travels slowly along the Fallopian tube, dividing into identical cells as it goes – first two, then four, then eight, and so on. By about day 4 it is a solid ball of cells and is called a morula. When it reaches the uterus it is a hollow ball of 50–100 cells and is called a blastocyst. It takes around 6 days for the blastocyst to reach the uterus and implant. Once implanted, it continues to grow and develop until it becomes an embryo.

2-cell zygote

morula

blastocyst

Fertilization usually takes place in the Fallopian tube. Once the egg has been fertilized, hormones prevent the endometrium from breaking down. The blastocyst burrows into the endometrium before sprouting finger-like projections that will develop into the placenta.

when an egg fails to implant

In some cases an egg can be successfully fertilized by a sperm but fails to implant in the uterus. This is usually because of an abnormality in the fertilized egg that means it cannot survive. If this happens, you usually will not even know that your egg was fertilized. You will just have a slightly later period than usual, possibly with heavier bleeding.

genes and inheritance

The genetic information that makes your baby the person she is comes from you and your partner. The sperm and egg each contain 23 chromosomes. When the sperm and egg fuse, the fertilized egg then contains 23 pairs of chromosomes. Each chromosome contains thousands of genes that determine everything from eye and hair colour to intelligence, personality and physical health.

what is a chromosome?

Chromosomes are elongated structures made up of thousands of genes, threaded together like beads. Every cell in your body contains 46 chromosomes, except for an egg cell or a sperm cell, which contain 23 chromosomes each. As a result, when the sperm and egg cells come together, they form a new cell that contains 46 chromosomes, in 23 pairs. This one cell then divides over and over again as it develops into a baby, and every cell in your baby's body contains the same genetic information as the very first cell.

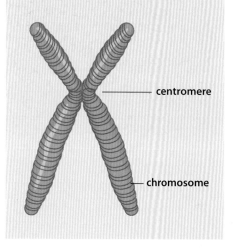

centromere

chromosome

genetic inheritance

Because your baby inherits half of her genes from you and half from your partner, she will have a unique combination of genetic material. As a result, your baby could inherit your eye colour but your partner's nose shape, your short legs but your partner's mathematical ability. Although the environment in which your child grows up, and the experiences she has, will contribute to the person she becomes, her genetic make-up is determined at the moment of conception.

dominant and recessive genes

In most cases, the two sets of genes, one from each parent, blend together so that your baby becomes a unique combination of genetic characteristics. However, some genes are 'stronger' and take priority over others: these are called dominant genes. Weaker genes are called recessive genes. For example, the gene for brown eyes is dominant while that for green eyes is recessive. As a result, if you have brown eyes and your partner has green eyes, your baby's eyes are more likely to be brown because your genes will dominate.

genetic surprises

To complicate matters, both you and your partner each carry genes from each of your parents, who carried genes from their parents, and so on. These genes are passed on from generation to generation, but may remain recessive for a long time until they suddenly pop up years later. For example, you may have blonde hair and your partner black hair, but you could still have a baby with red hair. How does this happen? At some time in the past, someone in each of your families must have had red hair. The gene for red hair is recessive so, although it is been passed from generation to generation, a more dominant gene, such as black or brown hair, has always dominated and no one has had red hair. Now, you and your partner both pass on a gene for red hair. The gene is recessive but when two recessive genes come together your baby ends up with red hair.

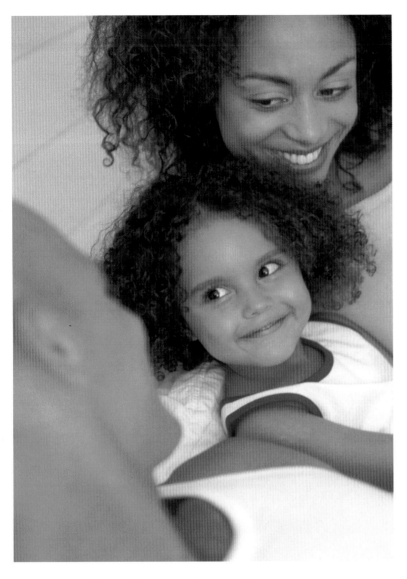

Your child will be a unique combination of your genes and your partner's genes and her genetic make-up is determined at conception.

genetically inherited conditions

Just like the genes that determine appearance, genes for inherited conditions can be dominant or recessive. Diseases such as cystic fibrosis, thalassaemia and sickle-cell anaemia are passed on through a recessive gene. This means that many people can carry the gene for the disease without actually suffering from the disease, as a dominant normal gene takes precedence over the disease gene. If two people who each carry a gene for a condition have a child together, that child has a 25 per cent chance of inheriting two disease genes, in which case they will suffer from the condition.

If you, your partner or any member of your family has an inherited condition, you should discuss this with your doctor before you try to conceive. You may be referred for genetic counselling or, if you are already pregnant, you may be offered tests to determine whether your baby is affected by the condition (see pages 126 and 128).

diseases that affect only one sex

There are some diseases, such as muscular dystrophy and haemophilia, which are carried on the X chromosome, the one that determines sex. In girls, the defective X chromosome is masked by a normal X chromosome, so they can carry the disease but will not be affected by it. Boys, however, have only one X chromosome and the other is a Y chromosome, so the disease cannot be masked and, if the defective chromosome is passed on, the child will be affected by the disease.

Because these diseases only affect boys, it may be possible for members of families who carry the gene for muscular dystrophy or haemophilia to opt for sex selection, so that they conceive only girls (see page 18).

how twins are formed

The discovery that you are expecting twins can be a shock. It is perfectly natural to worry about how you will cope with two babies, but you will also have a real sense of excitement. There is something different about expecting twins: other mothers to be will want to ask you what it is like, and you will receive extra care from medical professionals as well, adding to the feeling that something special is happening.

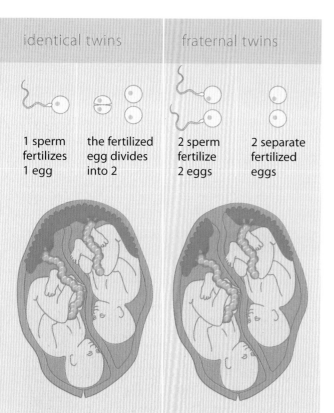

identical twins		fraternal twins	
1 sperm fertilizes 1 egg	the fertilized egg divides into 2	2 sperm fertilize 2 eggs	2 separate fertilized eggs

Although most sets of identical twins share a placenta, they do not share an amniotic sac. One of the pair may be bigger because he obtains more nutrition from the shared placenta.

About half of sets of fraternal twins will be of different sexes, and a quarter each boy-boy and girl-girl. They do not share a placenta, so each will be closer in size.

the likelihood of twins

If you have undergone fertility treatment, you will have a greater chance of conceiving more than one baby. Fertility drugs such as clomiphene (see page 28) make you more likely to release more than one egg at a time, while in the case of in vitro fertilization (IVF,) more than one embryo is usually implanted (see pages 30–31), so you may end up having twins or triplets. On average, 25 per cent of women using either fertility drugs or IVF conceive twins.

You are also more likely to conceive fraternal twins if there is a family tendency to do so, especially through the maternal side. Your age is also a factor in this: women who over 30 years old produce more follicle-stimulating hormones than earlier in life so they are more likely to release more than one egg at a time when they ovulate.

finding out if you have twins

If you have had no reason to suspect that you are expecting twins, you may not have a routine ultrasound scan until you are 12 weeks or more pregnant, by which time the two babies will be clearly distinguishable in the image. If you have had fertility treatment, you will probably have an early ultrasound scan at around 6 weeks into your pregnancy, and even at this stage of your pregnancy you will be able to see two tiny heartbeats on the monitor screen.

identical or not?

There are two types of twins: identical and fraternal (non-identical). Which type a woman has depends on how they were conceived.

Identical twins occur when one egg splits into two after it has been fertilized by a sperm. Because the twins develop from two halves of the same fertilized egg, they contain identical genetic information, so they will be the same sex, look very alike and even have similar personalities. Around one in three sets of twins are identical, and two-thirds of these will share a placenta while in the uterus. Each has their own amniotic sac.

Fraternal (non-identical) twins occur when a woman produces two separate eggs that are then fertilized by two different sperm. These babies will not be any more or less alike than any other pair of siblings, and each will be contained within their own amniotic sac and have their own placenta, although the latter may fuse during the pregnancy. Very rarely, a single egg may split before being fertilized by two different sperm. In this case, the babies are likely to be very similar although not identical because only half of their genetic information will be the same.

conjoined twins

If a single egg fails to split properly after fertilization, conjoined twins (sometimes known as Siamese twins) will develop. Conjoined twins occur only very rarely – about once per 200,000 live births. There are various types, depending on where the twins are joined. Although it may be possible to separate conjoined twins after birth, the condition carries serious health risks, especially if the twins are sharing vital organs or have a complex shared blood supply.

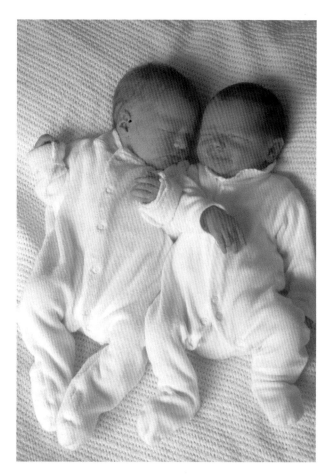

Like peas in a pod, these babies will have just as special a bond for life in the outside world as they did when they shared a uterus for 9 months.

Q **My mother has a twin brother. Does this make it more likely that I will have twins myself?**

A Identical twins do not tend to run in families but fraternal (non-identical) twins do, especially through the maternal side. So, because your mother has a twin brother, the chances of you conceiving fraternal (non-identical) twins are certainly higher than average. This would also be the case if you are a fraternal twin, have twin siblings or have already produced one set of twins yourself.

---

triplets

Triplets are becoming more common as a result of fertility treatments. However, in some countries, women under 40 can only have two embryos implanted with each IVF cycle, so the most they will conceive is twins. There are three types of triplets:

Three identical triplets if one egg splits into three after fertilization.
Two identical and one non-identical triplets if two eggs are released and only one splits in two.
Three non-identical triplets if three separate eggs are fertilized.

fertility problems

If you are struggling to conceive, it can seem as if the whole world is pregnant except you. The reality is that about one in six women has difficulty conceiving, and even women in fertile couples, who are having regular unprotected sex, have only a 20 per cent chance of getting pregnant each month. So, if you have been trying for a few months without success, do not despair.

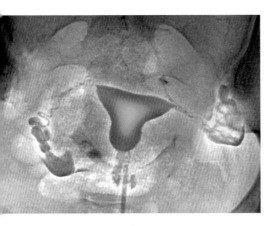

During a hysterosalpingogram blue-green dye is injected through the cervix, filling the uterus and Fallopian tubes.

when to look for help

If you have been trying for a baby without success for 12 months, it is worth talking to your doctor about your concerns. In some cases, it is worth seeking advice after only 6 months, for example if you are over 35 and do not have regular periods; if you or your partner have had a sexually transmitted disease (STD); a pelvic or abdominal injury or surgery; or if there is a tendency to fertility problems in your family.

what happens next?

Your doctor will take a medical history and ask you some questions about your menstrual cycle, how long you have been trying to conceive and your lifestyle. After some preliminary tests, he will probably refer you to a fertility specialist for further investigation.

There is no need to feel upset or embarrassed about talking through your fertility problems: every day, doctors and specialists see people with similar problems, which are a lot more common than you might think. It is important that you and your partner are emotionally prepared for the investigations you may have to go through. Some of the procedures are unpleasant, and waiting for results can be stressful. Remember that you want to have a baby together and there is no need to feel guilty if you discover that one or both of you have fertility problems.

tests by your doctor

You will be given a smear test and an internal examination and will have to provide urine and blood samples. Tests for hormone levels will show whether you are ovulating. Your blood will also be checked for STDs, as some, such as chlamydia, can affect fertility. Your partner's penis and testes will be examined, and he will be asked to go home and provide a semen sample to be sent to a laboratory for testing.

tests by a specialist

After these preliminary tests, you may be referred to a fertility specialist, who will carry out further investigations. These may include:

An ultrasound scan to look closely at your ovaries.

A biopsy, which will involve removing a tiny part of the endometrium. This procedure can be performed either with or without a local anaesthetic. The sample will then be checked in the laboratory to see whether it is becoming thick and spongy enough after ovulation to allow a fertilized egg to implant.

There are two main tests used for checking the correct functioning of the Fallopian tubes.

A hysterosalpingogram (HSG) involves injecting dye into the uterus, using a catheter passed through the cervix, so the fluid's progress up through your Fallopian tubes can be seen on an X-ray. There is no need for a general anaesthetic.

A laparoscopy and dye is performed under general anaesthetic and involves a telescope being passed through a small incision in your umbilicus (belly button). This enables the specialist to view your entire pelvis and reproductive organs. Dye can then be passed through the Fallopian tubes.

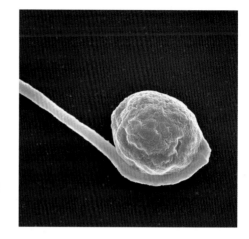

A deformed sperm may have no tail, more than one tail or – like the one shown here – a deformed head.

common causes of female infertility

Problems with ovulation A fine balance of different hormones is needed for the various stages of ovulation (the maturing and release of the egg) to occur. If any of these hormones is absent or not present in the right levels, ovulation may not happen. The ovaries may also be damaged, perhaps as a side-effect of radiotherapy or as a result of surgery or an infection.

Polycystic ovary syndrome (PCOS) Usually the eggs in the ovaries develop inside follicles until one is mature enough to be released. With PCOS, the follicles become cysts, so that the eggs cannot mature.

Endometriosis This condition occurs when the cells that normally make up the endometrium (the lining of the uterus) grow elsewhere inside a woman's body. They then bleed every month when she has her period, causing internal organs to become glued together with the blood and endometrial tissue.

The symptoms of endometriosis include painful and heavy periods. It can affect fertility if the ovaries, Fallopian tubes or uterus become damaged.

Damaged Fallopian tubes Damage or blockage by scar tissue can be caused by a previous ectopic pregnancy, by an infection such as chlamydia or by endometriosis.

Fibroids These benign tumours grow inside the uterus and do not usually affect fertility. Sometimes, however, they can press against the Fallopian tubes or interfere with the implanting of a fertilized egg. They can be removed surgically, if deemed necessary.

common causes of male infertility

Low sperm count This can range from none to a lower than average number; the normal range is 35 to 200 million per millilitre of semen.

Abnormal sperm The sperm may not be properly formed.

Bad sperm motility The sperm are neither fast nor agile enough.

Failure to ejaculate Some men suffer from retrograde ejaculation, where the semen goes backwards into the bladder during sex rather than into the vagina.

Blocked vas deferens The tubes that transport sperm from the testicles to the seminal vesicles ready for ejaculation may become blocked because of a defect or an infection.

Testicular failure Undescended testicles, that is, where the testicle is in the abdomen not the scrotum, injury to the testicles, chemotherapy, mumps after puberty or injury can all damage sperm production.

overcoming
fertility problems

If you have been trying to conceive a baby for a long time without success and have seen your doctor for investigations into your or your partner's fertility problems, the next step is to start treatment. There are four basic methods: drug treatment, sperm and egg donation, surgery and assisted conception, such as in vitro fertilization, or IVF (see page 30).

the stress factor

For many couples, the stress and anxiety involved in trying for a baby are to blame for difficulties in conceiving. It is easy to get hung-up on counting fertile days, filling in charts and having sex to order, but becoming obsessive about these things can often have the opposite effect to the one you are looking for. If conception is taking a few months, try to be relaxed about it. Remember that sex should be fun and a way of showing your love for each other, not just a way to make a baby. You may find that, if you stop counting, plotting and measuring and just try to have lots of sex without thinking too hard about the consequences, you will get lucky.

drug treatments

Drug treatments stimulate ovulation. They are often the first port of call for women with fertility problems, as they are relatively simple to use, very safe and have been used successfully for many years.

clomiphene

Ovulation is controlled by a finely balanced combination of hormones. Some of the hormones are collectively called follicle-stimulating hormone (or FSH). Clomiphene causes your body to produce FSH, which makes your ovaries produce the follicles in which the eggs can ripen.

One cycle of clomiphene treatment consists of a 5-day course of pills. You will be monitored while taking the drug so that your doctor can determine whether any mature eggs are being produced. However, it may be a couple of months after you take the drugs before you start to ovulate regularly.

sperm and egg donation

Some couples do not conceive a baby for the simple reason that the woman is not producing any eggs or the man is not producing any sperm. Treatments such as IVF rely on a couple's sperm and egg being fertilized outside the body, so if one of you is not producing sperm or ovulating, then your only chance of having a baby may be to accept sperm or eggs from a donor.

sperm donation

This procedure is a good option if the woman is fully fertile but the man is experiencing fertility problems and treatments used to boost his sperm count have failed. The donated sperm will have been frozen and are defrosted immediately before the procedure. The clinic will work out when you are ovulating and will sometimes recommend that you take fertility drugs, such as clomiphene, to make absolutely sure of this. The defrosted sperm are usually inserted directly into your uterus.

surgery

Women's fertility problems are often caused by damage to the Fallopian tubes (see page 27). If this is the case, there are two main surgical procedures that can repair the damage.

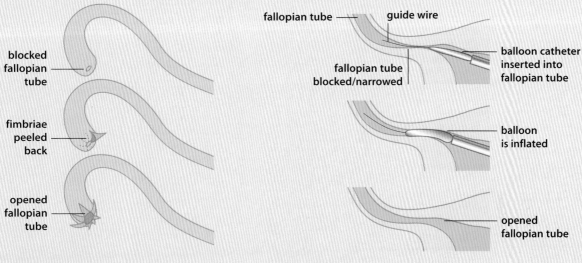

Fimbrioplasty is a procedure to open up a blocked Fallopian tube. The opening of the tube is made up of petal-like sections, called fimbriae, which sometimes fuse together and seal off the entrance. This operation peels back the fimbriae, opening up the tube so that the egg can pass through.

Tuboplasty is an operation to open up Fallopian tubes that have become blocked or narrowed. A catheter is inserted down the tube, and a balloon on the end is opened up to unblock the tube.

egg donation

If a woman is not ovulating and drug therapies, such as clomiphene, have not helped, but the man is producing healthy sperm, then egg donation could be a good option. The quality of the eggs that a woman produces declines as she ages, so this procedure can help women who choose to become mothers in later life. It can also help if your eggs have been destroyed by cancer treatments. You and your egg donor will take drugs to synchronize your cycles, so that she is producing eggs at the time your uterus is ready for an egg to implant. Once her eggs have been removed, they will be combined with your partner's sperm just as in normal IVF (see page 30).

embryo donation

Some couples who have extra embryos, created by IVF, donate them to other infertile couples. Receiving an embryo in this way is an option if there is a risk of you and your partner passing on a genetic disorder of which you are both carriers. It involves the same basic technique as IVF (see page 30).

handling reactions to childlessness

Anyone in a long-term relationship may have received comments from friends and relatives about 'the patter of tiny feet', the ticking of biological clocks or the wisdom of buying a large car. Such remarks can hurt if you are struggling to conceive, and it can be hard to know how to cope. One strategy is to plan your response in advance, deciding either to make light of it or to be completely honest and upfront about your situation.

in vitro
fertilization

In the process of in vitro fertilization (IVF), the part of conception where the egg is fertilized by the sperm takes place outside the body, in a glass dish – although many people imagine it is done in a test tube, which is the origin of the expression 'test-tube baby'. This process was first pioneered in the 1960s, and the first test-tube baby – named Louise Brown – was born in 1978.

the effects of IVF

The various stages of the in vitro fertilization process have different side-effects.

Taking drugs to suppress your ovaries may produce symptoms that are similar to those of the menopause. These can include hot flushes, sweating, night sweats, insomnia, dizziness, headaches and vaginal dryness.

Taking HCG (human chorionic gonadotrophin) to stimulate ovulation may produce symptoms similar to pre-menstrual tension (PMT), for example, anxiety, stress or tearfulness, bloating, sore ovaries or general aching and tiredness.

Collecting eggs may leave you feeling tired from the effects of the anaesthetic, and your ovaries and abdomen will ache.

Transferring embryos will leave you drowsy and you may feel emotional, and have sore breasts and a painful abdomen.

what it involves

Once you have been accepted onto a course of IVF treatment after tests and assessment, you will be offered counselling. IVF, like any fertility treatment, can be stressful and exhausting, and a counsellor can help with any emotional difficulties.

Next, you will be given drugs to suppress the activity of your ovaries. This involves 'sniffing' a hormone spray for about 21 days. After this, you will receive a course of injections to stimulate your ovaries to produce eggs. This is done so that the doctors can ensure that you produce a number of eggs at the same time. Your blood will be tested regularly and you will be given ultrasound scans so the doctors can check the progress of the eggs' development. It is important to get the timing right because the eggs will be collected within 2–3 hours of ovulation. When the follicles are almost ready to release eggs, you will be given an injection of human chorionic gonadotrophin (HCG), a hormone that will trigger the final maturing and release of your eggs.

what happens next

When your eggs are ready to be 'harvested' you will be given a local anaesthetic and, using an ultrasound scan as a guide, and a tiny needle, the doctor will remove several eggs. The needle is usually inserted through the top of your vagina but it can pass through your abdomen. You will be able to go home straight afterwards to rest.

Your eggs and your partner's sperm will be put together in a laboratory and left for a few days, by which time those eggs that have been fertilized will have divided many times and become embryos. Up to three embryos will then be placed into your uterus, using a catheter.

In some countries, such as the United Kingdom, if you are under 40, only two embryos will be used, to reduce the risk of your conceiving triplets. If you are over 40, you can have three embryos implanted if you wish, as it is less likely that all of them will implant. If more than three embryos have been produced, the extras can be frozen and used for another IVF cycle.

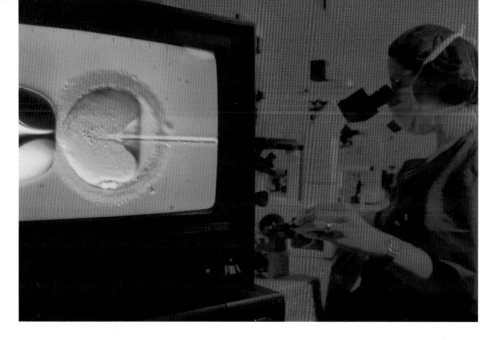

A single sperm is injected directly into an egg during this specialized type of IVF called ICSI – intracystoplasmic sperm injection.

the pros and cons

IVF has good success rates and means that a couple can conceive a baby using their own eggs and sperm. On the downside, it involves a lot of medical intervention, which at times can be painful and distressing, so if you need to have several cycles it can take its toll emotionally. Also, the drugs that boost ovulation can have unpleasant side-effects, and you will have to be monitored while you are taking them. It can also be expensive if you have to pay for it yourself.

tips for couples undergoing IVF

Decide early on who you are going to tell You may not want to tell the world what you are doing, but it can be stressful to keep it to yourselves, and it might help to have a friend or family member to whom you can talk. Also, you may need time off work for treatment, so confiding in a colleague can be useful in order to stop speculation about your frequent disappearances.

Consider donating eggs or sperm Some clinics give priority to couples who are prepared to do this for other couples with fertility problems, and it may mean a shorter wait for treatment.

Learn to give yourself injections In this way you will save yourself time and effort going to your doctor's surgery for the long course of hormones to suppress your ovaries. Remember that many people do not succeed at the first attempt; in many respects, it is a way for you and your doctors to find out how you respond to treatment.

Know when to stop It can be harder to give up than it is to begin – you may feel you are letting people down or being a quitter. But IVF is a hard slog, and it can be empowering to decide that it is no longer for you.

Keep communicating with each other If either of you feels in need of a break or is unable to cope with any more, do not be afraid to say: one partner may be soldiering on for the sake of the other. Keep talking about how long you want to continue, how you feel after each attempt and whether your desire for a baby makes it all worthwhile.

Q **How will I know if I'm pregnant?**

A As with a normal conception, you can do a pregnancy test after about 2 weeks – when your period is normally due – to find out if you have conceived. If IVF has been successful, at least one embryo will have implanted in the lining of your uterus and continued to develop.

It is difficult to say exactly what your chances of success are, as it depends on the nature of your fertility problems and your age. The average success rate across the United Kingdom is 17 per cent, while in the United States it is as high as 28–35 per cent. If you are pregnant, you will go on to be scanned and to have your antenatal care planned. If not, you may want to start considering another course of treatment, or take a break to think about what to do next.

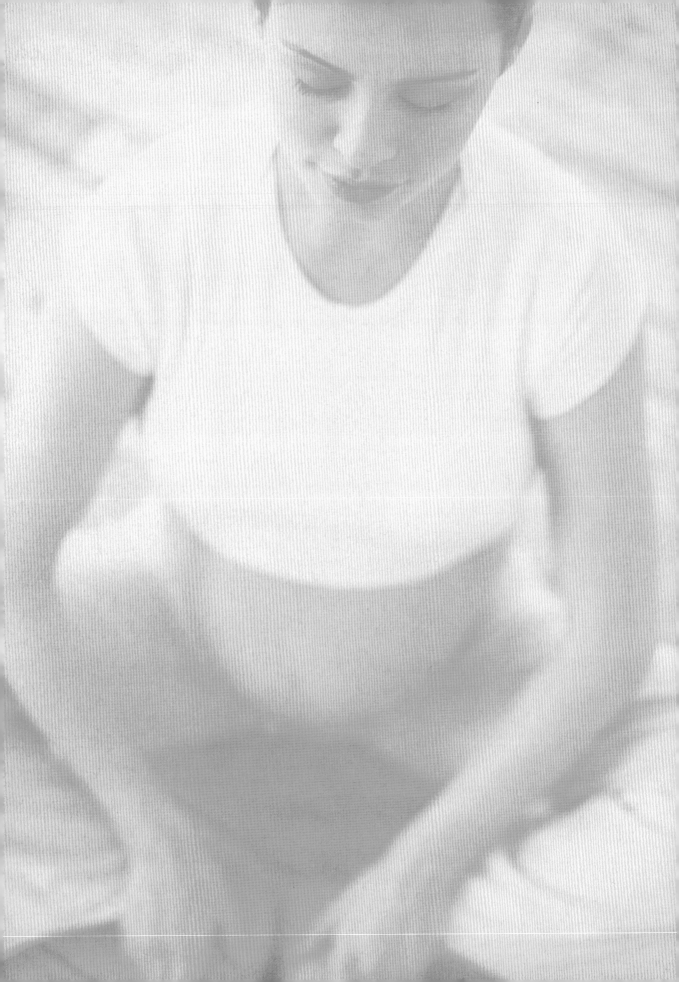

diet and
exercise

It is good to know there is so much you can do to promote the health and wellbeing of your baby during pregnancy – from eating oily fish to boost her brain power to brisk walking to top up energy levels. As well as the dos, though, there are a few don'ts. So, make sure you know exactly what foods you can and cannot eat and what exercises benefit both you and your growing baby.

diet during
pregnancy

A healthy diet is important for everyone but especially when you are pregnant. Your body needs the right fuel not only to function efficiently, but also to cope with the demands of your growing baby. The idea of eating for two means getting a balanced, healthy diet and increasing the nutritional quality of the food that you eat, not doubling the amount.

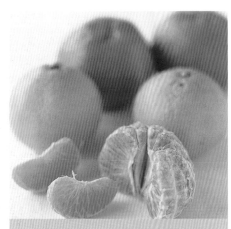

eating five portions of fruits and vegetables a day

This is not as difficult as it sounds. Try these suggestions.

- Add fresh fruit to your morning cereal.
- Drink a glass of fruit juice rather than a cup of tea (remember that any amount of juice you drink only counts as one of your five portions).
- Munch on carrot sticks during the day rather than crisps or cake.
- Add an extra portion of steamed vegetables to your evening meal.
- Eat a banana as part of your pre-bedtime snack.

On average, a pregnant woman needs to increase her daily calorie intake from 2000 to 2200 calories only in the last 3 months. You can obtain these extra 200 calories from any of the following:

- A 200 ml glass of semi-skimmed milk and one slice of wholemeal bread with cottage cheese.
- A large banana and a 150 ml glass of orange or other fruit juice.
- A small jacket potato with a little cheese.

The important thing is for you to eat as healthily as possible. In order to develop, your baby needs proteins, carbohydrates and the right fats, as well as vitamins and minerals. By eating the correct sorts of food in the right proportions, you will be sure of giving him the best possible start in life.

food groups

The following are the proportions of the foods you should be eating every day. Your daily food requirements include:

- Proteins: 2–3 portions.
- Dairy products: 2–3 portions.
- Complex carbohydrates (starchy foods): at least one third of your total calorie intake (As fats are more calorie-dense than complex carbohydrates, that is, 25 g of butter has far more calories than 25 g of brown rice, you would need to eat a lot less of the former to obtain the same number of calories).
- Fruits and vegetables: at least 5 portions.
- Fats: up to one-third of your total calorie intake.
- Simple carbohydrates (sugars): minimal.

proteins

Proteins, which are found in foods such as white and oily fish, meat, poultry, game, eggs, dairy products (see also opposite), lentils, pulses, beans, soya products, nuts and seeds, are essential for the maintenance and repair of every cell in your body and for the growth of new cells in your baby.

From the very beginning of your pregnancy your daily protein requirement increases by about 13 per cent overall.

Meat, fish and eggs are rich in iron and zinc, as well as vitamin B12, which works with folic acid to ensure that your baby develops a healthy nervous system. Oily fish is an excellent source of omega-3 fatty acids (see box below and pages 42–43) and vitamins A and D. Vitamin D helps the body to absorb calcium. Because you still need to be careful about how much, and what type of, fats you eat (see page 36), trim any excess fat from meat before cooking, and remove the skin from roast chicken, turkey or duck.

dairy products

Dairy products, such as milk, yoghurt and cheese, as well as containing small amounts of zinc and some B group vitamins, are rich in protein (see above) and calcium. Although your body becomes more efficient at absorbing calcium from foods when you are pregnant, you should include a variety of dairy products in your diet, especially towards the end of pregnancy.

complex carbohydrates (starchy foods)

Starchy foods, such as breads, grains, cereals and potatoes, should be the mainstay of anyone's diet, but it is particularly important during pregnancy that you obtain most of your energy from these foods rather than from fats or sugar. These carbohydrates are broken down and released into the bloodstream slowly, providing energy steadily throughout the day. This helps you to avoid feeling tired and may relieve the nausea of the first few months.

Grains and cereals also contain protein for growth and repair and B vitamins for cell development.

Choose from wholemeal or brown bread, potatoes, plantains, yams, couscous, brown rice and pasta, plus whole grains such as oats, barley and rye. Buy breakfast cereals that have been fortified with vitamins and minerals and are low in both sugar and fat. Starchy foods, especially wholegrain breakfast cereals, wholemeal bread and brown rice also provide fibre.

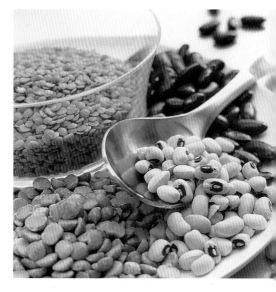

Eating a variety of foods is vital during your pregnancy. Legumes are a good means of adding extra protein.

omega-3 fatty acids

Omega-3 fatty acids are found in oily fish, such as mackerel, herrings, sardines, salmon, trout and fresh tuna, and in walnuts, soya beans, and rapeseed and linseed (flax seed) oils. They play a crucial role in the development of a baby's brain, nerves and eyes and have a beneficial effect on birth weight and length of pregnancy. Studies have shown that Inuit women, who eat plenty of oily fish, rarely give birth prematurely. (See page 42 for further information.)

did you know?
There are some suggestions that baby boys secrete a chemical that causes the mother to eat more during pregnancy!

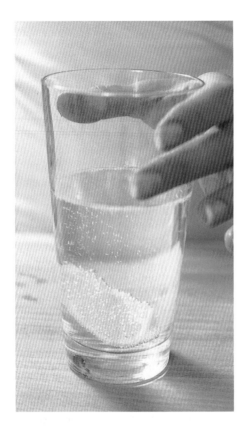

Try to drink at least eight glasses of water a day and watch how much tea, coffee and cola you drink.

fruits and vegetables

Fruits and vegetables supply valuable vitamins and minerals as well as dietary fibre, which helps to ease the constipation that a large proportion of women experience during pregnancy.

Fruits that are rich in vitamin C include citrus fruits, kiwi fruits, blackcurrants, and stone fruits, such as cherries, peaches and nectarines, mangoes and papaya. Vitamin C helps the body to absorb iron. Bananas are a good source of potassium, which is vital for cell growth.

Frozen vegetables are processed so quickly after picking that they often have more vitamin C than fresh vegetables, which often take days to reach the shops. Canned vegetables have already been cooked and may contain high amounts of salt so it is best to avoid them.

Green vegetables, such as spinach, kale, broccoli, watercress, green beans and brussels sprouts, provide folates (folic acid, see page 10), as well as vitamin K and iron. Leafy greens are also a good source of beta carotene (the safe, vegetable form of vitamin A) as are carrots, sweet potatoes, tomatoes and red peppers. Carotene and folic acid are lost in water and on heating, so prepare vegetables just before use. Wash them thoroughly, then steam or stir-fry them in a small amount of oil or, better still, eat them raw.

fats

Fats should provide up to one-third of the calories in your daily diet, which can be obtained from only minimal amounts of fatty foods. Beware of hidden fats in processed foods and try to replace saturated fats (for example, butter, cream and lard) with mono-unsaturated fats (for example, olive oil, and polyunsaturated fats, including sunflower oil). Fats found in oily fish, rapeseed oil and soya bean oil contain fatty acids, which are vital for your baby's development (see page 35).

simple carbohydrates (sugars)

Sugars are simple carbohydrates that are easily absorbed into the bloodstream and provide 'instant energy'. However, they contain few

Q **I am only 12 weeks pregnant and I feel hungry all the time – is this normal?**

A Lots of women feel hungry in the first few weeks, when their metabolism is increased, and often find that eating little and often helps to keep pregnancy nausea at bay. It is important that you eat a healthy, balanced diet. You should not worry about weight gain as long as you are eating healthily – pregnancy really is not the time to start dieting.

why iron is so important

Iron combines with protein to form haemoglobin in the red blood cells. This is the pigment that carries oxygen and carbon dioxide around your body. During pregnancy, the amount of blood in your body can increase by up to 30 per cent to meet the growing needs of your baby. Your body can store iron so, if you were eating healthily before conception, your iron stores should be sufficient. During pregnancy, your body can absorb more iron from foods, especially from red meat. Vitamin C increases iron absorption from vegetables and cereal sources, while tea hinders it.

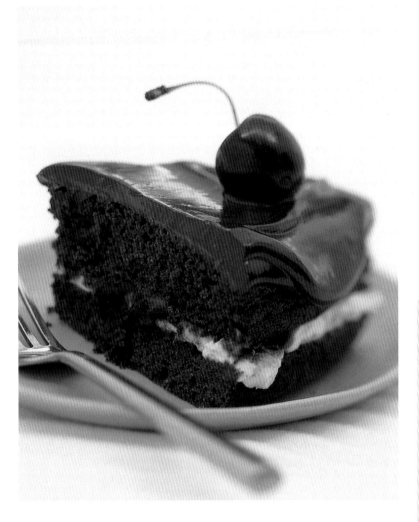

Foods that are loaded with sugars and fats, such as chocolate cake, are not complete no-nos, it is just best to indulge in a small amount once in a while rather than on a regular basis.

nutrients, if any, and may make you put on weight. You should avoid too many cakes, pastries, sweets and chocolate, and beware of the hidden sugars that are contained in many processed foods. Sucking on a mint occasionally may help to combat nausea, but be careful not to overdo it.

fluid intake

Your blood volume increases during pregnancy so it is important to keep up your fluid intake, even if you are feeling nauseous. Aim to drink eight 200 ml glasses of water a day – as well as fruit juice and other drinks, such as limited amounts tea, coffee or fruit squash. If you find that pregnancy sickness makes drinking even plain water unpleasant, try nibbling on moist fruits, such as watermelon, or sipping small amounts of fluid frequently.

‘ I am into kiwi fruit at the moment; before it was oranges. I don't find it hard to eat sensibly. I tend to listen to my body, and if it wants a Chinese takeaway every so often, I'll have one. I've put on about a stone, but it seems to be all babies. I can't eat a great big meal, so I try to eat about four or five small meals a day, when I'm hungry. I also eat a bit more than I want to, to make sure the babies are getting enough. I've read that since I'm carrying twins, I need around an extra 500 calories per day. ’

Sally, 18 weeks
pregnant with twins

shared experience

special
diets

If you have a restricted diet, either by choice or for medical reasons, you will probably be more aware than most people of what you eat. However, you may need to make some changes when you are pregnant in order to ensure that you are obtaining the correct nutrients in the correct proportions to meet the nutritional needs of both yourself and your baby.

vegetarian and vegan diets

It is not true that a vegetarian or vegan diet is bad for your baby. Like any pregnant woman, you need a balanced diet that supplies all the nutrition that you and your baby require, and you only need to make a few changes to your normal eating habits. Meat, fish and dairy foods supply protein, vitamins, minerals and essential fatty acids. To get the correct balance from a vegan or vegetarian diet simply takes a little ingenuity.

essential amino acids

Proteins are made up of substances called amino acids, eight of which cannot be manufactured in the body and are called essential amino acids. Vegetarians who eat dairy products and eggs will get all eight from these foods. Apart from buckwheat, quinoa, amaranth, soya beans and soya-based products such as tofu, no single plant source of protein contains all the essential amino acids, so non-dairy vegetarians and vegans need to ensure that they eat a mixture each type every day.

iron

You can boost your iron absorption from plant sources, such as beans, lentils, nuts, breads, fortified breakfast cereals, pasta, spinach, watercress and dried fruit, by eating them with foods rich in vitamin C, such as a glass of orange juice. Eggs also contain iron.

essential fatty acids

Sesame, sunflower and pumpkin seeds, linseed (flax seed) and walnuts are all rich sources of omega-3 fatty acids. Sesame and sunflower seeds, linseed and walnuts also provide omega-6 fatty acids.

vitamins and minerals

By eating a balanced vegetarian or vegan diet you should get enough vitamins and minerals. If you are unsure, ask your doctor, who may suggest a suitable supplement to take during pregnancy.

Choose cereals and breads fortified with vitamins and minerals. If you are not eating dairy foods, you must obtain sufficient calcium elsewhere – try fortified soya milk, soya yoghurts and tofu instead. Vitamin B12 is difficult to obtain in a vegan diet so eat foods such as yeast extract and fortified breakfast cereals and soya products, or ask for a supplement with vitamin B12.

food allergies

If you suffer from a food allergy or intolerance, you should avoid eating the food in question while you are pregnant or breast-feeding because you could pass on the allergy to your baby. If the baby's father, anyone in your immediate families or any of your older children has eczema, asthma, hay fever or a medically diagnosed food allergy, avoid peanuts and foods containing them while you are pregnant or breast-feeding.

diets for diabetes

For any person suffering from diabetes, managing blood-sugar levels is essential. In early pregnancy, this can be difficult because pregnancy sickness may prevent you from eating regularly. It is important to ask for advice about adjusting your calorie intake and eating habits to suit your changing requirements. If you develop diabetes during your pregnancy (see gestational diabetes, page 81), you should be referred to a specialist team that includes a dietician.

food safety

During pregnancy, changes take place in your immune system so that it does not reject your baby's DNA. This leaves you more at risk from food poisoning, which could put your baby at risk. As well as avoiding any foods that may be unsafe (see pages 40–43), you should also make sure that your own kitchen is a safe, hygienic place for food preparation.

hygiene

- Keep all food-preparation areas scrupulously clean.
- Change tea towels and dish cloths daily and wash them at the highest temperature possible.

buying and storing food

- Only buy food you will eat before its best-before date.
- Buy chilled and frozen foods at the last possible moment and bring them home in a cool-bag.
- Rewrap foods if needed and put them into the freezer or refrigerator as soon as possible. The coldest part of the refrigerator should be no higher than 5 °C and the freezer should be set to −18 °C or lower.
- Wrap raw meat and store it on a plate at the bottom of the refrigerator and keep eggs separate. Do not store milk and dairy products in the door.
- Store cooked and uncooked foods in different parts of the refrigerator and ensure that everything is covered.
- Throw away any food that has been in the freezer for longer than the manufacturer's guidelines.
- Always defrost food on a plate in the refrigerator.
- Never cook food that is not totally defrosted, unless the instructions say it may be cooked from frozen.

food preparation

- Use separate chopping boards for cooked meat, uncooked meat and vegetables.
- Wash all equipment in hot soapy water after use and knives between cutting meat and vegetables
- Wash your hands before and after preparing food and after handling raw meat or eggs.
- Always wash vegetables, fruit and salads.
- Rinse rice and pulses (dried and canned) before use.

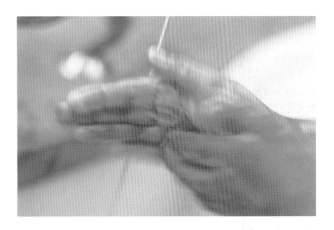

Pregnancy is not a time to be lax with personal hygiene and that applies to food hygiene, too. Wash your hands regularly to reduce the risk of infection.

cooking

Meat Make sure that meat and poultry are cooked thoroughly at oven temperatures of 180 °C or above. To test whether poultry is cooked, pierce the flesh through the thickest part with a skewer or a fork – the juices should be clear, never pink or red.

Fish The flesh should look opaque and flake easily when cooked.

Cook-chill foods Follow the manufacturer's recommended timings on packaged food. Make sure that the food is piping hot all the way through. If not, return it to the oven.

Barbecues Ensure the coals are white-hot before you start cooking. Check that meat is thoroughly cooked through. If it is still pink, put it back on the barbecue.

food guidelines

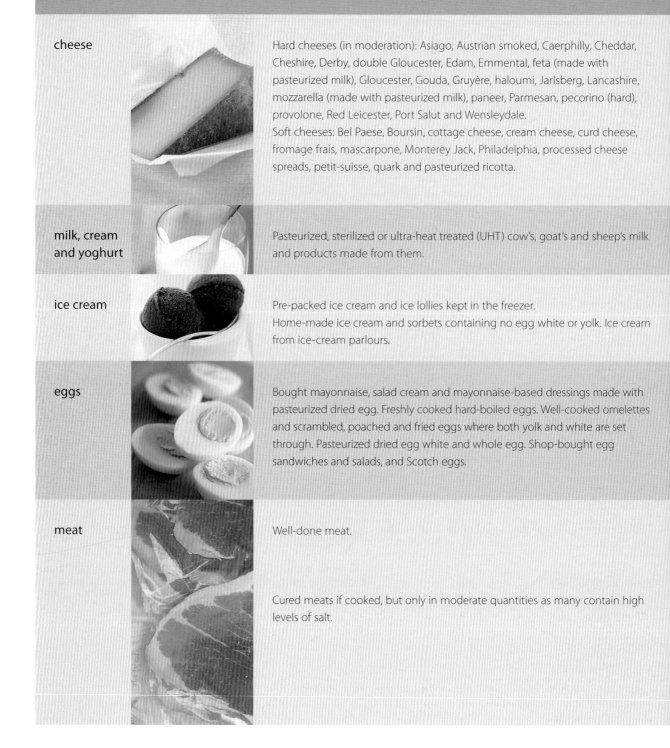

FOODS YOU CAN EAT

cheese

Hard cheeses (in moderation): Asiago, Austrian smoked, Caerphilly, Cheddar, Cheshire, Derby, double Gloucester, Edam, Emmental, feta (made with pasteurized milk), Gloucester, Gouda, Gruyère, haloumi, Jarlsberg, Lancashire, mozzarella (made with pasteurized milk), paneer, Parmesan, pecorino (hard), provolone, Red Leicester, Port Salut and Wensleydale.
Soft cheeses: Bel Paese, Boursin, cottage cheese, cream cheese, curd cheese, fromage frais, mascarpone, Monterey Jack, Philadelphia, processed cheese spreads, petit-suisse, quark and pasteurized ricotta.

milk, cream and yoghurt

Pasteurized, sterilized or ultra-heat treated (UHT) cow's, goat's and sheep's milk and products made from them.

ice cream

Pre-packed ice cream and ice lollies kept in the freezer.
Home-made ice cream and sorbets containing no egg white or yolk. Ice cream from ice-cream parlours.

eggs

Bought mayonnaise, salad cream and mayonnaise-based dressings made with pasteurized dried egg. Freshly cooked hard-boiled eggs. Well-cooked omelettes and scrambled, poached and fried eggs where both yolk and white are set through. Pasteurized dried egg white and whole egg. Shop-bought egg sandwiches and salads, and Scotch eggs.

meat

Well-done meat.

Cured meats if cooked, but only in moderate quantities as many contain high levels of salt.

FOODS TO AVOID	RISK
All soft, mould-ripened cheeses, even those made with pasteurized milk, such as Brie, blue Brie, Cambozola, Camembert, Chaumes, crottin, Lymeswold, Pont l'Evêque, Tallegio, vacherin, unless thoroughly cooked. Blue-veined cheeses, such as Bavarian blue, blue Cheshire, blue Shropshire, Blue Vinney, blue Wensleydale, Danish blue, dolcelatte, Gorgonzola, Roquefort and Stilton, unless thoroughly cooked. Avoid unwrapped cheeses from the delicatessen.	Listeriosis
All unpasteurized cheeses, such as fontina, especially soft ones.	Listeriosis or salmonellosis
Untreated cow's, goat's and sheep's milk, and products made from them.	Salmonellosis, E. coli 0157, toxoplasmosis, brucellosis
Home-made ice cream and sorbets containing egg white or yolk. Soft-whipped ice cream from kiosks or ice-cream vans.	Salmonellosis
Foods containing raw egg, for example, home-made mayonnaise, Béarnaise and Hollandaise sauces, mousses and uncooked home-made cheesecakes. Soft-boiled eggs and undercooked omelettes and scrambled, poached and fried eggs. Lightly cooked egg dishes, for example, tiramisu, zabaglione, crème brulée and soft meringues.	Salmonellosis
Raw and undercooked meat, including dishes such as steak tartare and carpaccio of beef.	Toxoplasmosis
Pre-cooked meat from the delicatessen.	E. coli 0157
Uncooked cured and smoked meats, such as bacon and hams, for example, Parma ham and other forms of prosciutto, sausages such as salami, mortadella and chorizo, and air-dried meat. Cold meat sold loose from the delicatessen.	Toxoplasmosis
Liver and liver-based products, for example, pâtés and liver sausage (Leberwurst).	High levels of retinol, a form of vitamin A considered harmful to unborn babies.

FOODS YOU CAN EAT

poultry and game	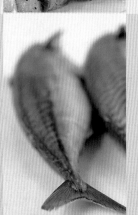	Thoroughly cooked poultry or game. Cooked and thoroughly reheated poultry or game. Pre-packed cooked chicken only if thoroughly reheated. Home-cooked chicken in sandwiches, salads and picnics, if kept chilled before eating.
fish		Properly cooked fish. Guidelines suggest no more than two portions of oily fish (mackerel, herrings, pilchards, sardines, salmon or trout) a week. Tuna – no more than two steaks or four cans per week. Shop- or restaurant-bought sushi and sashimi that has been frozen beforehand. Cooked smoked fish. Smoked salmon.
shellfish		Freshly and thoroughly cooked shellfish as part of a hot meal. Pre-cooked shellfish eaten cold, if kept chilled beforehand and used within sell-by date.
pâtés		
cook-chill foods		Foods that have been thoroughly reheated until piping hot all through. (Take extra care with dishes containing chicken, eggs or seafood.) Quiches, if reheated until piping hot. Pre-packed pies, pasties and pastry slices, if chilled and stored correctly.
fruits and vegetables		Raw or cooked, if peeled and rinsed or scrubbed clean under running water.
salads		Freshly made salads from well-washed ingredients. Dressed salads prepared immediately before eating (see mayonnaise under Eggs). Pre-prepared bagged salads if thoroughly re-washed just before eating and eaten before use-by date. Ready-made dressed salads, for example, bean or potato salads or coleslaw, if eaten within use-by date.

FOODS TO AVOID	RISK
Raw or undercooked poultry or game. Cold poultry or game if sold loose from the delicatessen.	Salmonellosis, Listeriosis
Raw or undercooked fish, for example, in dishes such as carpaccio of tuna, as well as home-made sushi and sashimi.	Toxoplasmosis
Shark, swordfish and marlin.	Excessive levels of mercury
Uncooked smoked fish, for example, mackerel pâté, taramasalata and gravadlax.	Toxoplasmosis
Fish oil supplements.	Contains too much retinol (see liver under Meat)
Raw shellfish, for example, fresh oysters.	Salmonellosis
Any shellfish with no sell-by or use-by date.	Campylobacter
Avoid all.	Listerioris
Foods that have not been reheated.	Listeriosis
Cold quiches.	Salmonellosis
Cold items from the delicatessen, for example slices of meat pie.	Listeriosis
Unwashed fruits and vegetables.	Toxoplasmosis
Pre-prepared bagged salads if not re-washed.	Listeriosis, Toxoplasmosis

exercise in
pregnancy

As well as helping your body to adjust to the changes imposed by your increasing bump and preparing you for labour, exercise can help you to avoid some of the common problems, such as constipation, swollen ankles, backache, aches and pains, varicose veins and haemorrhoids. Regular fresh air and exercise can also help you to feel better about yourself and can help you to sleep soundly.

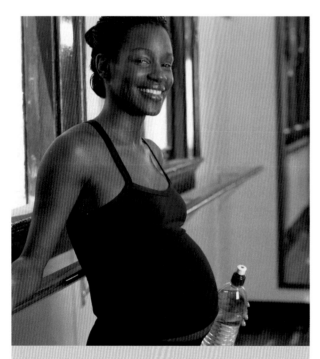

precautions

- Always warm up with gentle stretches before exercising and cool down again afterwards. A warm (but not hot) shower can help.
- Drink water before, during and after exercise, but take small, regular sips rather than a large quantity all at once.
- When exercising on the floor or on a straight-backed chair, make sure that you cushion yourself with pillows.

forms of exercise

The aims of exercise during pregnancy are general improvement or maintenance of fitness, increased stamina and improved muscle tone to help you during labour, so you should work on these aspects.

Walking, swimming, cycling, tennis, badminton and jogging all help with stamina, although you may find that your balance is affected after 5 months by the size of your bump. By 7 months, it is unlikely that you will be able to do more strenuous exercise.

Some of the more gentle yoga movements are ideal for improving muscle tone. Special yoga classes for pregnant women and water-based 'aqua-natal' exercise classes may be available in some areas. Always check that the trainer is fully qualified to teach women who are pregnant. When playing tennis or badminton, you may have to resign yourself to being less competitive than before.

starting out

If you have not exercised regularly before, you should take it gently at first. Talk to your midwife or doctor, who will be able to suggest an exercise plan. Do not suddenly take up a strenuous form of exercise, such as high-impact aerobics.

Walking, swimming and yoga are all good choices but, if you feel nauseous or very tired and do not have the energy for formal exercise, aim to get outside every day for a short walk and some fresh air.

If you already do regular exercise, you will usually be able to continue. Tell your midwife that you plan to do so. As your pregnancy progresses, you may need to slow down.

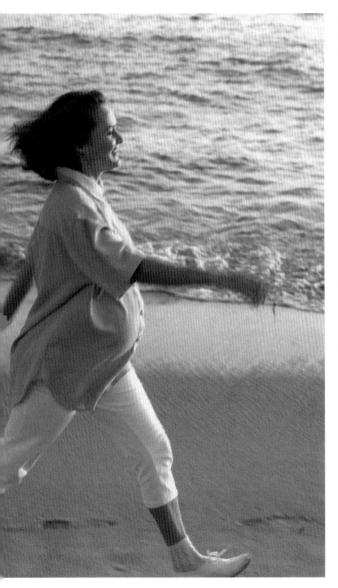

Stretching your legs every day, even for a short walk, is a safe and low-impact form of exercise, and it benefits both you and your baby.

and whenever you do it, you should not allow your heart rate to go higher than 140 beats per minute.

Although swimming is a great way to take the weight off your bump, do not swim if the water is too cold as you might get cramp. You should also stop swimming or doing aqua-natal exercises once your waters have broken. Also avoid breaststroke if you have symphysis pubis dysfunction (SPD) (see page 97).

In the last 12 weeks of pregnancy avoid any high-impact exercise, such as jogging or tennis, that increases the strain on the pelvic floor.

amount of exercise

It is best to exercise little and often, and to try to get some fresh air at least once a day. Do not exhaust yourself: it is not good for either you or your baby. Nor should you go for the burn when doing aerobics. If you cannot talk easily while you are exercising, you are overdoing it.

contraindications

Doctors may advise some women with certain conditions to do very little exercise, or even none at all. These include high blood pressure, a recent miscarriage, a threatened miscarriage, a multiple pregnancy or anaemia. If you have any of these conditions, you should always check with your doctor before starting any exercise programme.

You should stop exercising if you notice any of the following effects: breathlessness, feeling faint or dizzy, any bleeding or your baby being unnaturally still (although most do seem to stop kicking while the mother is exercising).

exercises to avoid

If you enjoy sports like horse-riding, water-skiing and skiing, or other sports where you might fall, such as squash, you can continue to do so, but you should be aware of the raised risk. Take extra caution cycling (except on an exercise bike firmly fixed to the floor) after week 28 because your growing bump will affect your balance and you might fall off. Pregnancy is not the time to take up an active sport.

For the first 12 weeks, avoid any exercise that makes you overheat. As your bump grows bigger, avoid exercises that involve either lying on your back or standing in one place for long periods, so reducing the blood flow to your baby. Whatever exercise you choose,

pregnancy exercise workout

The following simple exercises will improve your suppleness and muscle tone if done regularly.

pelvic mobility

These exercises will help to stretch and keep supple the ligaments of your pelvis and lower back and strengthen your pelvic floor.

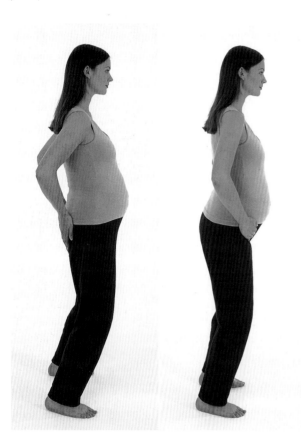

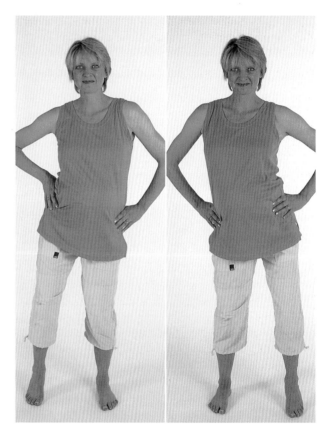

pelvic rocks

1 Stand with your feet apart and your knees slightly bent. Tighten your buttock muscles and tuck your 'tail' under.

2 Release your buttocks and swing your pelvis gently back, keeping your body upright and your knees in the same position throughout. Rock your pelvis backwards and forwards to loosen it and help prevent backache. When you feel comfortable with this, move your pelvis from side to side like a belly dancer.

hip circling

1 Put the two pelvic rock movements together, so that you rotate your pelvis first in one direction then in the other.

2 Try the rotation first with your legs straight, then with them bent. Move from your hips, not your legs.

kneeling pelvic tilt

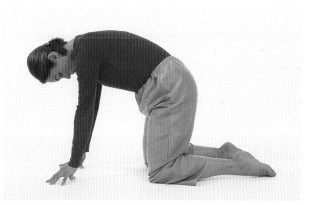

1 Kneel on all fours with your elbows slightly bent, then bring yourself up by extending your elbows and pressing your biceps forwards. Distribute your weight evenly and make sure the crown of your head is in line with your tailbone. When in this position, keep your elbows locked to maintain a strong body framework. Pause for two to three natural breaths. Repeat a further five times.

2 Inhale, then exhale for a count of five, lowering your head with your chin pointing towards your chest. Contract your buttocks and push your hips forward, curving your spine in a convex fashion. Then rise onto your fingertips to create the maximum stretch in your neck and shoulders. Inhale slowly as you release the posture, reversing the movement down to a flat-handed, straight-elbowed position. Pause for two to three natural breaths. Repeat a further five times.

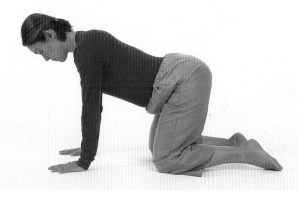

Wind down by sitting back on your feet, knees apart, and leaning on your elbows with your chin cupped in your hands. Hold the position for two to three natural breaths.

upper body

Suppleness in your upper body helps to prevent unnecessary aches and pains. Strong shoulders and arms make lifting, carrying and changing position easier, especially in late pregnancy or if you are recovering from a caesarean section. The first two exercises will strengthen your muscles and release tension in your neck and shoulders; the third will strengthen the pectoral muscles of your chest wall, which help to support your breasts.

neck and shoulders

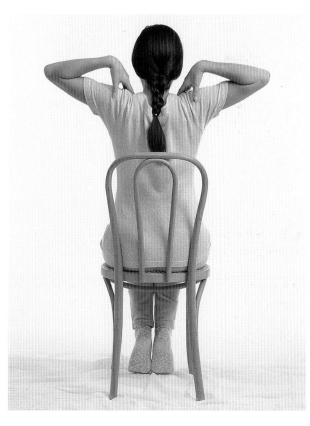

1 Sit up straight on an upright chair, with your hands on your shoulders.

2 Lengthen and widen your back, then sweep your elbows around in wide circles. Feel the stretch across your shoulders and upper back.

upper arms

1 Sit or stand with your arms stretched out to either side of your body and your fists clenched.

2 Rotate your arms quickly in small circles, and then more and more slowly as you make ever-wider circles.

3 When you reach the widest stretch possible, gradually return to small, fast circles.

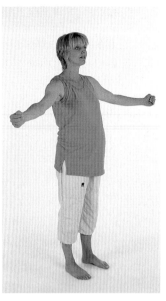

chest

1 Stand with your feet hip-width apart and your shoulders relaxed. Lengthen and broaden out your back.

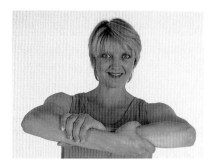

2 Grasp each forearm just above the wrist and lift your arms to shoulder height.

3 Without loosening your grip or letting your arms drop, push your hands towards your elbows in small jerks. Feel your breasts move with each little push. Repeat 20 times.

lower body and back

These exercises will strengthen your lower back and leg muscles. If you are not used to yoga, don't strain to get into these positions and stop if you are uncomfortable.

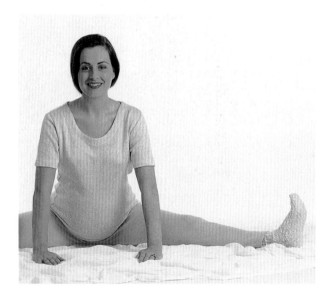

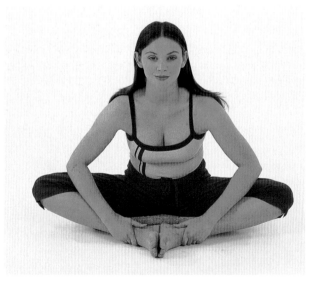

legs and back

1 Sit on the floor, with your back straight and legs apart. Lean gently forwards, pushing your heels away from your body. Feel the stretch in your back, thighs and calves. Then relax and rotate your ankles for a couple of minutes to improve your circulation.

inner thigh stretch

1 Sit on the floor, with your back straight and the soles of your feet together for a few minutes each day.

2 Rest your forearms on your knees and let your legs relax downwards without forcing or bouncing them.

looking after your back

If you use your body well, it will feel lighter and every movement will be easy and comfortable. At first you may not be aware that you have been moving badly and correcting your posture may feel slightly awkward. This is because muscles that you are not accustomed to using become weak and tire easily. However, if you persevere, they will quickly strengthen and, with practice, good movements will become a habit.

moving and lifting

Learning how to perform the following everyday actions properly will reduce your chances of muscle strain or injury whether or not you are pregnant.

standing

Keep your back upright with your shoulders relaxed, pelvis balanced and feet apart. Do not rest with your weight on one hip or stick out your bump.

sitting

Sit upright with your lower back supported. Try not to twist your body or cross your legs.

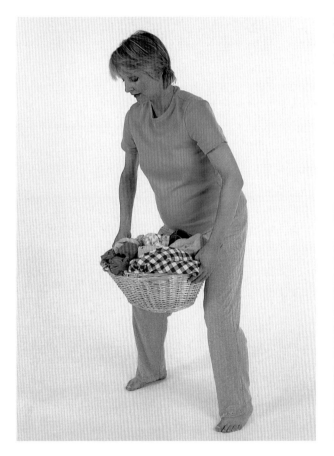

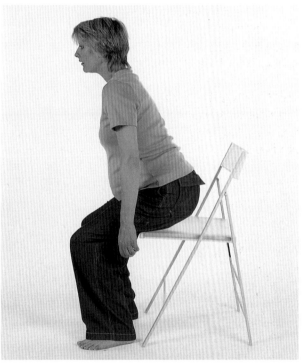

lifting

1 Position yourself close to whatever you are going to pick up, such as a bag of shopping or your toddler, so that you can keep the weight near to your body.

2 Bend from your hips, knees and ankles at the same time and keep your back straight but inclined, so that your thighs take the strain as you lift. Any form of exercise that helps to strengthen your thighs will make lifting easier.

getting up from a chair

1 Stop and think about the movement you are going to make. Lengthen and widen your back, then shift your weight to the edge of the chair and plant your feet firmly.

2 Lean forward slightly and get up smoothly, without letting your knees move towards each other or pushing yourself up with your hands. As you rise, think 'up' and lead with your head. (Imagine being pulled upwards by a thread attached to your head.) Notice how much lighter the movement feels.

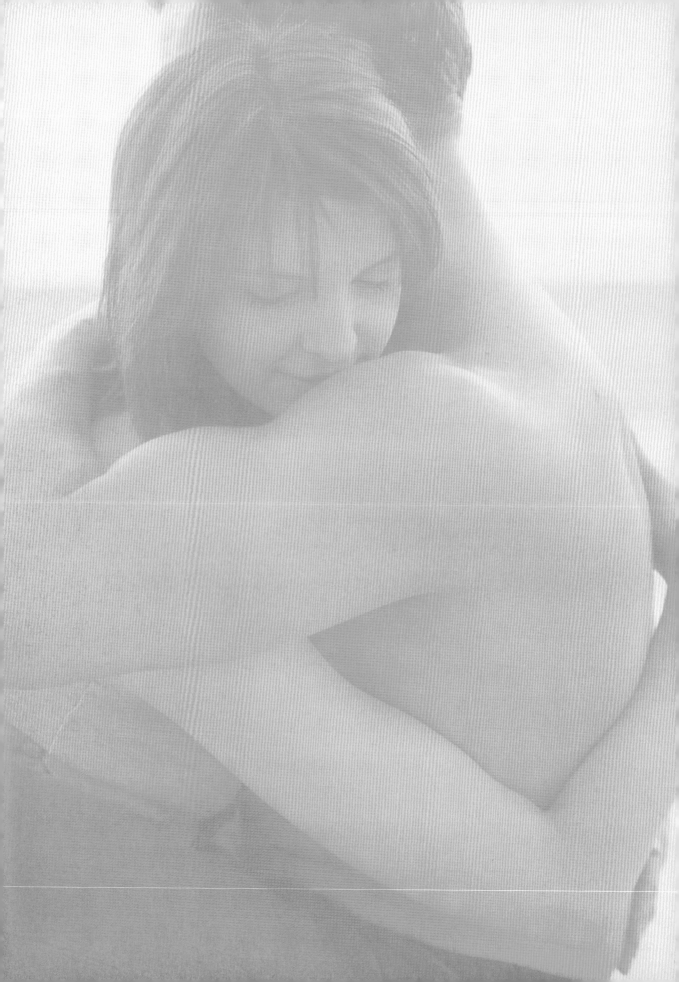

emotional
wellbeing

The initial euphoria of that positive pregnancy test may have worn off now, giving you time to concentrate on doing all you can to benefit your own and your baby's wellbeing. You are bound to have worries – all mothers-to-be have them – so share any concerns with your partner or friends. Calm and relaxation are the orders of the day – why not try an aromatherapy massage with your partner to boost your intimacy and talk about how the future will be?

rest and
relaxation

Inevitably there will be times during your pregnancy when your body tells you to rest. This may happen during the first few weeks, when tiredness can be quite overwhelming. To help you to cope with this, set aside times during the day when you can take the opportunity to take a brief nap. Even 10 minutes can help to replenish your energy stores and take the 'edge' off the tiredness.

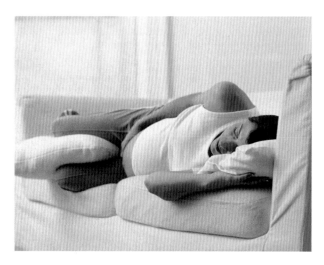

Take a nap whenever you get the chance, especially as trips to the toilet and your expanding belly can mean you're getting less quality sleep during the night.

relaxation

Relaxation is more than just resting. It is possible to rest physically but still be alert mentally, perhaps thinking about 'things to do'. It is important that you recognize how to clear your mind and truly unwind. Relaxing is a skill that can benefit anyone at any time of life, not just during labour.

Pregnancy is the ideal time to start learning relaxation techniques, as they will benefit not only you, but also your baby. They can lower your blood pressure and increase the oxygen supply to your baby, helping her to thrive. Tension can be caused by many different things: work, money, family or even worries about your pregnancy and it affects both the mind and body. Unfortunately many people do not realize when they are tense. Relaxation does not have to be structured – it can be as simple as taking time out every day to sit back, close your eyes and think about something peaceful.

sleep

Pregnancy can disrupt your sleep, sometimes almost as soon as you miss that first period. According to one theory, this is nature's way of preparing you for the sleepless nights to come, but that seems too cruel – you need all the sleep that you can get now, in view of what lies ahead!

during the early weeks

Your metabolic rate increases by 20 per cent during pregnancy, which means that your body is working harder and, although you might feel tired, it is hard to 'switch off' as your mind is still working overtime. In the early weeks, it is very common to wake during the night to go to the toilet, as the uterus is squashed against the bladder, but, as the uterus expands, it rises above the bladder, relieving the pressure.

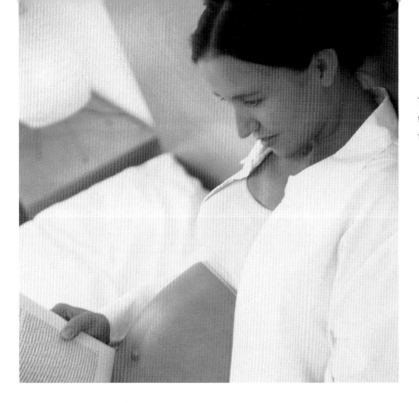

Try to take some time each day to put your feet up and read, watch television or listen to some music.

during late pregnancy

At around 30 weeks of pregnancy, women find it hard to get to sleep because their growing bump makes it difficult to get comfortable. There are things that you can try.

- Lie on your left side with one pillow underneath to support your bump and another between your knees.
- Taking some gentle exercise during the day can help you to sleep at night, so try going for an evening walk or a swim after work.
- Avoid stimulants, such as tea, coffee and fizzy drinks but have a drink of warm milk instead.
- Enjoy a soak in a warm, but not hot, bath before bed.
- Do not allow yourself to get overtired as this can make it even harder to fall asleep.
- Try to stay cool at night, particularly if you are suffering from frequent night sweats.

during the final weeks

Towards the end of your pregnancy, you may find that, when you are ready to sleep, it is time for your baby to be active, and this can keep you awake. It may be worth considering giving up work earlier than you originally planned if you are not sleeping well. At least you can then rest whenever you want to during the day.

As your baby gets bigger, her head will put pressure on your bladder and you will find that, as in the early weeks of your pregnancy, you are waking to go to the toilet several times a night.

There is nothing worse than lying in bed unable to get to sleep. It is far better to switch on the light and read a book or magazine, or get yourself a warm drink and wait until you feel sleepy, then try again. However, make time to rest the following day or the tiredness will inevitably catch up with you.

Q **I'm having the most vivid dreams about my pregnancy and baby. Is this normal?**

A It is normal to have vivid dreams in pregnancy, expressing fears and anxieties. We do not know for certain why this happens but it is most probably caused by hormonal changes, as well as the disturbed sleep that you experience during pregnancy – being woken up regularly by a full bladder or your baby deciding that it is time to kick. If you talk to other pregnant women you will find that most of them are experiencing the same thing. Try to relax before bed, with all the obvious things, such as a warm bath, gentle music and a milky drink. If you are worried about something but keeping it quiet, talk to your midwife – by expressing your emotions you may get a less disturbed night's sleep.

common
anxieties

During pregnancy, your body is being bombarded with a variety of hormones that can affect your mood, triggering a roller coaster of emotions. You may feel tearful but not know why. You may be deliriously happy one minute only to being gripped by a seemingly irrational fear moments later. Don't worry: you're not the only one. Most expectant mothers – and fathers – go through anxious moments.

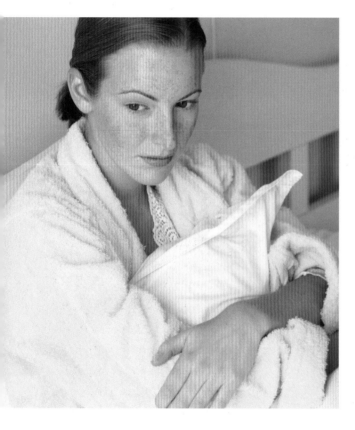

It is common to worry about your baby or how you are going to cope when he arrives. Share any worries with friends or family, or talk to your midwife to allay your fears.

am I really pregnant?

Pregnancy is a huge concept to grasp and one that many women struggle to accept. It is common for women to believe that they will never have a baby, despite a positive pregnancy test. They remain convinced that 'something will go wrong', even when they look at the car-seat and cot. It is important to discuss any worries with your partner or your midwife and, although the anxieties may not go away, you can be rest assured that you are not the first woman to have had them.

the birth

Couples often have fears about the birth, some of which stem from a lack of accurate information. Rather than avoiding the subject, it is a good idea for both of you to find out as much as you can about labour by attending antenatal classes. Here you will be encouraged to talk about your feelings and to discuss not only your fears but also your hopes.

attractiveness

As their shape changes during pregnancy, some women begin to worry that they will no longer be attractive to their partner. You may think you look fat rather than pregnant or get a shock when you catch sight of your growing bump in the reflection of a shop doorway or a mirror.

lifestyle changes

Becoming a parent involves adjusting to some huge changes in role and lifestyle, which can be difficult. If this is your first baby, you might worry that your partner will see you differently after the birth: not as a lover but in your new role as a mother. You may also have some regrets about the loss of freedom. If you already have an older child or children, you may worry about how they will adjust to the arrival of a new baby brother or sister.

There will probably be changes in your financial circumstances or in your housing as well. If your pregnancy was not planned, you may worry about being unable to support a baby financially or your house being too small. Of course, it is important to think through the practicalities of returning to work or enlisting your family to help out with childcare, but some people feel that they would never have enough money, enough bedrooms or a big enough car, and, with hindsight, do not regret an unplanned pregnancy.

Talking with other women with children can be a great support. It helps to learn how others have adjusted to motherhood and to see that, although the life changes involved in having a baby may be significant, the majority of people get through them and become good parents with happy children.

previous difficult pregnancies

Women with a history of difficult pregnancy, perhaps a stillbirth or miscarriage, can be particularly fearful about 'something going wrong'. If this is the case, it is important to talk about your worries. Speaking to others who have had a similar experience may provide you with the extra emotional support that you need. Alternatively, you might ask your midwife or doctor to see you more often, or have additional ultrasound scans if this gives you reassurance that everything is proceeding normally.

All care should be individualized, that is, suited to you and you alone. If, for instance, you have had a previous stillbirth, you may be given the option of having your baby early, as some women in these circumstances find the last couple of weeks of their pregnancy unbearable, worrying that something will go wrong again. Needs vary from person to person, not only physically but emotionally, so try to be honest with your midwife or doctor about how you feel and what it is that is worrying you.

concerns about your baby

Many women are afraid of something being wrong with their baby. They may feel guilty about having drunk alcohol in the weeks before they knew they were pregnant or worry that they have eaten the 'wrong' types of food.

There are screening tests available, including ultrasound scans, which can help reassure you about certain abnormalities. However, no one can ever guarantee that there will be no problems with your baby, no matter what you have eaten or not eaten, or whatever your lifestyle. But, if you have not done so already, do your best to adopt a healthy lifestyle as soon as you find out that you are pregnant. By stopping smoking, giving up alcohol and eating a healthy diet you will give your baby the best start possible.

'Throughout the pregnancy I was convinced that something would go wrong. At first being pregnant seemed too good to be true, but I never really enjoyed it. It was as if I was waiting for the bubble to burst. It was such a relief talking to other women in antenatal classes and finding out that I was not the only one who felt that way.'

Michelle, mother of 2-week-old Louise

shared experiences

'I was 7 months pregnant before I could bear to talk about labour. I felt so frightened that I would not cope. My midwife was brilliant and the more we talked about it, the better I felt. In labour my fears went. David was brilliant and kept reassuring me that I was doing well. I felt pain, but I did not feel frightened.'

Rhona, mother of 5-week-old Daisy-May

dealing with
stress

Having a baby is a huge life-changing event, which will inevitably cause some degree of stress, even if your pregnancy is planned and your baby is much wanted. It is natural that, at some point, you will have worries, feel emotional or be overtired because of the demands of everyday life. If you feel like this for any length of time, however, you may need to look at ways of reducing your stress levels.

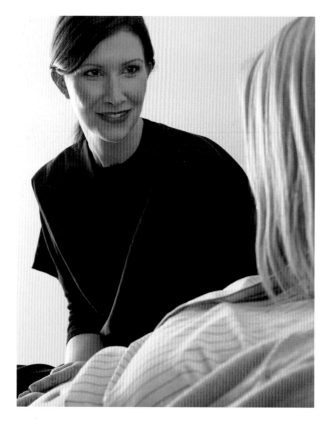

If you are feeling stressed, it may help to talk to your midwife, who will be able to suggest ways to relieve your stress.

Emotional stress can lead to physical and behavioural symptoms. Stress has a negative effect on your body and mind, and the problem is that you often do not even recognize that you are suffering from stress.

signs of stress

These can include:
- Reduced concentration
- Irritation
- Withdrawal
- Disturbed eating patterns, that is, reduced appetite or overeating
- Insomnia, fatigue
- Feeling low or anxious
- Inability to relax
- High blood pressure
- Aching muscles

There is some evidence that stress in pregnancy can cause lower birth-weight babies, as well as behavioural problems in children. Certainly we know that high blood pressure can have adverse effects on your pregnancy, including the growth of your baby, and it needs close monitoring.

coping with stress

Whether it helps to talk about things or simply switch off for a bit, there are ways to help yourself cope, including the following ideas.

accept help

If you feel stressed you will certainly benefit from more support and you should accept offers of help gladly. If you have other children and a friend or family member offers to have them for a couple of hours, seize the opportunity. If you have to stay in hospital for a few days after the birth, you will feel better knowing that they are comfortable being with someone else when you are not around.

talk

Talk to others about how you feel, including your midwife or doctor. As well as wanting to monitor how you are feeling they may be able to put you in touch with local women's groups.

exercise

You do not have to belong to a gym to get sufficient exercise – even taking a brisk walk in the fresh air is good for you. Exercise makes the body release endorphins, the natural 'feel good' chemicals, and also makes you feel more energetic.

make time for yourself

Treat yourself to a good book or a favourite magazine and be sure to make time for some quiet moments to yourself each day. If the prospect of an uninterrupted bath seems blissful, switch off the telephone, shut the door and relax. You could also try the relaxation detailed routine below.

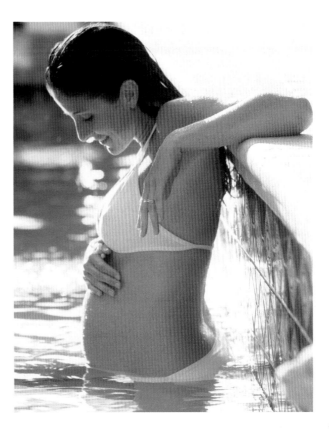

Get the swimming habit: it is great exercise for stress-busting and as your bump grows it offers fantastic support.

relax!

Try this routine wherever you get the opportunity.
- Lie back in a chair, or lie on your side on the bed, with pillows supporting your neck and shoulders.
- When you are comfortable, take slow, deep breaths.
- Concentrate on how your body feels with each outward breath.
- Start by tensing your feet, squeezing your toes tight, then let go. Feel the tension seeping out of your body.
- Work your way up your body, doing the same with your legs, pelvic floor, buttocks, stomach and so on in turn until you reach your forehead.
- Think about each part of your body and how it feels now.
- Your breathing should be even and slow, and you should feel relaxed.

massage

Ask your partner to give you a massage (see page 60). This has the added benefit that he will know he is helping you.

eat well

Your diet can have a huge influence on how you feel. Be sure to include fresh fruits and vegetables and do not snack on high-energy foods, such as biscuits and sweets. They may provide a 'quick energy fix', making you feel better for 10 minutes, but when your blood-sugar level sharply falls afterwards, you will feel no more energetic, and perhaps even more lethargic. Yo-yoing energy levels may also make any mood swings that you are suffering worse. You may find that it helps to have several small, healthy meals a day instead of three larger ones, as this will also keep your blood-sugar levels more even. If you find your energy levels are dropping between meals, snack on raw vegetables such as carrot sticks. Eating more, smaller meals may also help reduce pregnancy sickness.

alternative therapies

There are many alternative therapies for different conditions, such as the emotional ups and downs of pregnancy. During pregnancy it is important not to take any medication unless absolutely necessary so it is useful to try other approaches. Many midwives are now qualified in complementary therapies, such as aromatherapy, massage and reflexology, so ask when you go for your check-up.

yoga

Yoga combines movement and meditation to promote the wellbeing of body, mind and spirit. The exercises improve posture, muscle tone and breathing, and have the knock-on effect of improving the circulation.

Tell your yoga teacher that you are pregnant in case she needs to adapt some of the exercises. There may be

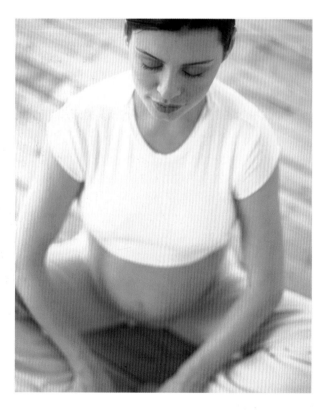

Yoga teaches you postures so you can find comfortable positions, how to breathe properly and how to relax.

yoga classes aimed specifically at pregnant women in your area, and these have the added advantage of enabling you to meet others in the same situation as you. The emphasis on breathing, concentration and visualization will benefit you not only during your pregnancy, but also during labour, helping you to relax and focus throughout the contractions.

reflexology

Reflexology can be beneficial for your emotional wellbeing and is safe during pregnancy, provided you are treated by a qualified reflexologist. It works on the principle that the feet are a map of the body, and different areas of the feet correspond to particular parts of the body. Therefore, 'treating' the feet benefits these areas of the body. A reflexology treatment is similar to having a foot massage – although your feet may feel tender at times, it should prove very relaxing.

Stress and anxiety cannot be alleviated by one session, so you may need regular sessions over some weeks. If you have a complicated pregnancy, reflexology should only be done by a member of your maternity team, such as your midwife or doctor.

breathing exercises

Imagine sinking into an armchair at the end of a day. Nobody has to tell you how to breathe when you do this – you automatically take a deep breath and 'sigh'. Breathing plays an important part in relaxation because, when tense, you breathe more quickly and take shorter breaths, your heart beats faster and your muscles tense. This uses up energy, which makes you feel more tired.

aromatherapy in
pregnancy

In aromatherapy, essential oils, which are extracted from plants, are applied to the skin or inhaled. These oils can have a beneficial effect on the mind and body: some are relaxing, while others are energizing. This is due not just to the scent of the oil but also to the chemicals that the oils contain. Usually, the oils are mixed with a 'carrier' oil, such as grapeseed oil, or added to water.

It is best not to use any essential oils during the first 3 months of pregnancy. Before using any oil you should do a patch test on your arm to check for any adverse skin reactions. Certain oils should not be used at all during pregnancy (see box below) and, if you have any doubts about the suitability of an oil, consult a qualified aromatherapist.

how to use essential oils

Always dilute oils in water or use them in a carrier oil and do not use them more than three times a week.

Footbath Add 2–3 drops to a bowl of warm water.

Inhalation Add 3 drops of essential oil to warm water and inhale the vapour. Alternatively, put a drop or two on a handkerchief and inhale.

Fragrance burner Heat 1–2 drops of oil, diluted in water.

Bath Stir 4–6 drops of oil into the warm water. Do not use soap and do not stay in the bath for more than 20 minutes.

Massage Mix 5 drops of essential oil with 25 ml of grapeseed oil.

Compress Add 3–4 drops of oil to a bowlful of warm water. Soak a flannel in the water then wring it out.

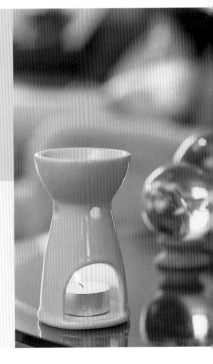

essential oils to use

From 12 weeks of pregnancy citrus oils in a fragrance burner for 'uplifting' your mood and revitalizing you, although you should avoid going out in the sunlight if they are applied directly to the skin.

From 24 weeks of pregnancy camomile oil for relaxation and insomnia.

From 28 weeks of pregnancy lavender oil for relaxation and insomnia.

In the final weeks neroli oil for stress and insomnia.

essential oils to avoid

During pregnancy cajuput, celery seed, cinnamon leaf, citronella, clary sage, fennel, jasmine absolute, lavandin, lavender (before 28 weeks), marjoram (sweet), may chang, myrrh, niaouli, rosemary, spike lavender, tagetes, yarrow.

If you have high blood pressure rosemary, thyme (red).

If you have a family history of allergy, asthma or eczema nut or wheatgerm oils.

massage in
pregnancy

Apart from having physical benefits, massage is a way in which your partner can help and feel involved in your pregnancy. Let him know what feels good, play some relaxing music and light some candles. Massage is not just for labour, it is a way of helping you to get in touch with your body, release tension and clear your mind. We express affection through touch, so massage can also be comforting.

positions for massage

As your pregnancy progresses, you will need to adopt different positions in order to receive massage, using pillows for support. For a back massage, you may feel more comfortable straddling a straight-backed chair (using a pillow to make yourself comfortable) but, by the fifth month, lying sideways is advisable, with plenty of pillows around your stomach area and under your upper legs. This position is also useful for massage during the early stages of labour.

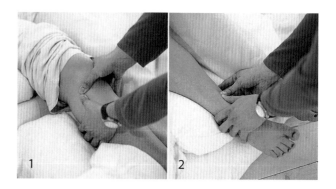

safety first

Always observe the following safety precautions:
- Do not give body massage during the first 12 weeks of pregnancy.
- Do not use intense pressure or vigorous strokes, especially on the abdomen, inner thigh and groin.
- Do not apply pressure around and across the top of the ankles, because these points relate to the ovaries and the womb.
- Up to week 12, do not use essential oils in any form. Certain oils are not suitable at any stage of pregnancy, so either use a pre-mixed blend designed especially for the purpose or consult a qualified aromatherapist (see also page 59).
- Do not massage varicose or spider veins.
- Use less pressure over joint areas and work along either side of the spine, not directly over it.
- Avoid lying on your back in late pregnancy.

leg and ankle massage

During pregnancy, leg massage can be an excellent means of reducing water retention and relieving that 'heavy leg' feeling.

1 Make sure that your partner's back and legs are well supported and that she is comfortable. Place the pads of both thumbs at the top of her shin on the outer edge of the leg, where the bone widens. Apply gentle but firm pressure three to five times.

2 Moving down her leg, support her foot with one hand and place the thumb pad of your other hand about four finger-widths above the inner ankle bone, again applying gentle but firm pressure three to five times.

3 Move down to her toes and, with one hand supporting her foot, take her little toe between your index finger and thumb. Pull and squeeze in a downward movement, rotating the toe very slightly from the base to the tip. Do this to each toe in turn. Repeat these steps with the other leg, finishing by holding your partner's feet gently for at least 30 seconds.

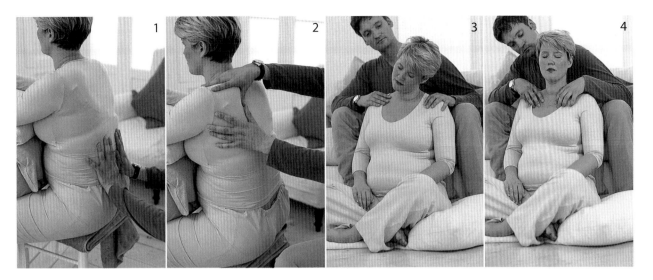

neck and lower back massage

This area is often the weakest and most troublesome, and muscle tension here leads to the shoulders being held unnaturally high by the end of the day.

1 Starting at the lower back, with your hands flat on either side of her spine, glide them up her back, across her shoulders and return to the starting position. In all back massage, the pressure is on the up stroke. Repeat this three to five times. Work up her back again, making small circles in opposite directions, until you reach the shoulders. Return as before. Repeat three to five times.

2 Working on one side at a time glide across her shoulder blade. Then separate your hands, bringing one around the shoulder and the other around the armpit, pulling back gently as you return to your starting position. Repeat this three to five times and then move to the other side.

3 Bring your hands gently down to your partner's shoulders and rest them there for about 30 seconds. Then, with your thumbs on the muscle at the back of the neck and your fingers over the front of the shoulders, begin to squeeze the shoulder muscles between the heels of your hands and your fingers, working outwards towards the tops of her arms and then back in. Repeat this three to five times.

4 Splaying your fingers slightly, rest them on either side of her breastbone (sternum), at the top of the breast tissue. With the pads of your fingers, massage the muscle between the upper ribs, working outwards from the breastbone to the edge of the ribcage. Repeat each stroke three to five times then move up to the next rib muscle. Ask your partner to take a few deep breaths between strokes.

when and where to massage

Concentrate on areas other than your bump, which should be given no more than a light stroking.
Weeks 1–12 Head or face massage can soothe away headaches. Do not massage the body.
Weeks 13–28 Indigestion and insomnia are common, and massage of the back, shoulders and buttocks will aid relaxation and sleep. The abdomen can be massaged but only with light, gentle strokes.
Weeks 29–40 Massage should concentrate on the back, neck, shoulders and particularly the legs to relieve fatigue. The lower back and buttocks can be massaged during labour to help the process along.

you, your partner
and fatherhood

During your pregnancy, you and your partner will start to think about your new roles as parents. So far you may only have thought of each other as 'partners' or 'lovers', but now you may be wondering if you will be a good mother and your partner a good father. He will probably be having the same feelings and doubts about his role in the months and years to come.

' I have never felt so excited as when I found out that I was going to be a dad. I was bursting with pride and wanted to go and tell everyone, but Mandy pleaded with me to wait until she was 12 weeks pregnant! '

Will, father of
3-week-old Jane

shared experiences

' When I held my baby in my arms for the first time I can remember gazing at her, thinking that I had finally 'grown up'. The feeling of love and also responsibility felt overwhelming. '

Mark, father of
3-week-old Poppy

involving your partner

Your partner may feel detached at the beginning of a pregnancy, because he has none of the signs or symptoms that, for you, make the pregnancy real. It is as if your partner needs something more tangible before he can accept the pregnancy. You will not look any different and so, in some cases, it is only when he has seen an ultrasound image of the baby, or heard the heartbeat, that the reality will hit him.

Although you may be feeling tired and nauseous, until you have an obvious, if small, bump or he feels the baby move, he may find it hard to accept that anything has changed. Parenthood is a journey together and it can help to involve your partner from the start, getting him to accompany you to antenatal checks whenever possible.

You may become so preoccupied with the pregnancy and growing baby that your partner feels pushed out and lonely. He may have his own worries about becoming a father, so find time when you can talk together about the way that you both feel. He may be anxious about providing financial security, particularly if you are planning to give up work, and so you need to plan together for the months ahead.

changes in your relationship

Women often feel more sexual at certain times during their pregnancy. It is normal to go off sex at times during your pregnancy, and you may find that your desire peaks and troughs over the 9 months. Some men are reluctant to make love during pregnancy for fear of hurting the baby. For most women, it is perfectly safe to have sex throughout their pregnancy (see page 64), and your partner may need to be reassured that his penis does not go further than the vagina, and that the baby will not be affected. The arrival of your baby will inevitably change your relationship in some way and, for some couples, it is important to spend some quality time together before they become a family. If possible, plan a holiday together before the birth.

Remember that your partner will have his own concerns about the pregnancy and birth, or even about the idea of becoming a parent,

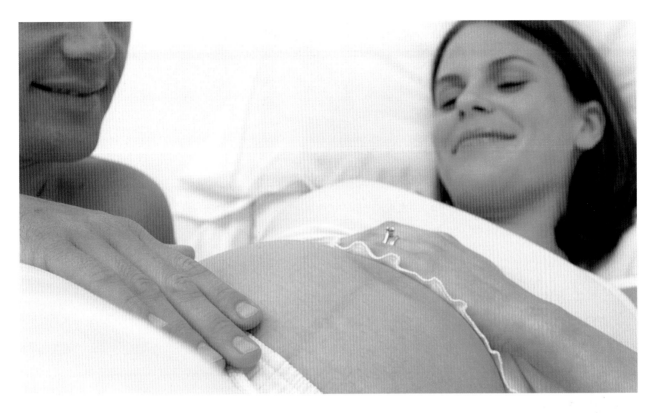

Your pregnancy may seem more 'real' to your partner as your bump gets bigger and he can feel the baby moving inside you.

and he also needs someone to talk to. By attending antenatal classes with you, he will get the opportunity to talk with other men about their feelings. Some men might worry about whether they will be a good father, perhaps because they had a difficult relationship with their own father.

Q **I really want my partner to be at the birth but I am worried in case he sees me 'differently' afterwards.**

A Women tend to fret about this more than men but, if you are concerned about your partner's reaction, talk to him about it. If you are still concerned, ask him to stay with you at the 'top end'. We are all different, and some women feel more comfortable if their partner does not actually witness the delivery but stays where he can provide support. Most partners describe the birth as the most amazing thing they have ever seen and, if they see their partner differently, it is with wonder and respect at what they have managed to produce!

how your partner can help

There are a number of ways in which your partner can help, all of which will make him feel more involved. These include:

- Running a warm bath for you before bedtime.
- Massaging your back and shoulders (see page 61).
- Trying to be understanding of your mood swings – pregnancy can be a roller coaster of emotions.
- Listening to what you want from him.
- Coming with you to antenatal classes and ultrasound scans.
- Offering to be your birth partner (see page 120).

sex during
pregnancy

If you have a history of miscarriages, premature labour or bleeding in pregnancy, it may be advisable not to have sex, so check with your midwife or doctor first. It is also advisable not to have sex if you have a condition called placenta praevia, in which the placenta is lying close to the cervix (see page 114). However, for the majority of women, it is perfectly safe to have sex throughout the pregnancy.

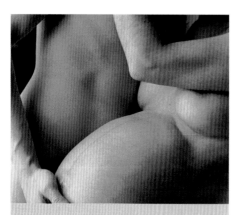

positions for sex

- As your bump grows you might find it more comfortable being on top of your partner.

- He can be on top but with his weight off your abdomen.

- If you lie side by side, with your legs over your partner, there is no pressure on your bump but you are still able to face each other.

- If you kneel on all fours, with your partner entering you from behind, there is no pressure on your bump, but there is still an opportunity for foreplay.

sex drive

It is normal to feel more sensual at certain times in your pregnancy than others and most women have a sexual peak during mid-pregnancy. This is partly the result of hormones and not having to worry about contraception, and partly because their bodies are more voluptuous. Continuing to have sex during pregnancy is healthy: it helps to exercise your pelvic floor, relaxes you and, if you orgasm, exercises the muscles of the womb. Your baby is safe in the bag of fluid and neither you nor your partner can hurt her.

Because orgasm can make your uterus contract, you may feel slight pain, but this will not harm your baby. Also increased discharge may make your vagina slippery so your partner may find it harder to reach orgasm. In early pregnancy, your breasts may be tender so tell your partner about this so that he can avoid touching them when you are having sex.

Q **Is it normal to go off sex during pregnancy?**

A We are all different and, for every woman who goes off sex while she is expecting a baby, there will be another one who feels particularly sensual. Your feelings might change at different stages of your pregnancy, too. In the early stages, women sometimes feel too tired and nauseous to enjoy sex and then, later on, when they are feeling better, they find that their bump becomes uncomfortable and not conducive to an active sex life. There are other ways for the two of you to make love apart from sex. Give each other a massage or a cuddle. You will both want to feel loved and give love, so find other ways of being intimate together.

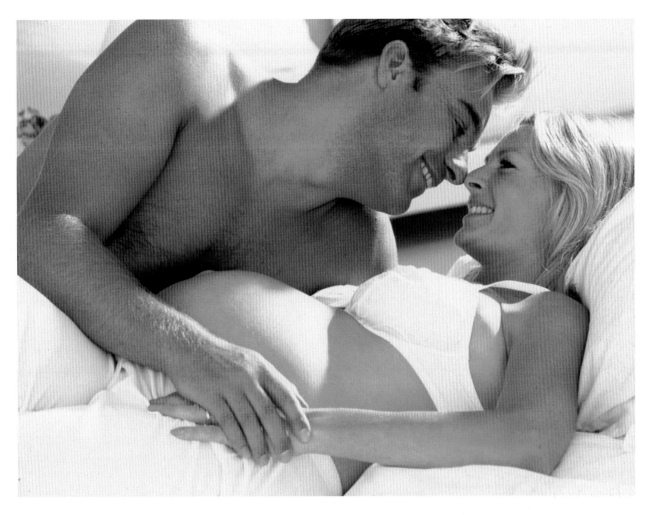

positions

As you get bigger, you will probably need to experiment with positions because you will not want your partner resting on your bump or breasts. Pregnancy is the perfect opportunity to become more adventurous. It is important to keep a sense of humour because your baby may become active at the most inappropriate moment!

The joy that you share about the baby on the way can bring you closer together as a couple.

Q **Is it true that sex can trigger the start of labour?**

A Sex can help to get you into labour towards the end of your pregnancy, but only if your body is ready to do so. Sperm contains the hormone prostaglandin, which is the same as the synthetic hormone used to induce labour. Also, when you are aroused, your body releases the hormone oxytocin, which helps to stimulate your uterus and can start contractions.

single
mothers

Whether you are a single mother by choice or by chance, there is no reason why having a baby should be any less fulfilling, although it is important that you have some support. Everyone needs someone to talk to at certain times in their lives, and becoming a parent is one of them. Such a change in your life will provoke questions or doubts, and it is helpful to have someone with whom to share your feelings.

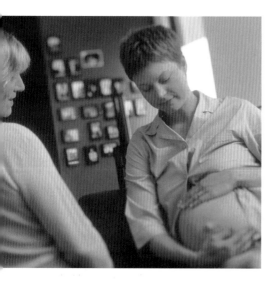

A close support network is even more important if you are facing pregnancy on your own. Talk to good friends or your sister or mother if you would like them to be more closely involved.

networking

Other women with children can be a wonderful source of support. Pregnancy is the ideal time to start building up a network for after the baby is born. By going to aqua-natal or antenatal classes, you will meet other pregnant women with whom you can keep in contact. Getting together with other single women can be helpful, and many areas have a network of groups aimed at single parents.

reactions to your pregnancy

If you are not in a permanent relationship, you may worry about announcing your pregnancy to your family. Although being a single parent is by no means unusual, there are still many people who find it unacceptable. Some women are rejected by their parents, although this often blows over once they realize that nothing they can say or do will change your decision to have the baby. They might not 'approve' but many proud grandparents, who cannot imagine being without their grandchildren, started off as disapproving parents.

Give people time to accept your decision. Often parents are disapproving only because they are concerned about you and how you will cope, and they express their concerns as anger. If your family or friends are not prepared to support you, it may be time to move on and find someone who is happy to do so. As a parent you will probably find that your new responsibilities make you more assertive. Your new baby is a part of your family now and will become your priority.

choosing a birth partner

You do not have to be on your own in labour just because you do not have a partner. You are just as entitled to have a birth partner – perhaps your mother, a friend or a family member (see page 120). Choose someone you can rely on and with whom you feel comfortable. This person could also attend antenatal classes with you, although there may be classes aimed specifically for single women in your area – ask your midwife.

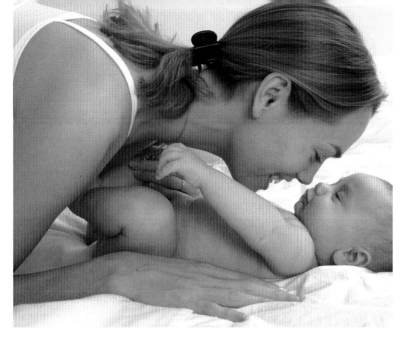

You may sometimes find it hard work being a single parent, but having a beautiful baby does have its good side too!

family and friends

Family and friends tend to offer well-meaning but sometimes unwanted advice. You may feel that they are trying to take over and make decisions for you, when all you need is someone to bounce ideas off. It is important to establish clear boundaries from the beginning. If you are on your own, they may assume either that you will not be able to cope, that you will be staying with them or that they can move in with you for the first few weeks. This is fine if it is what you want. However, if you are at all worried about offending people or about their reactions to you having the baby, it makes sense to let them know your plans well in advance in order to avoid any misunderstandings.

after the birth

Nobody knows for certain how they will cope after the arrival of a new baby, whether they are a single parent or one member of a couple. However, looking after a baby can be lonely, particularly when you feel tired and your baby is crying.

If you are lucky enough to have family or friends who offer help, do not be too proud to accept it. This does not mean that you are not coping. In fact, new mothers often cope so well as they do precisely because they do have help and support.

getting help

If you have no one to support you, tell your doctor or midwife who can recommend sources of additional support. In this way, you should be able to find out if you are entitled to any benefits or if you can get any help with housing. Help is often available but it is also a question of knowing where it is and how to find it.

'After I had Josh, I felt so lonely, and desperately wanted my mother to come and stay. She told me afterwards, she had stayed away so that I did not think that she was taking over. If we had only been honest with each other from the beginning it would have been a much happier time for both of us!'

Alison, mother of
1-year-old Josh

shared experiences

'It was terrifying when all my friends had gone and I was alone with my baby for the first time since leaving hospital. I remember thinking "this is for real, I'm not babysitting now" and I felt so scared.'

Caroline, mother of
10-week-old Beth

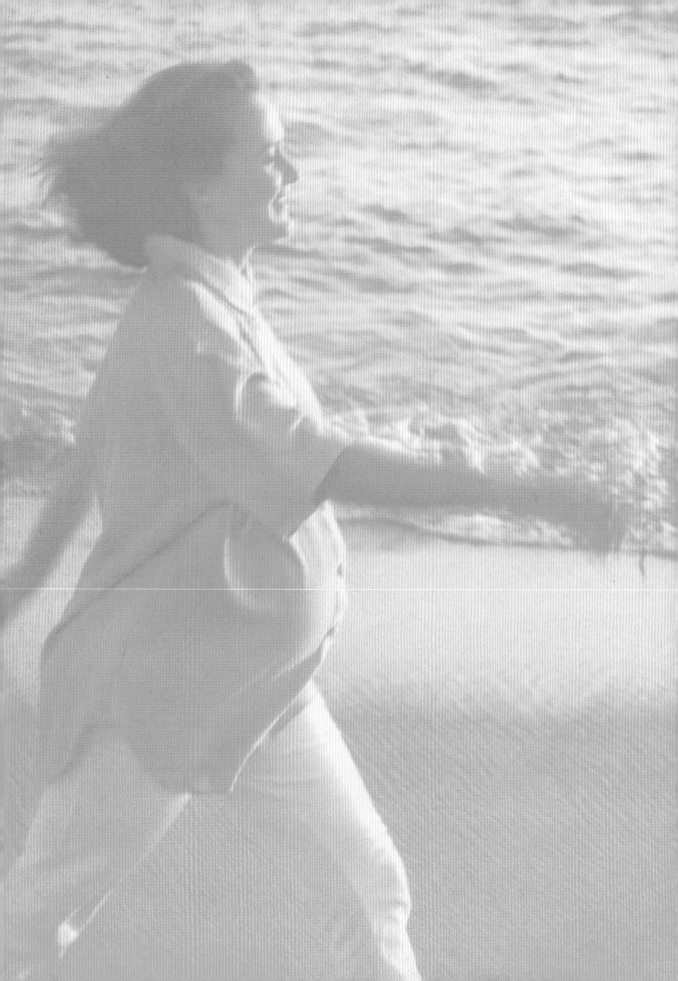

health

It is good to know that most pregnancies are healthy and normal. Even so, like many women, you may also want to know what can go wrong so that you can be super-vigilant about your health and protect your growing baby. Most common complaints are minor, ranging from itchy skin and constipation to lower-back pain and headache, but do read on and be aware of anything out of the ordinary, as it could mean something more serious.

avoiding
risks

Being pregnant makes you suddenly aware of all the everyday things that might be hazardous to your baby while he is at such a crucial stage of development. This is obviously a good thing, but if you become too anxious about everything, you will not be able to relax and enjoy your pregnancy. The lists below give general guidelines and suggestions.

chemicals

We use an enormous number of chemicals at work and at home and they are not usually harmful if we follow the manufacturer's instructions. However, they may have a cumulative effect, so it is best to restrict their use during pregnancy, especially during the first 3 months.

- Use natural cleaning agents, for example, bicarbonate of soda, salt, vinegar and lemon juice, or eco-friendly products.
- Avoid coming into contact with chemicals. Wear rubber gloves or wash your hands thoroughly.
- Avoid inhaling vapours from, for example, glue, petrol and paint, oven-cleaners, cleaning fluids, air-fresheners, and use pump-action sprays rather than aerosols.

You should also be aware of the less obvious chemicals in the environment.

- Avoid exposure to toxic wastes or polluted water.
- Avoid polluted air, for example, noxious fumes or smoky atmospheres.
- If your house still has lead pipes, always run the tap for a few minutes before using the water.

infectious diseases

You should avoid coming into contact with infectious diseases, especially rubella, chickenpox and mumps. Apart from fever affecting your baby's development, these diseases carry a number of particular risks

Chickenpox may cause fetal malformations in early pregnancy and problems in the newborn (see page 175).

Mumps is associated with a slight risk of miscarriage in the first 12 weeks.

Rubella is associated with malformations, such as deafness, blindness and heart disease, especially in the first 3 months of pregnancy. This is why your doctor or midwife will always check your immunity to rubella.

recreational drugs

Avoid these at all costs because of their potential side-effects. For example, cannabis affects the production of male sperm for up to 9 months after use, and hard drugs (for example, cocaine and heroin) can damage the chromosomes in the sperm and egg, leading to abnormalities in the baby. Sharing syringes also increases the risk of contracting HIV or hepatitis. Use of recreational drugs during pregnancy can cause such problems as miscarriage, low birth weight, congenital abnormalities and even babies born with addictions.

over-the-counter and prescription drugs

You are just as likely to get everyday illnesses, such as coughs, colds and tummy upsets, when pregnant than at any other time, and knowing what over-the-counter or prescription drugs are safe can be confusing. If you are in any doubt, check with your pharmacist or doctor, who will be able to give you the most up-to-date advice. Always tell them that you are pregnant, particularly in the early stages, when your pregnancy may not show or may not yet be in your medical notes.

The following is a guide to what you can and cannot take during pregnancy.

Antibiotics Certain antibiotics are safe – your doctor will be able to prescribe something appropriate.

Aspirin can affect how your blood clots and is therefore best avoided unless specifically prescribed in low-dose form by your obstetrician.

Codeine and medicines containing it, such as some cold or flu remedies as it has been linked with certain birth defects. Always check with your doctor.

Cough/cold/flu remedies often contain codeine, aspirin or ibuprofen, so check with your pharmacist or doctor before using any of them.

Cystitis remedies are not safe because of their high salt content.

Diarrhoea remedies are not safe because they slow down the action of the stomach and the intestines, which has already been slowed down by pregnancy hormones. However, you can use rehydration sachets, which help replace lost nutrients.

Ibuprofen is best avoided because it has been associated with problems in fetal heart growth.

Laxatives containing senna, cascara or bisacodyl are not safe. These ingredients may cross the placenta and also stop your bowels working normally so that your baby may be deprived of nutrients. Bulk-forming laxatives are safe.

Migraine remedies often contain codeine, so ask your doctor if there are any that are safe for you to take.

Paracetamol is safe in small doses, but large doses can harm your baby's kidneys and liver.

Supplements Only take those specially designed for pregnant women.

Thrush remedies are not safe if taken by mouth, but you can use creams or pessaries.

Vapour rubs are safe.

drug treatments for ongoing conditions

With many conditions, for example, diabetes, epilepsy or depression, the most important thing during pregnancy is that your health should be as good as possible because this is vital to the health of your baby. For this reason, your doctor will always weigh up whether it is better for you to continue with your current medication, to change drugs, or to come off them entirely, and he will make the best decision for your particular situation.

diabetes

Babies born to women with insulin-dependant diabetes are at greater risk of heart defects so, if you are diabetic, it is important to monitor your glucose levels and manage your diet carefully, both before you conceive and throughout your pregnancy (see page 80).

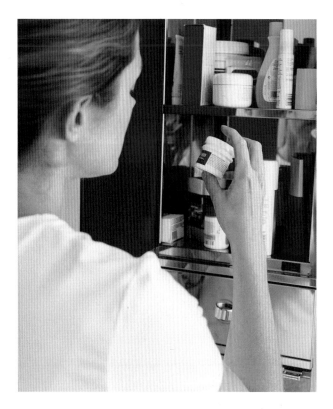

Paracetamol, in small doses, is the only safe painkiller to take during pregnancy, but many women prefer to avoid all unnecessary medicines during this precious time.

epilepsy

If you are epileptic, it is vital to see your doctor for advice before you try to conceive. He may advise a change of medication because some drugs have been more thoroughly tested for pregnant women. However, the most important thing for you and your baby is to keep your seizures to a minimum, so he will take this into consideration when giving you advice. He will also advise you to take extra folic acid, as epilepsy drugs can affect your ability to absorb it. You will be carefully monitored throughout your pregnancy to ensure that both you and your baby are alright.

depression

The majority of women who take anti-depressants during pregnancy go on to have healthy babies, and there are now drugs available that are considered safe for use during pregnancy. Your doctor will be able to advise you on the best way to change or manage your medication to ensure that both you and your baby are as safe as possible.

listeriosis and toxoplasmosis

When pregnant, you must be extra careful about hygiene and food preparation in case you pick up viruses or bacteria and pass them on to your baby. Small numbers of the bacteria that cause food poisoning usually produce minor symptoms in adults, ranging from a slight temperature to a touch of sickness or diarrhoea, but some strains can be very harmful to a developing baby.

did you know?

Even if you do not own a cat, local cats may have visited your garden, so wear rubber gloves when gardening in case you come into contact with any cat faeces – and wash your hands thoroughly afterwards.

Listeria cannot survive high temperatures, so if food is piping hot and cooked through, it is safe. This also applies to soft cheeses, like Brie or stilton, if they are grilled or cooked in sauces.

listeriosis

This is a type of food poisoning caused by the Listeria bacterium. Symptoms include a high temperature, aching muscles, back pain, sickness and diarrhoea, rather like those of flu or an ordinary stomach upset. However, they often appear some time after you have been exposed to the bacterium, so it is often tricky to spot that you have had listeriosis. If it is not treated, listeriosis can lead to miscarriage or stillbirth, or make your baby more likely to suffer from breathing problems, hypothermia or meningitis after birth. Follow the basic food safety rules (see page 39) and avoid foods that commonly carry the bacterium (see pages 40–43). If you suspect that you have contracted listeriosis, speak to your doctor, who can arrange a blood test to find out. If necessary, she will prescribe antibiotics that are safe for use during pregnancy.

toxoplasmosis

Toxoplasmosis is caused by Toxoplasma, a parasite that is carried in raw or undercooked meat and cat faeces. Symptoms include swollen glands in the neck, aching muscles, headaches and fatigue, again rather like those of flu.

Although not serious in adults, toxoplasmosis can have major implications for your unborn baby. It can cause miscarriage or stillbirth, and babies born to infected mothers often have eye problems or 'water on the brain' (hydrocephalus).

If you own a cat, you may already have developed an immunity by coming into contact with toxoplasmosis in its faeces. However, to be safe, you should avoid emptying or touching your cat's litter tray throughout your pregnancy. If there is no one else who can empty the tray for you, use a new, clean pair of disposable rubber gloves each time. You should also get someone to clean your cat's litter tray every day and fill it with boiling water for 5 minutes to kill off bacteria and wash your hands after throwing the gloves away. Again, it is important to be particularly aware of food safety (see page 39).

travel during pregnancy

The thought of a holiday appeals to many pregnant women because this may be the last chance of time alone together with their partner for some years. Most women feel at their best during mid-pregnancy, when fatigue and nausea are less likely. Wherever you are going, take a copy of your antenatal records with you. Travel in loose clothing and wear shoes that will allow your feet to swell while travelling.

driving

It is safe to continue driving during pregnancy but, as always when travelling long distances, take a break after a couple of hours and walk around. The seatbelt might feel more uncomfortable but it is still important to wear it. Make sure that the diagonal strap goes between your breasts and the lap strap goes across the lower part of your hips, flat on your thighs – not across your bump.

air travel

Most airlines will not accept women after 34 weeks of pregnancy onto flights, but check with the individual airline. In some cases it may not be advisable to fly during pregnancy, for example, if you have a history of high blood pressure or premature labour, so check with your doctor first. Also, it is unwise to fly in an unpressurized aircraft because this can significantly reduce the oxygen supply to you and your baby.

Pregnant women are at increased risk of deep vein thrombosis (DVT, see page 77) so on a long flight you should get up and walk around every couple of hours. Ask for an aisle seat if possible, so that you can stretch your legs and leave your seat easily. You can also wear supportive flight socks that reduce the risk of DVT. Drink plenty of water to prevent dehydration and wear slipper socks, as your feet will inevitably swell during the flight. If you are suffering from pregnancy sickness, ask for a seat over the wings as the ride is less bumpy there.

travel sickness

Although some travel sickness medicines are safe for most pregnant women under medical supervision, you may prefer to do without them. 'Travel bands' – stretchy bands worn on the wrists – work on the acupressure point to reduce nausea. Children's travel bands stretch to fit most wrists and are available from pharmacies.

foreign travel

You should take extra precautions if you are travelling to a foreign country.
- Ask your doctor whether you need any vaccinations and which ones are suitable during pregnancy.
- Make sure that your travel insurance covers you for pregnancy-related cancellation and health problems.
- Take a record of your notes, including your blood group, any allergies and contact numbers for your midwife or doctor.
- Where food and drink are concerned be scrupulous about hygiene. Drink bottled water if you have any doubts about the tap water – and remember to avoid ice for the same reason.
- You may not be able to tolerate the heat as much during pregnancy, so stay in the shade and drink plenty of water to prevent dehydration and keep your body temperature down.

work and
pregnancy

Choosing the right time to tell your employer that you are pregnant is always tricky. She may be delighted for you personally, but less happy professionally as she still has to arrange cover while you attend antenatal appointments or decide how to cope while you are away. However, on no account should you feel guilty: your employer has obligations towards her employees, including the pregnant ones!

Q I am 10 weeks pregnant and get stressed at work. Will this affect my baby's growth?

At this stage in pregnancy stress will not affect the growth of your baby, but it can make you feel very tired and also spoil the excitement of these early weeks. Find some way of tackling the stress, either at work or after work – such as swimming, yoga or a massage.

Q I'm 30 weeks pregnant. When can I start my maternity leave?

The earliest you can start your maternity leave is the start of the 11th week before your baby is due. Your employer has the right to start your maternity leave early if you are absent with a pregnancy-related illness during the last 6 weeks of your pregnancy.

The first few months, when pregnancy sickness is at its worst, can be a problem. However, there is no need to announce the news as soon as you find out that you are pregnant, unless your occupation might affect your baby. Women in low-risk jobs often wait until they are around 3 months pregnant.

Once you have told your employers, you can claim any entitlements in terms of time off for antenatal appointments or risk assessments of your job. You do not immediately have to tell them exactly when you are intending to give up or return to work.

It is important to find out what benefits you are entitled to in your pregnancy. Read your contract of employment, contact your union if you are a member, get in touch with a benefits agency – and, of course, ask your midwife, who can provide you with information.

safety at work

Once you have told your employers, they should carry out an assessment to see whether any aspects of your work pose a risk during your pregnancy, for example, if your work involves X-rays, chemicals or heavy lifting. If this is the case, you should be offered alternative work.

Some women worry about the effects of printers, photocopiers and computer display terminals (particularly if they spend long hours sitting in front of one), but there is no evidence to suggest that these pose a risk to your unborn baby.

Another consideration is the environment in which you work:
• Is it smoky or excessively noisy?
• Does your chair support your back properly?
• Is the room well ventilated or stuffy, making you feel drowsy?
These factors can usually be remedied quite easily.

taking a rest

If you feel very tired in early pregnancy work can be tough, but most people can find a short time to 'switch off'. Some women listen to a personal stereo at lunchtime while they close their eyes and relax. Try

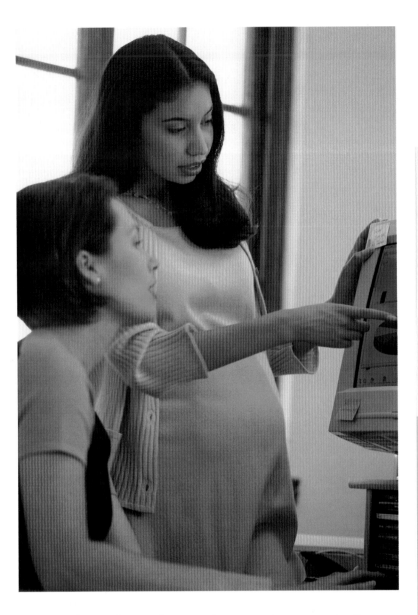

Your work life won't have to change just because you're pregnant, but if you think your job poses any risks to your baby, speak to your employer right away.

to find somewhere quiet during your lunch break to read a book or a magazine. Ask if there is a place to go for a 10-minute nap at some point during the day – after all, you will perform the better for this.

reducing stress
There may be small changes that you can make to reduce stress.
- Take breaks – 'power nap' if you can.
- Do not take on more work than you can cope with.
- Avoid travelling to and from work at peak times – ask if you can alter your working hours slightly.
- Do not stand for hours on end without a break.

'I felt awful at the beginning of my pregnancy and great at the end. I felt that it would have made more sense to have maternity leave in the first 2 months rather than the last 2!'

Janine,
39 weeks pregnant

shared experiences

'I worked until I was 37 weeks pregnant and at 38 weeks I gave birth to Simon. I wish that I had stopped work earlier as I am convinced it is one of the reasons that I developed postnatal depression. It was such a shock to be a professional working woman one week and the next to be at home full time with a baby. I wish I'd had a few more weeks to gradually adjust.'

Nicola, mother of
14-month-old Simon

special-care
pregnancies

Pregnancy imposes many stresses and strains on healthy women. However, if you already have a condition such as high blood pressure, heart disease, thyroid disease or asthma, you will be naturally concerned about the effect of the condition on your pregnancy and also about the effect of your pregnancy on the condition. Discuss such problems with your midwife or obstetrician at the first opportunity.

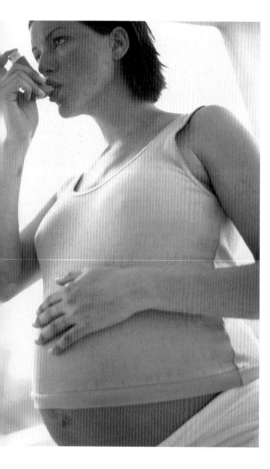

Common treatments for asthma, such as inhaled bronchodilators, are safe to use during pregnancy, under medical supervision.

asthma

During normal pregnancy, the demand for oxygen increases: breathing (ventilation) increases by about 50 per cent, usually as a result of breathing more deeply rather than more quickly. As a result, you may feel slightly breathless. On the other hand, respiratory diseases, such as asthma, can also cause breathlessness, and this can lead to difficulties in diagnosis. Asthma also causes coughing, wheeziness and chest tightness, often in response to allergens, such as pollen, or after exercise. Asthma does not usually cause any significant harm to the pregnancy, although severe asthma may restrict the baby's growth or cause premature labour.

management

Common drugs, such as inhaled or oral steroids or inhaled bronchodilators (for example, salbutamol), are safe to use during pregnancy and should be continued to ensure effective treatment.

thalassaemia

Thalassaemia is a genetic order that causes abnormality of the proteins making up the respiratory pigment haemoglobin. There are two types: **Alpha thalassaemia** which is common in women from southeast Asia. **Beta thalassaemia** which is common in women from Cyprus and Asia. If only one of the genes for haemoglobin is faulty, this is known as a thalassaemia trait. This may be detected for the first time during pregnancy, during a routine blood test for anaemia.

management

If you have the thalassaemia trait, you may need iron and folate supplements throughout your pregnancy, particularly if your ferritin levels (a measure of your iron levels) are low. If your partner also has the trait, you should be referred for further tests because there is a risk that your baby may have the more serious condition, known as thalassaemia major.

high blood pressure

Some women already have high blood pressure (or hypertension) when they become pregnant. Others may be diagnosed as having hypertension during the first 3 months of pregnancy. These women probably already had a blood pressure problem, such as pre-eclampsia (see page 110), which does not usually present until much later in the pregnancy. In most cases, the cause of the hypertension is unknown (referred to as essential hypertension) while a minority of women have an underlying cause, for example, kidney or heart disease.

The main problems associated with hypertension during pregnancy are the increased risks of developing pre-eclampsia (see page 110), reduced blood flow through the placenta, affecting the growth of your baby, or having a placental abruption (see page 114).

management

If you are already taking anti-hypertensives, your obstetrician will advise you whether to continue your medication. If you are not, he will decide whether your blood pressure is high enough to warrant starting medication. The drug that is most commonly used to treat high blood pressure in pregnancy is methyldopa, although beta blockers are also widely used. A close eye will be kept on your blood pressure throughout your pregnancy, and you will be given extra scans to monitor your baby's growth.

deep vein thrombosis and pulmonary embolism

In a normal pregnancy, the mother's blood clots more easily. This is designed to reduce the amount of blood loss at delivery. Having slightly thicker blood puts all pregnant women at risk of clots in the legs (deep vein thrombosis, or DVT) or lungs (pulmonary embolism, or PE). Other factors, as well as pregnancy, increase the risk of blood clots. These include obesity, greater age, having a caesarean section, a history of a previous blood clot, pre-eclampsia, immobility (for example, during long-haul flights), and thicker blood caused by a tendency to excessive blood clotting (or thrombophilia).

The symptoms of a DVT are swelling, redness, pain and tenderness in the calf muscle, while breathlessness, chest pain on breathing in, a cough and coughing up blood may indicate the presence of a PE.

management

DVTs and PEs are potentially life-threatening complications so, if you are at particular risk, your doctor may advise you to take blood-thinning drugs during and immediately after your pregnancy to prevent a clot developing.

If your doctor suspects a blood clot, he will refer you to hospital for tests to confirm the diagnosis. If a clot is found, you will be given drugs (usually by an injection into the skin but sometimes through a vein) to prevent the clot worsening.

'I did know that there could be side-effects from my epilepsy medication – it carries a high risk of spina bifida – but Natasha was born perfectly healthy. I did worry that she'd have epilepsy too and my doctor says there's a one in ten chance that she'll develop it.'

Liz, mother of
14-week-old Natasha

shared experiences

'I've had asthma since I was a small child. I use inhaled steroids twice a day and I also have a ventolin inhaler. When I became pregnant my doctor lowered my dose but at 20 weeks I caught a chest infection, which meant I had to go back onto my normal dose. I was worried Ben would be affected but he was perfectly normal.'

Sam, mother of
2-year-old Ben

Your midwife or doctor will keep a closer than normal eye on your blood pressure if early readings are high, to minimize any effects on your baby.

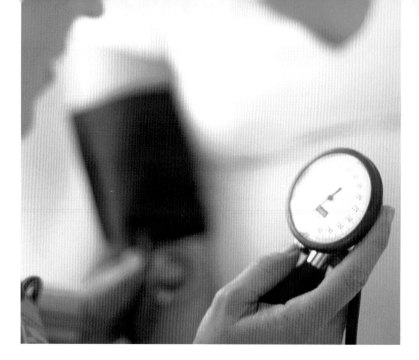

HIV

Pregnant women are encouraged to have HIV screening. If a woman accepts screening, she is talked through the procedure and the possible consequences, and asked to give her consent. If the results of the test are positive, she will be offered counselling. The aim of treatment is to lower the chances of HIV infecting the baby. Giving the mother anti-retroviral drugs during the last few months of pregnancy reduces the risk of the baby acquiring the infection. HIV-positive pregnant women will normally be advised to have an elective caesarean section and to bottle- rather than breast-feed. All babies born to HIV-positive mothers start life with HIV antibodies, but this does not automatically mean that they are infected, as these are the mother's antibodies. The baby will be given a series of tests over the ensuing months to monitor the levels of the virus in the bloodstream.

heart disease

In a normal pregnancy, significant changes occur in the cardiovascular system. These include:
- An increase in heart output of almost 50 per cent.
- An increase in heart rate of up to 20 beats per minute.
- A lowering of blood pressure in early and mid-pregnancy, with a return to normal by late pregnancy.

These changes are quite normal but often lead to the discovery of an innocent heart murmur, which can be heard through a stethoscope because of the increased blood flow. Labour places an additional strain on the heart.

management

Ideally, all women with heart disease should be given pre-conceptual counselling by a heart specialist to address the potential risks of any future pregnancy. They include, for example, women who received corrective heart surgery as children (for example, repair of a hole in the heart) and are now of child-bearing age, women who have problems with their heart valves, for example, narrowing of the aortic or mitral valves (aortic or mitral stenosis), and women with artificial heart valves.

If you become pregnant and have significant heart disease, your doctor will refer you to a specialist clinic where you can receive the best advice and the appropriate tests, for example, an echocardiogram (an ultrasound of your heart) or an ECG. Your condition will also be monitored regularly.

thyroid disease

It is normal for the thyroid gland, which is situated at the front of the neck, to increase in size during pregnancy because of the increase in blood flow. However, the gland can cause problems if it is overactive (hyperthyroidism) or underactive (hypothyroidism). Uncommonly, thyroid disease is a cause of infertility.

management

If you have hyperthyroidism, your doctor will prescribe anti-thyroid drugs, such as carbimazole and propylthiouracil. These can cross the placenta and cause fetal hypothyroidism, so the lowest possible doses of the drug must be used. Your paediatrician should be made aware of your condition so that he can check your baby once it is born. It is usually safe to breast-feed.

Hypothyroidism is treated with thyroxine, and very little crosses the placenta so your baby would not be at risk of side-effects.

sickle-cell anaemia

Sickle-cell anaemia is a genetic disorder that mainly affects people of Afro-Caribbean origin, but also some people from the Mediterranean region, the Middle East and Asia. People with sickle-cell anaemia have abnormal haemoglobin that becomes distorted (sickle-shaped) under conditions of stress, blocking small blood vessels and causing severe pain and sickle-cell crises. The stress of pregnancy is sufficient to trigger a sickle-cell crisis.

In addition, pregnant women with sickle-cell anaemia have an increased risk of miscarriage, premature labour, stillbirth and pre-eclampsia, as well as DVT and PE (see page 77), urinary tract infection and puerperal sepsis. The baby is also more likely to suffer from growth restriction and fetal distress.

management

If you have sickle-cell anaemia, you should be referred to an antenatal clinic that is used to dealing with high-risk pregnancies, where there are obstetricians and haematologists at hand.

cholestasis

Obstetric cholestasis (OC) is characterized by severe itching that normally affects the arms and legs, particularly the palms of the hands and soles of the feet, and the trunk. It develops during the last 3 months of pregnancy.

Blood tests usually show abnormalities in liver function and an increase in bile acids, but other causes of itching, such as hepatitis or gallstones, need to be excluded. In OC, the mother is at increased risk of bleeding after the delivery and the baby is more likely to be stillborn or suffer from fetal distress.

management

If you are diagnosed as having OC, your baby should be monitored at regular intervals. You will be given vitamin K to reduce the chance of bleeding. You may also be given antihistamines to relieve the itching, although ursodeoxycholic acid, which reduces the level of bile acids circulating in the blood, is more effective. It is usually advisable to induce labour at 37–38 weeks. The likelihood of OC recurring in future pregnancies is about 90 per cent.

fetal problems and surgery

New surgical techniques mean that it is becoming possible to correct some abnormalities while the baby is still in the womb. Some techniques are available only in a few centres worldwide and may not be appropriate for all babies with the specified condition, depending on the severity of the case.

spina bifida In this surgery, the tube around the spinal cord is closed to reduce further damage in cases where the fetus is not thought to be severely affected already.

twin-twin transfusion syndrome (TTTS) Identical twins who share a placenta (see page 24) have a small but significant risk of developing TTTS. One twin receives more blood than the other because of abnormal blood vessels that connect across the placenta. Treatments include destroying these vessels with a laser and draining excess amniotic fluid.

hernia of the diaphragm A weakness in the diaphragm allows the baby's intestines to move up into the chest and prevent the lungs from developing properly. A clip or balloon catheter is used to block the baby's airway, so that fluid can build up inside the lungs and help them to expand and grow more normally.

heart valve problems Progressive narrowing of the valves in the fetal heart can be life-threatening and has recently been treated in the uterus. Using ultrasound to guide it, a tiny balloon is guided into the defective valve and then inflated. This enlarges the valve, allowing more blood to flow through it.

diabetes in
pregnancy

Diabetes is a disorder that prevents the body from using food properly. Normally, the body's main source of energy is glucose. After being digested in the stomach, sugars and starches enter the bloodstream in the form of glucose, a sugar that becomes a source of energy. The body uses the hormone insulin to get the glucose from the bloodstream to the muscles and other tissues of the body.

the role of insulin

Insulin is manufactured by the pancreas, a gland lying behind the stomach. Without insulin, glucose cannot get into the cells of the body, where it is used as fuel. Instead, high levels of glucose accumulate in the blood, from where it spills into the urine via the kidneys. This is known as diabetes.

types of diabetes

If you have diabetes before pregnancy (that is, pre-existing diabetes), it will be one of two types:

Type I, or insulin-dependent diabetes mellitus (IDDM) formerly called juvenile onset diabetes. This results from the failure of the pancreas to produce enough insulin.

Type II, or non-insulin-dependent diabetes mellitus (NIDDM) formerly called maturity onset diabetes. This is caused by the body becoming resistant to insulin so that it cannot use it efficiently.

Common symptoms include frequent passing of urine, exceptional thirst and a dry mouth.

diabetes and pregnancy

Pregnancy itself makes the body resistant to insulin because of the anti-insulin effects of the pregnancy hormones released from the placenta. In normal pregnancy, the body produces almost double the amount of insulin. However, if the pancreas fails to produce enough insulin, pre-existing diabetes can become worse or diabetes can develop for the first time (gestational diabetes, see opposite).

All antenatal clinics routinely test urine for the presence of glucose. Pregnant women normally excrete glucose in their urine, particularly after eating a sugary snack or meal. Therefore, almost all women have glucose in their urine at some stage. Further tests are necessary to reliably diagnose diabetes.

risks of poorly controlled diabetes

Poorly controlled diabetes during pregnancy can have adverse effects on both mother and baby.

risks to the mother

There is a greater risk of miscarriage, pre-eclampsia (see page 110) and infection, particularly of the urinary tract and respiratory system. In addition, the high-risk nature of these pregnancies increases the likelihood of a caesarean section being necessary.

risks to the baby

Excess glucose from blood of a mother with pre-existing diabetes can cross the placenta and enter the fetus, causing abnormalities, particularly during the first 3 months, when most of the organs are forming. Common abnormalities include heart, skeleton and neural tube defects (for example, spina bifida). Fetuses of diabetic women are often larger but their growth may be restricted. There is also an increased risk of the baby dying during late pregnancy and the few weeks after the birth by 5–10-fold. In addition, newborn babies sometimes suffer from complications, for example, respiratory distress syndrome and jaundice.

pre-existing diabetes

If you have diabetes and are planning to become pregnant, you should talk to your doctor first. He can explain about any possible risks and can arrange for you to receive the best advice and care both before and throughout your pregnancy.

pre-conceptual counselling
It is very important to get counselling about good diabetic control when you are planning to become pregnant. This can significantly reduce the risk of your baby having a congenital abnormality, as well as improving the outcome of your pregnancy. Talk to your doctor about improving the management of your diabetes and, as in all pregnancies, take folic acid to reduce the risk of spina bifida.

management
Your doctor should refer you to a specialized clinic, where you can see an obstetric/diabetic team, that is, an obstetrician, midwife, diabetic physician, diabetic nurse, dietician and ophthalmologist (to check for any diabetic damage to the retina of the eye).

The main aim is to achieve near-normal glucose levels. This entails:
- Frequent monitoring of your blood glucose, which you do at home.
- Changes in your insulin dosage if necessary.
- Avoiding oral diabetic drugs in pregnancy because these can cause low blood-glucose levels in your developing baby.
- Paying particular attention to your diet: a low-sugar, low-fat, high-fibre diet with regular snacks can prevent your blood-glucose levels falling too low.

You will also be given a series of scans:
- An early scan to date the pregnancy.
- A detailed anomaly scan at 20 weeks to check your baby for structural abnormalities.
- Serial scans to check your baby's growth and the amount of amniotic fluid surrounding your baby. (This is sometimes raised in diabetic pregnancies, a condition known as polyhydramnios.)

Delivery will usually be planned for 38–39 weeks, with the options of:
- Induction of labour.
- caesarean section.
You may be given intravenous infusions of insulin and dextrose during your labour to control your blood-glucose levels.

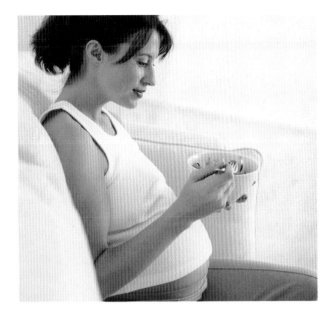

If you suffer from diabetes during your pregnancy, it is vital that you eat the right foods.

gestational diabetes
About 5 per cent of women, especially those from the Indian subcontinent and southeast Asia, develop diabetes for the first time in pregnancy. As well as the implications for the pregnancy, women with gestational diabetes have a 50 per cent risk of developing Type II diabetes within the next 10–15 years.

management
Many units screen women who are at particular risk, for example, those with a personal or family history of gestational diabetes, a previous large baby or a large baby in the current pregnancy, unexplained stillbirth, obesity, high levels of glucose in the urine (glycosuria) and excess amniotic fluid (polyhydramnios).

Different screening tests are available. If your doctor suspects that you have gestational diabetes, he will arrange for you to have a formal 'glucose-tolerance test' to establish the diagnosis. This test measures your blood-glucose levels after you have taken a sweet glucose drink.

In most cases, gestational diabetes will respond to a low-fat, increased fibre and altered carbohydrate intake. Avoiding sugary foods can lead to improvements, although insulin may become necessary. Regular scans to check your baby's growth are advisable.

rhesus disease

Everyone is born with a certain blood type (A, B, AB or O) and Rhesus factor (Rh positive or Rh negative). If you are Rh negative and your baby is Rh positive, you may become sensitized to the Rhesus factor in your baby's blood, in which case you will produce antibodies to your baby's red blood cells. If this is your first pregnancy, this is not usually a problem.

However, in subsequent pregnancies, if your baby is again Rh positive, these antibodies can cross the placenta and destroy your baby's red cells, causing fetal anaemia. After the birth, the destruction of red blood cells results in high levels of bilirubin (a yellow pigment produced by the breakdown of the blood cells). As well as making your baby appear jaundiced, this can be harmful to his brain.

If both you and the father are Rh negative, there is no danger because your baby will also be Rh negative.

prevention

One of the greatest success stories in obstetrics is how rare Rhesus disease has become. This is due to the use of Anti-D injections – a blood product – in Rh negative women at risk of Rhesus disease. Anti-D injections prevent Rhesus disease by destroying any fetal cells that enter the mother's circulation before she has a chance to produce any antibodies. Anti-D is routinely given to the mother after the birth (within 72 hours) if a baby is shown to be Rh positive. In recent years, Anti-D

the cause of rhesus incompatibility

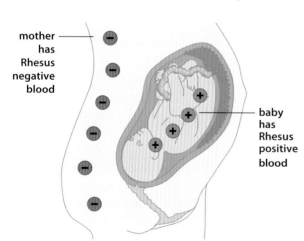

mother has Rhesus negative blood

baby has Rhesus positive blood

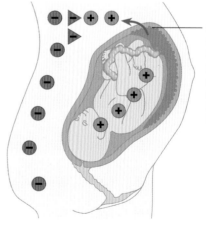

during the birth some fetal blood cells cross into the mother's blood and she creates antibodies to Rhesus positive blood

If a Rhesus negative mother (that is, with no Rhesus factor in her blood) has a Rhesus positive first baby, there are usually no complications during that pregnancy.

During the birth, some of the baby's blood may cross the placenta into the mother's bloodstream. If she is not given an Anti-D injection within 72 hours of giving birth, she may develop antibodies to the Rhesus factor. This may also occur during a miscarriage or an abortion.

injections have also been given at 28 and 34 weeks. Anti-D is recommended for pregnant Rh negative women after certain events (for example, miscarriage, threatened miscarriage – if this occurs after 12 weeks, or 'trauma' to the abdomen, such as a fall or car accident), or after certain procedures that have a risk that fetal blood could cross the placenta (for example, amniocentesis or chorionic villus sampling, see page 128).

symptoms and diagnosis
The severity of Rhesus disease depends on how many of the baby's blood cells have been destroyed. It ranges from mild disease, where the baby is found to be mildly anaemic at birth, to severe disease, where the baby suffers heart failure in the uterus.

A warning sign of Rhesus disease is the presence of Anti-D antibodies in the mother's blood. If you have high levels of Anti-D antibodies, your obstetrician will recommend regular ultrasound monitoring of your baby to keep an eye on his progress. In the past, if there was any suspicion that a baby might be suffering from anaemia, an amniocentesis was performed. Nowadays, this procedure has largely been replaced by looking at the blood flow to the baby's brain. A very high blood flow is an indication that the baby may be anaemic.

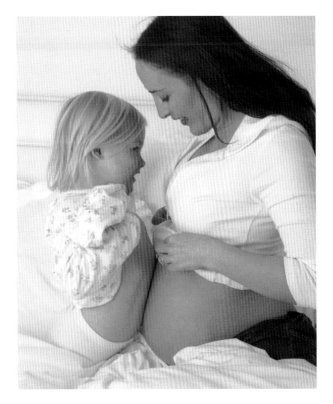

Rhesus disease is now rare, thanks to anti-D injections, which will protect you when you become pregnant again.

Recently, it has become possible to tell whether a baby is Rhesus positive or negative from a blood sample taken from the mother. If, for example, Rhesus disease is suspected, finding that the baby is Rhesus negative is very reassuring.

treatment
If your baby has Rhesus disease, he can be treated either while he is still in the uterus or after the birth.

in the uterus
If your baby seems to be anaemic, a fetal blood sample can be taken. If this confirms anaemia, he can be given a blood transfusion. This procedure may need to be repeated until he is developed enough for delivery.

after the birth
Treatment depends on the severity of your baby's jaundice and anaemia. In mild cases of jaundice, bilirubin levels may respond to light therapy (phototherapy). In more severe cases, an exchange blood transfusion may be necessary.

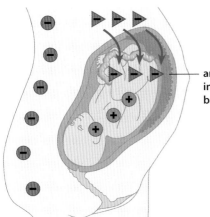

antibodies cross into a subsequent baby's bloodstream

In a subsequent pregnancy, some of these antibodies will cross into the fetus's bloodstream. If the baby is Rhesus positive, the antibodies will attack his red blood cells and cause a condition called fetal anaemia.

common complaints
during pregnancy

During pregnancy, your changing hormone levels and your growing baby can have effects on your appearance and how you feel, some of which may be unexpected. The following chart features brief descriptions of common (and some less common) complaints that women experience during pregnancy, together with practical suggestions for coping with them. Do not worry: you will not get all of them!

Remember that this is only a guide. If you experience any unusual symptoms, or are in any doubt, always consult your doctor or midwife.

COMPLAINT	DESCRIPTION	ACTION
SKIN CONDITIONS		
itchy stomach	Nearly all women get an itchy stomach. This is caused by your skin stretching over your bump and becoming thinner, resulting in loss of moisture, dryness and progressively more itching. Other common skin conditions that may coincide with pregnancy, or be aggravated by it, include eczema, urticaria and scabies.	Use gentle soap and massage your skin with a mild moisturizing lotion to soften it. If the itching is intolerable, try a simple moisturizer or a safe anti-itching remedy. A cool bath may help. If you feel itchy, particularly on your hands and feet, tell your midwife or doctor (see cholestasis, page 79).
pigmentation changes – general	A general increase in pigmentation is quite normal. This is more marked in dark-haired women and mostly affects the nipples, genital area and the centre of the abdomen. Some changes are permanent. It is also normal for freckles and moles to get darker during pregnancy. They often fade back to normal soon after the birth. There may also be an increase in the number and size of moles.	If you notice any new mole, or any change in the appearance of existing moles, including size, shape and colour, or itching or bleeding, see your doctor immediately.

COMPLAINT	DESCRIPTION	ACTION
pigmentation changes – chloasma	Also known as the 'mask of pregnancy', this butterfly-shaped pigmentation appears on the face of 70 per cent of pregnant women. It sometimes appears as small blotches but almost always fades after the birth. The marks are usually lighter, and therefore most apparent, in dark-skinned women and darker in fair-skinned women. Chloasma is caused by a combination of oestrogen, other hormones and sunlight.	If the marks bother you, use a concealer make-up that matches your skin tone. Do not try to bleach dark marks: it is unlikely to work and it is best to avoid chemicals during pregnancy.
pigmentation changes – linea nigra	This is a dark line that appears down the centre of the abdomen and usually fades after the birth. It is caused by increased levels of hormones and is nothing to worry about.	None.
rashes – heat rash	Heat rash, especially under the breasts and in the groin, is common. Most pregnant women sweat more and the sweat gets trapped in the glands, giving rise to these itchy pimples.	Wear a support bra. Wash the affected areas regularly and dust them lightly with unscented talcum powder. Try moisturizers and avoid excessive weight gain if possible.
polymorphic eruption of pregnancy (PEP)	Some women get itchy pimples in their stretch marks. This usually occurs in the last 3 months of a first pregnancy or, more rarely, shortly after delivery. The pimples disappear after delivery and are less severe in subsequent pregnancies, if they recur at all.	Your doctor may prescribe a cream to ease the problem.
red or itchy palms or soles of the feet	Most women develop red, itchy palms and some get red itchy soles to their feet. This is a side-effect of oestrogen in the blood (but see also cholestasis, page 79).	Tell your midwife or doctor so they can rule out the possibility of cholestasis. Moisturize your hands regularly and wear rubber gloves for housework.

COMPLAINT	DESCRIPTION	ACTION
skin dryness	Many women with dry skin find that it gets even drier during mid-pregnancy. This is an effect of increasing oestrogen levels. Ultimately, changes to the skin will depend on your individual response to the different pregnancy hormones.	Drink plenty of water. Air conditioning and central heating can be very drying to the skin. Hang humidifiers from your radiators and make sure that you get fresh air every day. Use a gentle face wash instead of soap. At night, use a rich moisturizer specifically designed to work on your skin while you sleep. Apply a face mask, made by mixing 2 tablespoonsful of oatmeal to a paste with rosewater, and apply it to clean skin, avoiding the eyes. Cover a pillow with a towel and lie down and relax for 20 minutes. Gently rub the mask with your fingertips (over a basin) then rinse your face in warm water.
skin oiliness	It is fairly normal to suddenly develop spots during mid-pregnancy. This is due to pregnancy hormones increasing the production of sebum (an oily substance with antibacterial properties that is secreted onto the skin's surface), which can make your skin oily and prone to spots.	If you are already taking any oral drugs for acne, you should stop because they could affect your baby's development. Some topical treatments are safe but always check with your doctor or pharmacist. Drink plenty of water. Eat a balanced diet containing plenty of fresh fruit and vegetables. Dab spots with dilute tea tree oil whose antiseptic properties should help to reduce the inflammation. Use a gentle cleanser and toner regularly. Change to a light, unperfumed moisturizer designed for oily skin. Exfoliation can help. Apply a face mask of whipped egg white to clean skin. After 10 minutes, wash it off with lukewarm water and pat your face dry.
skin tags	These tiny, floppy growths develop on the underarms, face, neck and breasts in mid- to late pregnancy. They are nothing to worry about and usually shrink after the birth. They are probably caused by hormones.	Show your doctor or midwife at your next visit. Unsightly skin tags can be removed by simple surgery.

COMPLAINT	DESCRIPTION	ACTION
stretch marks 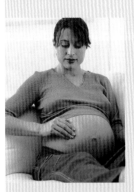	Approximately 50 per cent of women develop these pink or red marks, which fade to a shiny silver after the birth. They may be itchy (see rashes, page 85). Stretch marks seem to be more common in younger women and in women who are overweight, although they also occur in women who gain very little weight. They are thought to be caused by the skin stretching rapidly as you gain weight and causing ruptures in your skin structure. There may also be a genetic element involved.	There are no treatments to prevent stretch marks but, if your skin is supple and you do not gain too much weight, you may find them less of a problem. Moisturize your skin, particularly on the sides of your bump, your breasts and thighs. Try using 4 drops of mandarin oil in 20 ml of carrier oil, such as baby oil. (Avoid creams that claim to prevent stretch marks because they have no scientific basis.)

HAIR

COMPLAINT	DESCRIPTION	ACTION
changes in texture	Women often find that their hair appears to be thicker than usual during pregnancy, and that individual hairs become coarser. This is because pregnancy hormones slow down the rate of hair loss, although the hairs will eventually fall out after the baby is born. Their hair may also become dry, unmanageable and limp, or curly hair may frizz out of control. In late pregnancy, many women find that their hair becomes greasier. This probably results from increased production of sebum (see skin oiliness, page 86).	Experiment with different shampoos until you find one to suit your hair condition. Do not have a perm or a relaxer because the chemicals may be absorbed through your skin. Do not use bleach or have highlights. Hair dyes will not harm your baby, but your hair may absorb the dye differently. Also your skin may be more sensitive, resulting in an allergic reaction. Try a different hair style to make your hair more manageable before your baby arrives.
extra facial or body hair	Some women notice more hairs on their body and face, and these may be darker and thicker than normal. Conversely, others find that they have less body hair. Both depend on the individual woman's response to pregnancy hormones.	Do not bleach dark hair growth because the chemicals may be absorbed through your skin. Pluck any hairs that bother you. Consult your doctor if extra hair growth is excessive.

COMPLAINT	DESCRIPTION	ACTION
BREASTS		
blocked milk ducts/mastitis	Blocked milk ducts are more common after the birth but can occur beforehand. They take the form of small, painful lumps, often with red streaks radiating out from them – a condition known as mastitis. Blocked milk ducts can be caused or aggravated by wearing an under-wired bra or one that presses on the underside of the breast, or by pressure from car seat belts on a long journey. Mastitis is the result of infection.	Wear a correctly fitted bra. Talk to your midwife, who can advise you how to get rid of the lump. See your doctor if you develop mastitis. This must be dealt with promptly to avoid infection spreading further.
leaky nipples	From the fourth to fifth month of pregnancy onwards, your breasts may begin to secret colostrum. This is quite normal.	Buy some breast pads to slip inside your bra if the leakage is marking your clothes.
prominent glands in the areola	This is a sign that your breasts are preparing for breast-feeding and is quite normal.	None.
prominent veins	Spider veins, or thread veins, are quite normal and often disappear after the birth.	They are caused by the action of oestrogen on the blood vessels. Use concealer make-up if these veins bother you.
tenderness	Tender breasts are one of the early signs of pregnancy. The tenderness is caused by stimulation of the milk-producing glands and, as the pregnancy progresses, expansion of the milk ducts as they prepare for lactation.	Wear a support bra throughout your pregnancy. This will also help to prevent your breasts sagging when you stop breast-feeding. (Always be fitted for bras and replace them as your breasts grow.) Try wearing a sleep bra if you are uncomfortable at night.

COMPLAINT	DESCRIPTION	ACTION

DIGESTIVE SYSTEM

constipation and wind 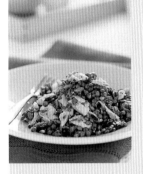	Constipation (the passing of hard, infrequent, dry stools) can occur from conception onwards and may be accompanied by other digestive disturbances, such as wind. From early pregnancy, the hormone progesterone relaxes your muscles, including those of the large intestine. This makes your digestive system sluggish, so that you may not have a bowel movement for several days. In addition, your bowel absorbs more water than usual, adding to the problem. Taking iron tablets may make the symptoms worse.	Drink up to 3 litres of water and fruit juice a day. Eat more fruit, vegetables and high-fibre foods (for example, wholemeal bread, baked beans and healthy cereals). Take light exercise, such as walking or pregnancy yoga, to improve your general circulation. Remember that some over-the-counter laxatives are not safe to use because they reduce the amount of nutrients that you absorb. Always ask your doctor or pharmacist for advice. Consider massage: a reflexologist can apply pressure to the arches of the feet, which are related to the intestines. Or your partner could massage this area of your feet in a clockwise direction, which should help to encourage movement of the bowel.
dental problems	Pregnant women can suffer from bleeding or swollen gums and loose teeth. This is caused by the action of the oestrogen hormone on the tissues of the mouth.	Brush your teeth at least twice a day, using a softer toothbrush if your gums bleed. Floss regularly to remove any food that has settled between your teeth. See your dentist during pregnancy because your teeth and gums may need extra attention.
food aversions	Many women develop an aversion to certain foods during pregnancy. This may be associated with a changing sense of taste. Some of these aversions may be protective because certain naturally occurring bitter substances can be harmful to the developing baby.	If you cannot bear to eat certain foods, be sure to eat other foods that provide the same nutrients, for example, if you cannot stomach red meat, eat more poultry, fish and dairy products instead.

COMPLAINT	DESCRIPTION	ACTION
food cravings	Some women develop cravings for particular foods, regardless of how healthy they are.	If you crave unhealthy foods, prepare a plan of daily meals and stick to it as far as possible. Buy fewer unhealthy foods so you cannot easily snack on crisps and biscuits when in the house. Always have some fruit, yoghurts, chopped carrot, and similar, as an alternative snack.
food cravings – pica	Pica is the technical term for the desir o eat strange things, for example, coal, rubber bands – even mud! It may be caused by a nutritional deficiency.	Tell your doctor, who may prescribe a nutritional supplement.
heartburn	This unpleasant burning sensation occurs when stomach acids leak into the oesophagus. This is common during pregnancy because progesterone relaxes the valve that normally prevents this happening. This pregnancy hormone also reduces the tone and activity of the stomach muscles, so that it takes longer to empty the stomach of its contents. Also, in late pregnancy, the uterus presses upwards on the stomach, squeezing out the stomach acids.	Eat little and often, and never late at night. Avoid spicy foods if you are not used to them. Drink milk or peppermint tea, and have a glass of milk at bedtime. Avoid drinks with a high sugar content, which may slow down the emptying of the stomach. Improve your posture because slouching can make the problem worse (see page 94). In bed, either prop up your shoulders with pillows or prop up the head of the bed on a couple of bricks. If these measures do not help, ask your doctor to prescribe suitable medication.
pregnancy sickness and nausea – 'morning' sickness	This is often one of the first symptoms of pregnancy and affects roughly 70 per cent of women. It occurs mostly in the morning. Altered taste and smell sensations can make nausea worse. The sickness usually improves at around 14 weeks but sometimes continues throughout pregnancy, or disappears but then reappears towards the end. It is thought to be linked to the pregnancy hormone human chorionic gonadotrophin	Eat little and often. Choose foods that are high in protein and complex carbohydrates (for example, brown rice, pasta) and avoid fatty foods. Have a snack at bedtime and another at least 20 minutes before you get up. Take snacks (for example, packets of dried fruit or rice cakes) with you when you go out. If you are vomiting, you must replace lost fluids. Avoid caffeinated drinks, for example, coffee, tea and cola, which are dehydrating.

COMPLAINT	DESCRIPTION	ACTION

(HCG). Levels in the blood drop at around 12 weeks, when other hormones begin to take over, which is why it is more common in early pregnancy.

The hormone oestrogen can lower blood pressure, as well as slowing the action of the digestive system, which in turn can cause nausea.

Normal pregnancy sickness will not harm your baby, who will still get what he needs from you – even if you can only eat small amounts – as long as your diet is balanced.

Some evidence shows that nausea and vomiting are associated with a better pregnancy outcome, that is, miscarriage is less common – which may be of some reassurance to women who are otherwise feeling dreadful!

Instead, drink vegetable or fruit juices as well as water, and eat fresh, juicy fruit. If drinking water makes you feel ill, try sipping water between meals, sucking ice cubes or eating ice lollies. Some women find that fizzy drinks help.

Fresh ginger can help to reduce sickness. Pour some hot water over freshly grated root ginger, and add a teaspoonful of sugar, honey or lemon juice. Strain after a few minutes and drink it either hot or chilled from the fridge. Also try non-alcoholic ginger beer, adding ginger to stir-fries and sauces, or nibbling ginger biscuits.

Avoid smells and foods (usually strong-smelling ones) that trigger your nausea.

Try to get more sleep and relax for short periods during the day. Morning sickness is often worse when you are tired or stressed.

Wear loose clothing. Many women feel more bloated at the end of the day.

Take your mind off the nausea as much as possible by keeping occupied.

Ask your doctor whether you need a general vitamin supplement (some women with pregnancy sickness lack vitamin B6). Always ask your doctor before taking any vitamin supplements.

Consider complementary therapies:

- Acupuncture is a form of Chinese medicine that can be used to treat sickness, but only by a qualified practitioner.
- Try acupressure bands (or 'travel bands'), which are readily available and are worn on the wrists. These work on the same principle as acupuncture: a plastic button on the band presses on an acupressure point that is thought to reduce nausea and vomiting.
- Try aromatherapy: (see page 59). Citrus oils (lime, grapefruit, bergamot, orange and mandarin) are safe to use, as are peppermint, spearmint and ginger – or consult a qualified aromatherapist.

COMPLAINT	DESCRIPTION	ACTION
pregnancy sickness – severe	Approximately 2 per cent of women suffer from a severe sickness (hyperemesis gravidarum) that is very different from normal pregnancy sickness. They are unable to keep down fluids and can become dehydrated. Severe sickness during pregnancy can also be a sign of a urine infection so this should always be excluded. Symptoms include extreme weight loss, passing of small amounts of very concentrated urine, and dry, less elastic skin. This sickness can also be a feature of a twin pregnancy or a 'failed' pregnancy or a rare condition known as a hydatidiform mole when there is distorted growth of the placenta. In this case, the nausea and vomiting may be accompanied by vaginal bleeding, excessive enlargement of the uterus, increased HCG levels, early raised blood pressure and lack of fetal movement or heartbeat. Consult your doctor who can find out whether the sickness is due to a urine infection.	If you become very weak, you may be admitted to hospital for intravenous fluids and regular injections of anti-emetics to prevent further vomiting. If your doctor suspects a failed pregnancy, he may recommend an early ultrasound scan. Consult your dentist for advice on effects of the acid from vomiting and the possiblity of the erosion of tooth enamel.
salivation or drooling	Increased salivation or drooling seems to accompany pregnancy sickness and should diminish after the first few months. On rare occasions, it is caused by an increase in the amount of saliva.	Sometimes it is due to a reluctance to swallow as a result of nausea. Chew mint-flavoured gum or use a mint-flavoured mouthwash.

COMPLAINT	DESCRIPTION	ACTION
RESPIRATORY SYSTEM		
breathlessness	Breathlessness in early pregnancy is usually caused by progesterone hormones stimulating the brain's respiratory centre, increasing your rate of breathing. In late pregnancy, your baby is pressing on your diaphragm, which restricts your breathing: your lungs are unable to expand fully because of the increasing size of the uterus and the fact that carrying around the combined weight of the developing baby, the placenta, amniotic fluid and uterus is hard work! If breathlessness is accompanied by fatigue and palpitations, this may be a sign of anaemia (see page 99).	Sit up straight, not slumped. Try propping yourself up with a couple of pillows at night. If you show signs of anaemia, see your doctor or midwife. If you develop unexpected and severe shortness of breath, rapid breathing, blue lips and fingers, and a rapid pulse or chest pain, get medical attention immediately.
enhanced sense of smell	Some women find that they develop an increased sensitivity to smell. This is probably related to hormones causing congestion and swelling in the tissues lining the nose. This alters the signals reaching the nerves that are responsible for the sense of smell.	None.
sinusitis	Sinusitis affects the mucus membrane lining the cavities around the eyes, cheeks and nose (see also nosebleeds, page 101). Symptoms include pain above and below one or both eyes, apparent toothache and thick, discoloured mucus. It often follows a cold and is caused by an infection.	If you think you have sinusitis, tell your doctor, who may prescribe a safe antibiotic or decongestant. Do not use over-the-counter decongestants as some may have adverse effects on your baby.

COMPLAINT	DESCRIPTION	ACTION
stuffy or blocked nose	Many women feel particularly 'snuffly' during certain stages of pregnancy, for example, from 9 to 12 weeks. This can also cause headaches. General 'snuffliness' is the result of nasal congestion caused by swollen mucus membranes.	There is little that you can do apart from hanging humidifiers over your central heating radiators or putting a bowl of water on the window sills above them. Avoid getting dehydrated as, in theory, this can make nasal secretions even thicker. Try using nasal strips to hold your nostrils open if you are having problems breathing at night. These may also help if you snore. Do not use over-the-counter decongestants as some may have adverse effects on your baby's development.

ACHES AND PAINS

COMPLAINT	DESCRIPTION	ACTION
backache 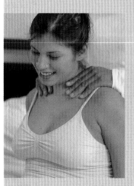	As your pregnancy progresses, you may become more susceptible to back pain, especially if you are already prone to it. This is usually the result of poor posture. As your baby grows and your uterus expands, you may find you are not standing so upright. This can increase the curve in the small of your back, adding to the strain in an area that is already carrying more weight than normal.	Watch your posture (pregnancy yoga can help with this) and try not to arch your back. Avoid standing for too long or sitting hunched over your desk. Be careful when lifting objects and always carry them close to your body. Regular exercise, for example, walking and swimming, can help. Gentle massage of the back may alleviate pain (see page 61). It is also worth considering a visit to a chiropractor or osteopath. Replace your mattress if it is very old. If back or pelvic pains are severe, see a specialist pregnancy physiotherapist who may give you a 'bump support'.

COMPLAINT	DESCRIPTION	ACTION
braxton hicks tightenings	These mild, irregular tightenings are present from the beginning of pregnancy but you do not usually become aware of them until about the beginning of late pregnancy. These tightenings are named after the doctor who discovered their purpose, and they are a normal part of pregnancy. They squeeze blood out of the uterine veins, enabling them to fill with fresh blood, and help to stretch the lower part of the uterus, preparing it for labour. They may be triggered by having sex or an orgasm, but this does not mean that you are going into labour.	If contractions become frequent, regular or painful, contact your midwife or doctor to rule out the possibility of an early labour.
carpal tunnel syndrome	These pains in the hands generally occur in mid- and late pregnancy and usually disappear within a couple of weeks of the birth. The thumb, index and middle fingers and half of your ring finger may feel numb and/or get pins and needles, and there may be pain in the fingers that travels up to the wrist and forearm. The symptoms tend to be worse at night and may be accompanied by a weakness in the movement of the thumb. The condition is caused by swelling in the part of the wrist through which the median nerve to the fingers runs.	Rest your hands on a separate pillow rather than sleeping with your head on your hands. Try to disperse the swelling by gentle exercise, for example, circling and flexing your wrists and putting them in cold water. Drink plenty of water. Ask your doctor to refer you to a physiotherapist, who can give you some exercises that may help. If the condition does not improve, you may be given a splint to support your wrist. An osteopath may be able to manipulate the wrist to help with the drainage. Occasionally, a steroid injection around the nerve can be given in pregnancy.
headache	Many pregnant women get headaches. These are usually the result of hormone changes but can also be caused by anxiety and tiredness, low blood sugar or dehydration. They can also be a sign of high blood pressure, particularly after 24 weeks of pregnancy (see page 100).	Wrap some ice in a flannel and hold it against your forehead (or buy cooling gel strips from your pharmacist). A few drops of lavender oil on your pillow, or on a hanky, is an effective headache cure. Rub a headache stick on your forehead. This combination of natural soothing oils is safe in pregnancy and handy to carry around. Try a head massage to relieve tension. Have a snack or a drink.

COMPLAINT	DESCRIPTION	ACTION
leg cramps and restless legs 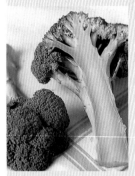	About 50 per cent of pregnant women suffer from night cramps in their legs at any time from 14 weeks of pregnancy. According to one theory, this is related to iron deficiency in certain areas of the brain, so iron supplements may help. Restless legs (Ekbom syndrome) is a relatively common feature of pregnancy but usually settles down after the birth. This burning or twitching feeling in the legs is accompanied by an irresistible urge to move the legs, which can bring some relief. It can be very distressing and may severely interfere with sleep.	Make sure you are getting enough fluids. Increasing the amount of calcium in your diet may help. Good sources include milk, yoghurt, cheese, canned fish, tofu, green leafy vegetables and baked beans. Wear support tights and rest several times a day with your legs raised. Try leg stretches (see page 48) a few times during the day, or take several short walks. If you often get cramp at night, during the evening massage your legs with a carrier oil with 2 drops of lavender oil or soak your feet in a bowl of water with 2 drops of lavender. To relieve leg cramp, straighten your leg and point your toes towards your head, or pull your toes up towards your ankle to stretch the leg muscle. Breathe deeply to encourage the muscle to relax. If these work, apply gentle heat and gentle massage. If they don't work, do not heat or massage the leg, tell your midwife or doctor because there is a slight risk of a thrombosis (see also varicose veins, page 102).
ligament pain	Ligaments are the tough bands of fibrous tissue that connect bones and cartilage, control movement in the joints and support the muscles. These loosen and stretch during pregnancy and can cause a variety of aches and pains, particularly around the sides of your stomach and your pelvis. This is usually nothing to worry about unless accompanied by other symptoms.	Mention the problem to your doctor or midwife at your next appointment.
pins and needles (see also carpal tunnel syndrome, page 95)	Pins and needles or numbness in the hands and feet are common and will disappear within a few days of the birth. The problem is thought to result from the pressure of excess fluid (oedema) on nerve endings (see swelling, page 102).	Sit with your feet up whenever possible.

COMPLAINT	DESCRIPTION	ACTION
rib pain	This is usually caused by your baby's feet lodging between your ribs.	Try persuading her to move with a very gentle prod.
sciatica	This is a sharp pain that starts in the lower back, buttock or hip and radiates down one leg, usually during late pregnancy. It is caused by the uterus pressing on the sciatic nerve that runs from the middle of the back, through the buttocks and down each leg.	Gentle stretching exercises and heat therapy may ease the symptoms.
stomach cramps	See Braxton Hicks tightenings and ligament pain (pages 95 and 96)	If cramps are accompanied by bleeding, fever or chills, increased vaginal discharge, faintness or other unusual symptoms, see your doctor immediately. If cramps become more painful or occur frequently, contact your midwife or doctor.
symphysis pubis dysfunction (SPD)	This condition can cause a lot of discomfort during pregnancy. The pain can be at the front, around the pubic area, or sometimes in the lower back, and can start as early as the twelfth week of pregnancy. The pain may continue postnatally but will eventually get better. It is caused by the joints in the pelvis parting slightly, because of hormones stretching and softening the ligaments (see ligament pain, page 96).	Your midwife should refer you to a physiotherapist, who can assess the extent of the problem and may give you a support belt to wear around your stomach. Rest is often advised and you should be taught how to get in and out of bed, keeping your knees together, and on how best to go up and down stairs.

URINARY SYSTEM

COMPLAINT	DESCRIPTION	ACTION
urinary tract infections – urine infections	Pregnant women are at risk of urine infections and this is increased if they have diabetes. During pregnancy, progesterone relaxes the muscles of the bladder and of the ureters that connect the bladder and kidneys. This allows urine to collect and stagnate in the bladder, and it sometimes passes back into the kidney, increasing the risk of infection.	See page 98.

COMPLAINT	DESCRIPTION	ACTION
urinary tract infections – cystitis 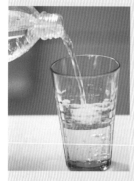	The bladder is the commonest site affected by a urinary tract infection. Infection causes inflammation of the bladder (cystitis), which, depending on its severity, causes symptoms including a burning sensation when urinating, a frequent urge to urinate that only produces a small amount, and general pain in the pelvic area. Sometimes the urine is cloudy, with traces of blood and an unpleasant smell. The condition can be recurrent. Sometimes there are no symptoms and the infection is diagnosed during a routine screening.	Drink plenty of water, as well as barley water and cranberry juice, in order to flush out your kidneys, ureters and bladder. Pass water immediately after sexual intercourse and wipe from front to back after using the toilet. Avoid over-the-counter remedies, most of which contain high amounts of salt. Consult your doctor because antibiotic treatment is essential to avoid the infection progressing to the kidneys (see below).
urinary tract infections – kidney infections	Kidney infections are more serious. The symptoms are similar to those of cystitis but may be accompanied by fever, backache, chills and nausea or vomiting. If untreated, high fever can lead to premature labour.	If you develop these symptoms, call your doctor immediately. Depending on the severity of the infection, you may need to be admitted to hospital for intravenous antibiotics.
urination problems – increased urination	This is a common feature of early and late pregnancy. In early pregnancy, pregnancy hormones cause changes in your circulation and muscle tone, leading to a feeling of congestion in your pelvic area. Also your bladder is squashed by your growing uterus until the twelfth week, when it rises above the pelvic cavity. It occurs again in late pregnancy, when the engagement of your baby's head places more pressure on your bladder. If there are no signs of urinary tract infection (see above), this is perfectly normal.	In late pregnancy, avoid standing for prolonged periods.
urination problems – stress incontinence	During the last 12 weeks of pregnancy, you may leak urine when you cough, sneeze or laugh. This is caused by the pressure of your uterus and baby on your bladder, and possibly by the effects of hormones on the pelvic floor.	Practise pelvic floor exercises (see page 272).

COMPLAINT	DESCRIPTION	ACTION
REPRODUCTIVE SYSTEM		
bleeding/spotting	There are many causes, from the minor (cervical erosion, where the surface of the cervix becomes fragile under the influence of hormones) to the serious (sexually transmitted diseases, ectopic pregnancy, miscarriage or cervical cancer). In late pregnancy, bleeding may indicate problems with the placenta (see page 114).	Tell your midwife or doctor about any bleeding immediately, especially if it is accompanied by pain.
candida (thrush)	Pregnant women tend to be prone to this infection, which is caused by a yeast (candida). Symptoms include a white, itchy discharge and vaginal soreness, and sometimes itching of the anus and pain on urination. Recurrent thrush can be a nuisance but is not harmful to the baby. However, it may be an indication of diabetes (see page 80).	Your midwife will take a swab to confirm the cause of the discharge. Candida is easily treated with pessaries and creams. If your partner also shows signs of infection, it may be worthwhile for him to be treated, too. Reduce the chance of recurrence by washing the affected area only with plain water. Avoid scented bath products and tight clothing.
increased/ changed vaginal discharge	An increased vaginal discharge is normal during pregnancy and is usually caused by the effects of hormones on the tissues of the cervix and vagina. More serious causes are sexually transmitted diseases and candida (see above).	If the discharge is excessive, itchy, smells bad or is coloured, tell your midwife or doctor. Vaginal infections must be treated as some can provoke labour or be transmitted to the baby. Tell your doctor or midwife if you have any unusual discharge.
BLOOD AND CIRCULATION		
aching legs		See swelling and varicose veins, page 102.
anaemia	Women are usually checked for anaemia at their first midwife appointment, but iron-deficiency anaemia may develop at any time during pregnancy, particularly after the twentieth week. After this time, the amount of iron required by your baby soars. Symptoms include pallor, exhaustion, breathlessness, palpitations and fainting.	Eat plenty of iron-rich foods (but not liver) and fresh fruit and vegetables (the vitamin C they contain will aid iron absorption). Ask your doctor or midwife whether you need an extra iron supplement. They may offer you another blood test and give you iron supplements if they suspect anaemia.

COMPLAINT	DESCRIPTION	ACTION
blood pressure – high (hypertension) 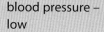	About 10 per cent of women experience high blood pressure, especially towards the end of their pregnancy. Blood pressure is recorded as two measurements, systolic and diastolic. Systolic is the pressure as the heart beats and diastolic the pressure as it relaxes.	Make sure that your midwife takes your blood pressure regularly. Have periods of rest and use breathing exercises as an aid to relaxation. Avoid too much salty food and eat more fruit and vegetables.
blood pressure – low	In early pregnancy, blood pressure falls as your circulatory system expands to include that of the enlarging uterus and placenta. Hormones, particularly oestrogen, play a part by reducing the elasticity of the blood vessels and dilating them. Blood pressure is lowest in mid-pregnancy and gradually increases towards pre-pregnancy levels at term. The most noticeable symptom is light-headedness or dizziness when you stand up rapidly. You may also notice that your fingers are trembling and your heart rate is raised (see also anaemia, page 99). Fainting is a defence mechanism that comes into play when the brain is not getting enough blood. Falling down restores the brain's blood supply because blood no longer has to flow 'uphill'.	Stand up slowly, especially after sitting for a long time. Do not go for too long without a meal or snack as hunger can make the problem worse. If you feel faint, lie flat on the floor and raise your legs above hip level. If you are very pregnant, lie slightly to one side rather than flat because the weight of the uterus can squash the large blood vessels in the abdomen, causing further faintness. If lying flat is not practical, sit down so that you cannot fall and hurt yourself. Put your head between your knees as low as possible until you recover. A drink or a light snack may help at this point. Never prop up anyone who is about to faint – this could be very dangerous. If you have not fainted before, ask your doctor to check that there is no other reason for this blackout.

COMPLAINT	DESCRIPTION	ACTION
haemorrhoids (piles)	Piles are similar to varicose veins (see page 102) but they occur in the anus. They are painful, especially during or after opening your bowels, when they sometimes bleed, and often itchy. In most cases, piles disappear a few weeks after the birth, although they may worsen in the short term after labour. Piles are aggravated by the weight of the baby and uterus on the pelvic veins and by constipation with straining.	To allow the piles to shrink and settle, try to avoid constipation by drinking plenty of fluids to avoid dehydration and eating plenty of fruit and fibre-rich foods. Try not to strain when passing a stool: relax your pelvic floor muscles and breathe deeply. If necessary take a recommended stool-softening laxative. Soothe the pain and irritation by using an aqueous cream (readily available over the counter or on prescription) as a soap substitute, taking a cool bath, or applying a cold compress made by soaking a flannel in a bowl of cold water to which 2 drops of witch hazel have been added. Avoid standing for too long, especially in late pregnancy. Lie on your side rather than on your back. Take regular gentle exercise to improve your circulation: swimming is very good. If the piles are uncomfortable or have prolapsed (that is, are outside the anus), ask your doctor for a cream to reduce the swelling. If piles persist and cause discomfort, they can be surgically removed.
nosebleeds	These may occur more frequently during pregnancy due to dilation and congestion of the fine blood vessels causing the lining of the nose to become fragile and bleed more readily. This is especially the case if you are already suffering from a stuffy nose (see page 94).	Do not blow your nose too hard because this may damage the walls of the blood vessels. Gently clear your nostrils alternately. To stem a nosebleed, lean forward slightly and pinch just below the bridge of your nose for 5 minutes. If necessary, repeat twice more or until the bleeding has stopped. Avoid blowing your nose. If the bleeding does not stop, recurs or is heavy, tell your doctor or go to the outpatients department of your local hospital.

COMPLAINT	DESCRIPTION	ACTION
swelling 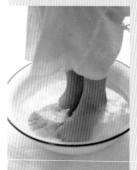	Puffiness of the ankles and wrists is common during pregnancy and is caused by the accumulation of fluid (oedema). This is probably related to expansion of the blood vessels near the skin, which increases the blood flow and encourages fluid to move into and remain in the tissues. In most cases this is uncomfortable rather than serious. However, any new or rapidly worsening swelling, particularly later in pregnancy, may be an indication of pre-eclampsia (see page 110), so you should tell your midwife or doctor. In the legs, the pressure of the pregnant uterus slows the rate of blood flow in the small blood vessels, effectively squeezing out fluid into the tissues.	Drink plenty of fluids. To alleviate discomfort, wear support tights or stockings and avoid tight shoes. Take short brisk walks and put your feet up when sitting down. If possible, lie down for short periods on your left side during the day. Wear open-toed flat sandals, low mules or loosely laced trainers rather than tight shoes. Avoid wearing tight socks, which can restrict your blood flow – wear loose socks or support tights instead. A pedicure will refresh your aching feet. Treat your legs and feet with a body or facial scrub. Or you could refresh tired feet by soaking them in a cool footbath containing 2 drops of peppermint oil. After a warm, but not hot, bath, sit on a chair and roll your feet backwards and forwards on a rolling pin.
varicose veins	Varicose veins vary in severity from faint bluish lines to bulging veins that protrude from the skin. They ache and are sometimes very painful, as well as producing a feeling of heaviness. They are caused by a restriction in the flow of blood back to the heart. The veins dilate to accommodate the extra blood. The problem seems to be hereditary and may be exacerbated by excess weight. Any tenderness in your calf or thigh, accompanied by swelling, inflammation, an increased heart rate or a raised temperature may indicate a thrombosis.	Prevention is the key. Do not sit with your legs crossed and raise your legs while you are seated. Avoid standing for long periods of time. Massage the area gently to reduce the likelihood of getting varicose veins, but do not massage the area once they appear. Daily exercise, such as swimming, walking or yoga, helps to improve circulation. Wear support tights. Ideally, put them on before you get up. To ease aches, spray your legs with alternate blasts of hot and cold water from the shower. If veins are painful and itchy, apply an ice pack or a bag of frozen peas. Tell your doctor immediately if you suspect a thrombosis.

COMPLAINT	DESCRIPTION	ACTION
vulval varicose veins	Varicose veins (see opposite) sometimes develop in the vulva during pregnancy, particularly as the baby becomes heavier. They can cause an uncomfortable feeling of heaviness that aches, particularly towards the end of the day.	Wear a thick sanitary towel to support the affected area. Apply an ice pack or a bag of frozen peas to reduce the swelling. Avoid standing for long periods.

ENERGY AND SLEEP

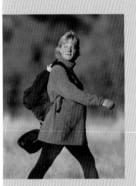

COMPLAINT	DESCRIPTION	ACTION
fatigue	Extreme fatigue is especially common during early and late pregnancy. In early pregnancy, it is caused by increased amounts of hormones, particularly progesterone, which also helps you to sleep. Also, your metabolism is working overtime, your heart is beating faster and your baby is developing at an amazing rate. All this, combined with nausea, can make you feel completely drained. In later pregnancy, especially during the last few weeks, the extra weight that you are carrying will make you tired and a variety of factors (for example, pressure on your bladder, heartburn, aches and pains) may make sleeping difficult. Excessive tiredness may be due to anaemia (see page 99).	Do what your body tells you and get as much rest as you can. Learn how to relax (see page 52) and set aside times each day to do this. Pace yourself: when you have the energy, use it. Drink plenty of water and do not go too long without food (see pages 34–37). Eat little and often to maintain your blood-sugar level. Avoid sweet food and drinks. Try exercise (see pages 44–49), which will give you more energy and improve your circulation. Try aromatherapy (see page 59). Citrus oils are revitalizing and can easily be inhaled by putting 2 drops onto a handkerchief. If you have any symptoms of anaemia, tell your doctor.
vivid dreams	Most pregnant women express their fears and anxieties by having vivid dreams. Some also have very erotic dreams. This is quite normal and is most probably caused by disturbed sleep or changes in hormone levels. From 25 weeks the quality of sleep changes to include more rapid eye movement (REM) sleep, which may explain changes in dreaming.	Relax before going to bed: taking a warm bath, listen to gentle music and have a milky drink. If anything is worrying you do not keep it to yourself. Talking to your midwife, or friends and family may help you get a good night's sleep.

COMPLAINT	DESCRIPTION	ACTION
EMOTIONAL AND MENTAL		
depression	Mild depression is common – perhaps more common than postnatal depression – and it is just as important as physical complaints.	Ignore anyone who tells you to 'snap out of it'. The sooner you get help, the quicker the symptoms are likely to improve.
	The symptoms include mood swings, lethargy, irritability, lack of interest in anything and an inability to concentrate.	Look after yourself: eat as healthily as you can, get enough sleep and ask friends and family to help out if things are getting on top of you (for example, housework, the children).
		Make time to do the things you enjoy, for example, going to the cinema or eating out.
		Talk to your doctor, who should be able to refer you to a therapist with whom you can discuss treatment options.
memory loss	Many pregnant women suffer from short-term memory loss.	Relax and do not get frustrated – this will only make the problem worse.
	The effect may persist until a few weeks after the birth.	Make lists and try to adjust to being less efficient than usual.
mood swings	Although mood swings, irritability and weepiness may be difficult for you and those around you to deal with, they are very common during pregnancy. If you talk to other women they will tell you that they have the same problem.	Avoid foods that give an initial high, then have a rebound effect, which might make you feel down, for example, sugar and coffee.
	They are simply the result of the natural rollercoaster of emotions that accompanies pregnancy.	Indulge yourself: spend some quiet time alone; try a pedicure or massage; take up relaxation techniques and yoga, Pilates or gentle exercise.
MISCELLANEOUS		
blocked ears	Women may get partial deafness (as if they have cotton wool in their ears), and 'popping ' (due to changing pressure, as in an aircraft). This is due to congestion of the tissues lining the Eustachian tubes, which run between the back of the throat and the inner ears.	Block one nostril with your finger and blow gently through the other nostril. Repeat with the other nostril. Do not stick cotton buds into the ear canal.

COMPLAINT	DESCRIPTION	ACTION
eyesight changes	Many women find that they become either short- or long-sighted during pregnancy. This is because extra fluids in the body cause the eyeball to change shape. The tear ducts secrete less fluid and the eyes are drier. These changes may make hard contact lenses uncomfortable and result in tired eyes or headaches after watching the television, reading or working at a computer, but should return to normal within a few months. Headache and visual disturbances (for example, blurring, dizziness, floaters or spots), late in pregnancy in particular, may indicate high blood pressure (see page 110).	Get your eyes tested to see whether you need a pair of glasses for a while. If you wear hard contact lenses, you may have to switch to soft lenses or glasses. Tell your midwife or doctor if you have any unusual symptoms.
dizziness	Feelings of light-headedness often occur during early or mid-pregnancy because of low blood pressure (see page 100). Later, it may be caused by the pressure of the uterus on the vessels carrying blood back to the heart. Other possible causes include anaemia (see page 99) and low blood-sugar levels.	Avoid standing for long periods and never take hot baths. Tell your midwife or doctor if you get recurring dizziness.
changes to fingernails and toenails	Some pregnant women find that their nails grow more quickly. Others find that their nails become softer, develop grooves and break or split easily.	Keep your nails short, wear gloves to wash up and moisturize your nails at least once a day. If you notice any signs of discoloration, you may have an infection and this should be treated by your doctor.
raised temperature and increased sweating	Many women find that they are constantly warm, particularly in their hands and feet, and have a permanently shiny face. This is because your basal metabolic rate increases by about 20 per cent during pregnancy. This increases the amount of body heat that you generate. Some of this heat is dissipated through the skin by means of increased blood flow, which makes the hands and feet warmer.	Wear loose clothing made from natural rather than synthetic materials. In winter, wear layers so that you can peel them off as necessary. If your underarms are working overtime, have wipes and an antiperspirant to hand. You'll be more aware of it than people around you, so do not get stressed as this will make it worse.

understanding
miscarriage

The term 'miscarriage' refers to a pregnancy that is lost before 24 weeks of gestation. Miscarriage occurs after approximately 50 per cent of conceptions. In many cases it is not recognized because it happens very early on, within a fortnight of conception, and is interpreted as a late period. Miscarriage is clinically diagnosed in only 15 per cent or so of pregnancies.

'I had a feeling something wasn't quite right on the day of my first antenatal check, when I noticed some bleeding. It was only a few spots but I told the midwife. She was reassuring and said it was probably breakthrough bleeding as my period would have been due. I wasn't convinced – I felt achy, as if I was having a period. About a week later I started bleeding heavily and was taken to hospital because I was miscarrying. It was a horrible time and I was so happy when I became pregnant six months later. The first months were tense – I was so worried about losing another baby. It was a while before I could relax.'

Jane, mother of
11-month-old Frances

shared
experience

types of miscarriage

There are several types of miscarriage, and these are classified according to the manner in which they occur.

Threatened miscarriage In this situation, bleeding occurs at some point during the first few months of pregnancy but there is minimal pain, the cervix remains closed and an ultrasound scan confirms a viable pregnancy.

In more than 90 per cent of cases the pregnancy will continue normally and a repeat scan to check the fetal heart will provide reassurance for the mother.

Inevitable miscarriage This involves a considerable amount of bleeding and the cervix will be open. There are two types:

- Complete miscarriage in which the products of conception are completely expelled.
- Incomplete miscarriage in which some of the products of conception are retained. In rare cases, they will become infected (septic) and the infection may spread, causing peritonitis and septicaemia.
- Delayed (missed) miscarriage is commonly diagnosed when an early pregnancy scan identifies a fetus but no fetal heart is seen on the monitor. In this case there are often very few symptoms to indicate that the baby has died.

causes

Over 50 per cent of miscarriages in early pregnancy are a result of the baby having abnormal chromosomes. Less common are maternal factors, such as:

- Infection, for example, listeriosis, cytomegalovirus or rubella
- An underlying medical disorder, for example, thyroid disease or systemic lupus erythematosus
- Smoking
- Alcohol
- Late age of the mother

In rare cases, miscarriage is caused by a congenital abnormality of the uterus or cervix. A miscarriage in mid-pregnancy may be due to the cervix dilating unusually early (cervical incompetence), possibly caused by previous cervical surgery, for example a large cone biopsy after abnormal smear tests.

treatment
In some cases, miscarriage can be allowed to progress on its own with no further intervention. If treatment is required or requested, this can be either by the use of drugs to encourage the uterus to expel the products of conception or by an operation (called an evacuation of retained products of conception, or ERPOC).

recurrent miscarriage
This term is used when three or more consecutive miscarriages occur. This happens in 1 per cent of women and will need further investigation to try to identify the underlying cause.

causes
Possible causes of recurrent miscarriage include:
- Genetic abnormality in either parent
- Abnormality of the uterus (for example, bicornuate uterus)
- Chronic illness, for example, thyroid disease or diabetes (see page 80)
- Polycystic ovary syndrome (see box, right)
- Raised levels of testosterone or luteinizing hormone (LH)
- Cervical incompetence (see above)
- Antiphospholid syndrome. This is a very rare disorder in which antibodies from the mother are directed at the placenta, causing blood clotting and other damage.

prevention
Up to 80 per cent of women who have had recurrent miscarriage will go on to have a successful pregnancy with just supportive treatment, such as an early scan followed by serial scans for reassurance. Often no specific therapy is necessary. In the rare case of antiphospholid syndrome (see above), evidence shows that taking aspirin and heparin early in pregnancy can improve the outcome of the pregnancy.

trying again
There are no strict rules about when to try for another baby after a miscarriage. Many women are advised to wait for a few months, mainly so that their cycle can return to normal and to make it easier to know how pregnant they are when they manage to conceive.

support groups
After the sadness of a miscarriage, women need both emotional and physical care. The hospital or doctor can give advice on counselling, and support groups.

polycystic ovary syndrome

PCOS is common (affecting 1 in 10 women at some stage) and is characterized by multiple small cysts within the ovary (seen on ultrasound scans) and features such as period problems, reduced fertility, excessive hair growth and acne. Many women with PCOS are also overweight.

ectopic
pregnancies

An ectopic pregnancy occurs when a fertilized egg implants outside of the uterus. The incidence of ectopic pregnancy varies enormously between countries, for example, 1.24 per cent of pregnancies are ectopic in the United Kingdom compared with 4 per cent in Ghana. The method of conception also has an effect, for example, after in vitro fertilization (IVF), the incidence is as high as 4–11 per cent.

Q **Will a pregnancy test show positive in ectopic pregnancy?**

A A urine home pregnancy test will be positive in almost all instances of ectopic pregnancy, but it might be only weakly positive. Where there is any doubt, a blood test will always be positive in an ectopic pregnancy.

The most common site for an ectopic pregnancy is the Fallopian tube (see page 12). More rarely, an ectopic pregnancy occurs in the ovary or abdominal cavity.

Risk factors for an ectopic pregnancy include:
- A previous ectopic pregnancy
- A history of pelvic inflammatory disease (for example, chlamydia infection)
- Previous tubal surgery (for example, reversal of a sterilization procedure)
- Conception while on the mini-pill or with a coil in place
- Fertility treatment (for example, ovulation induction or in vitro fertilization).

symptoms

Most women with an ectopic pregnancy complain of a missed or abnormal last period, vaginal bleeding or abdominal pain. However, not all women have these classic symptoms. Therefore an ectopic pregnancy should be suspected in any woman of reproductive age who has abdominal pain.

Ectopic pregnancy can be life-threatening. The main danger occurs when the pregnancy occurs in the Fallopian tube and causes a rupture in the Fallopian tube, in which case major internal bleeding can occur, resulting in shock and collapse.

diagnosis

Early diagnosis is vital whenever an ectopic pregnancy is suspected, for example, when the uterus is found to be empty or, in some cases, when a mass is seen next to the uterus.

Investigations such as an ultrasound scan (see page 124) – which is often performed transvaginally – and blood tests are useful in diagnosis. A laparoscopy (see page 27) will enable the obstetrician to inspect the Fallopian tubes and pelvis and will confirm the diagnosis.

ectopic pregnancy

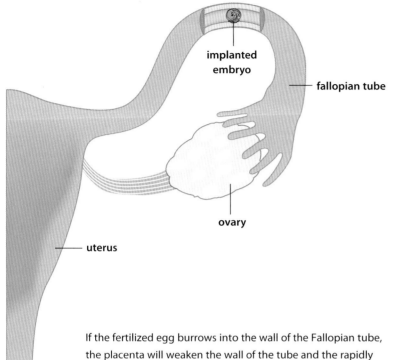

implanted
embryo

fallopian tube

ovary

uterus

If the fertilized egg burrows into the wall of the Fallopian tube, the placenta will weaken the wall of the tube and the rapidly expanding embryo will stretch it, causing pain and bleeding.

treatment

The treatment of an ectopic pregnancy is aimed mainly at preventing major haemorrhage and most commonly involves an operation on the affected Fallopian tube. It may be necessary to remove the tube, or the ectopic pregnancy itself can be removed while preserving the tube. Nowadays, this can often be done by using keyhole surgery, but it may be necessary to make an incision (usually just below the bikini line) in the abdomen, particularly if the ectopic pregnancy has ruptured the Fallopian tube. If the tube ruptures, a blood transfusion may be necessary.

In some cases, it may be possible to treat a small ectopic pregnancy with powerful drugs designed to stop it growing, thereby avoiding the risk of it rupturing or the need for surgery.

consequences

The conditions that originally gave rise to the ectopic pregnancy, and its treatment, may affect subsequent fertility. Only about one third of women trying to become pregnant after an ectopic pregnancy will be successful. A significant number (15–20 per cent) will have another ectopic pregnancy.

In subsequent pregnancies women who have had a previous ectopic pregnancy will usually be advised to have an early ultrasound scan at about 7 weeks gestation to determine whether the pregnancy is within the uterus or not.

'Having reported a minor pain in my abdomen and the passing of a little blood to my doctor, I was referred to hospital. Following an internal scan and a blood test I was told that I had an ectopic pregnancy and that I would have to have it surgically removed that day. The procedure itself was relatively simple – keyhole surgery under general anaesthetic to remove the pregnancy and part of my now damaged Fallopian tube, but I was not prepared for the shock of emergency surgery, losing part of my reproductive system (would I be able to conceive again?) and of going into the hospital six weeks pregnant and coming out not pregnant the following day.'

Sally, mother of
3-year-old Sam

shared
experience

pre-eclampsia and eclampsia

Pre-eclampsia occurs only during pregnancy (generally after 20 weeks) and during the period immediately after the birth. It can affect both mother and unborn baby. It is a complication of 2–3 per cent of all pregnancies and 5–7 per cent of first pregnancies and is a major cause of growth restriction in the uterus and perinatal mortality. Pre-eclampsia is also a major reason for delivering babies prematurely.

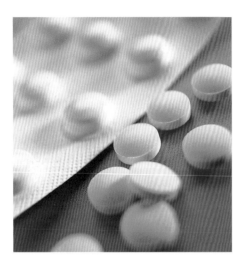

Women who are particularly at risk of pre-eclampsia may benefit from a daily dose of aspirin, calcium, folic acid or vitamins C and E.

A small proportion of women with pre-eclampsia (2 per cent) go on to develop convulsions, known as eclampsia. Risk factors for pre-eclampsia include:

- A first pregnancy
- Being pregnant with twins or triplets
- A new partner
- Previous pre-eclampsia or a family history of pre-eclampsia (for example, a sister or mother)
- A pre-existing medical problem, for example, high blood pressure (see page 78) or diabetes (see page 80).

causes

Although the exact causes of pre-eclampsia are not fully understood, current understanding suggests that the placenta is mainly responsible. Failure of the fertilized egg to implant properly in the uterus results in the placenta receiving less blood from the mother's uterine arteries. This triggers a sequence of events that can harm the mother, especially her cardiovascular, urinary and central nervous systems and her liver. It also affects her blood-clotting mechanism, can adversely affect the growth of the fetus and increases the risk of placental abruption (see page 114).

symptoms and diagnosis

Early symptoms of pre-eclampsia include visual disturbance (such as flashing lights), headache, upper abdominal pain, vomiting and rapidly worsening swelling (for example, of the legs and ankles). However, most women do not complain of any symptoms when the condition first arises, so diagnosis depends on the vigilance of the midwife or doctor. Therefore, pre-eclampsia is more commonly diagnosed when classic signs of high blood pressure, high levels of protein in the urine (proteinuria) and swelling appear. Pre-eclampsia is an enigmatic condition that presents itself in a great variety of ways, so it is not always easy to spot. Blood tests are also useful in diagnosis.

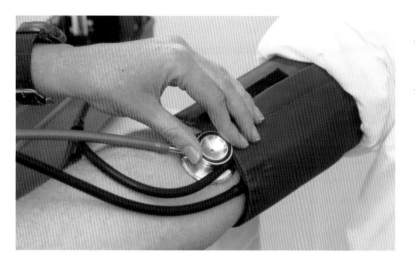

Blood pressure is measured routinely at every antenatal appointment – you will soon get to know what your average reading is. Any high readings can alert your midwife or doctor to the possibility of pre-eclampsia.

Eclampsia is diagnosed when convulsions (fits) occur alongside symptoms of pre-eclampsia. Of these seizures, 44 per cent occur postnatally, 38 per cent before birth and 18 per cent during birth.

screening

All pregnant women should have their blood pressure monitored regularly and their urine tested. Women who are at particular risk of developing pre-eclampsia should be given extra tests, for example, blood tests to check kidney and liver function, and blood counts. Ultrasound scanning of the uterine artery (by Doppler measurements) can detect abnormalities in blood flow at 20–24 weeks. Women with a decreased blood flow are at greater risk of developing disease.

treatment

The only cure for pre-eclampsia is delivery of the fetus and placenta. However, for women with only mild disease, the plan is usually to continue the pregnancy until it is safe to deliver the baby. On the other hand, if the condition is severe or life-threatening, which unfortunately can occur very early in pregnancy, there may be only a few hours in which to act. Treatment therefore depends on the severity of the disease and the how long the baby has been developing.

Blood pressure treatment is sometimes advisable, either in the longer term in mild disease (for example, with oral medication such as methyldopa or a beta blocker) or in the short term (often with intravenous drugs), as part of an intensive treatment regime aimed at stabilizing the mother's condition before delivery. In severe cases, intravenous magnesium sulphate is commonly used in order to prevent eclampsia occurring.

prevention

Low doses of aspirin (75 mg/day) – or calcium, vitamins C and E and folic acid – may help to prevent pre-eclampsia in women who are particularly at risk.

'At 36 weeks a check-up showed my blood pressure was dangerously high. I had to go into hospital to be monitored. "You won't go home before the babies are born," I was told. All I could think was that the kitchen needed decorating.'

Sandra, mother of 4-week-old Ellie and Sofia

shared experiences

'I went to see my midwife because my legs were so swollen I couldn't get my shoes on. I had no other symptoms, so was horrified when she said that I had pre-eclampsia and would need to be admitted to hospital immediately.'

Angela, mother of 6-month-old Matthew

your baby's
life-support system

Normally, the development of the fetus, from a tiny group of just a few cells to a fully grown baby, ready for life in the outside world, occurs inside the uterus with the help of the placenta, the umbilical cord and the straw-coloured amniotic fluid. The main functions of these important elements of your baby's support system are explained below.

the placenta

The placenta is a disc-shaped structure that is attached to the wall of your uterus and is connected to your baby via the umbilical cord. Essentially, it consists of a network of arteries and veins, from your baby, that interfaces with your circulation. At term, it weighs approximately one sixth as much as your baby.

Blood vessels from your baby (the umbilical arteries) enter the placenta, where they divide into fine blood vessels (capillaries) that enter tiny finger-like projections of the placenta (the placental villi). These villi increase the surface area of the placenta and are bathed in your blood, which is transported to the uterus by branches of your uterine arteries (the spiral arteries). This means that your blood and your baby's blood can come very close to each other without actually mixing.

The placenta is usually situated well out of the way of the cervix but occasionally remains in the lower part of the uterus, a condition known as placenta praevia (see page 114). This may be noted at the 20-week scan, but in nine out of ten cases, it will have moved out of the way before you are due to give birth.

functions

The placenta has two main functions:
- It enables carbon dioxide and waste products to cross from your baby's blood into your blood.
- At the same time, it enables oxygen and nutrients to cross from your blood into your baby's blood.

In addition, the placenta manufactures a number of hormones:
- Human chorionic gonadotrophin (HCG), which is important for sustaining the pregnancy during the first few weeks (and is responsible for making your pregnancy test positive).
- Human placental lactogen (HPL), which is important for fetal growth.
- Oestriol (a type of oestrogen).
- Progesterone, to maintain the lining of the uterus.

Throughout your pregnancy, your uterus expands to accommodate your growing baby. Food and oxygen are obtained and waste materials returned via the placenta and umbilical cord. The amniotic fluid keeps the baby safe from bumps and at a constant temperature.

total support

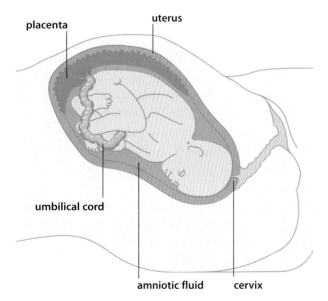

placenta

uterus

umbilical cord

amniotic fluid   cervix

The placenta also protects your baby in the following ways:
- It prevents your baby being rejected by your antibodies.
- It blocks the passage of many (but unfortunately not all) potentially harmful substances, for example drugs and other chemicals.

the umbilical cord

The cord is usually about 50 cm long, 1–2 cm wide and contains two arteries and one vein, which coil around each other in a spiral fashion. Inside the cord is a jelly-like substance called 'Wharton's jelly', which cushions the blood vessels of the umbilical cord. Occasionally there is a knot in the cord. In most cases this does not cause any problems because blood is still able to pass through it.

the amniotic fluid

Throughout pregnancy, your baby is surrounded by a pool of fluid (see also page 143). For most of the pregnancy, this amniotic fluid comes from your baby's urine. The quantity of fluid increases from 150–200 ml at 16 weeks to 1000 ml at 36 weeks.

Amniotic fluid is constantly being recirculated: your baby swallows it as she practises breathing and then passes it out as urine. Any process that interferes with your baby swallowing or passing urine can produce too much amniotic fluid (polyhydramnios) or too little (oligohydramnios). The quantity of amniotic fluid can be measured by ultrasound: a normal amount is one indication that she is thriving.

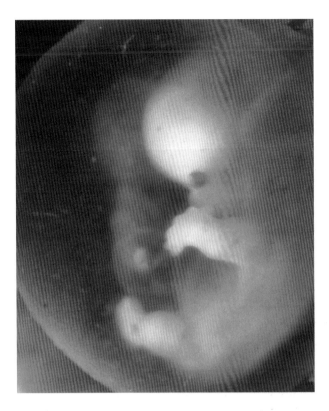

The amniotic sac provides a safe, protective environment in which your baby can develop and grow.

functions

The amniotic fluid has several functions:
- It allows your baby to move around freely.
- It protects her from knocks.
- It keeps her at a constant warm temperature.
- It helps her lungs to develop normally.

nuchal cord

In a small number of pregnancies, the cord winds around the baby's neck (referred to as a nuchal cord). This rarely causes any complications. However, as the baby descends during labour, the cord may tighten, particularly if it is wrapped more than once around the neck. This may lower the baby's heart rate, resulting in signs of fetal distress. Once the baby's head is out, the midwife can usually gently loop the cord over it. Because it is the baby's lifeline, it is not usually advisable to cut it at this stage.

when your waters break

When your waters break, before or during labour, it is amniotic fluid that is expelled. This is usually clear and straw-coloured, but can be greenish in colour, indicating that your baby has opened her bowels in the womb, producing meconium (a mixture of waste secretions, cells and pigments). This is often a sign of fetal maturity, but may also indicate fetal distress.

placental problems

The placenta, which is eventually discharged from the mother's body as the afterbirth (during the third stage of labour, see page 242), is vital to the baby's continuing wellbeing in the uterus (see page 112). Problems concerning the placenta can therefore have important consequences for the baby, during both the pregnancy and the birth.

placenta praevia

This condition occurs when the placenta is situated in the lower part of the uterus. The main danger is major bleeding which normally occurs after about 30 weeks. However, although the 20-week scan often shows the placenta to be 'low lying', in most cases the placenta moves upwards, out of the way of the cervix. As a result, by late pregnancy, fewer than 1 per cent of pregnancies show placenta praevia.

Risk factors for placenta praevia include:
• Previous placenta praevia
• A previous caesarean section
• Pregnancies where there is a larger than usual placenta (for example, twin pregnancies).

symptoms

Classic symptoms include recurrent episodes of painless, heavy vaginal bleeding. Why this should happen before labour is a mystery, but during labour it is the result of the placenta lying over the dilating cervix and coming away from the uterine wall.

diagnosis

Ultrasound is usually a straightforward means of diagnosis. In some instances, particularly when the placenta is at the back of the uterus, a transvaginal scan will show how close the leading edge of the placenta is to the cervix. Another indication of placenta praevia, apart from bleeding, is the failure of the baby to engage into the pelvis – instead he adopts a variety of positions (referred to as 'unstable lie') because the placenta is preventing him from adopting the normal 'head-down' position of late pregnancy.

treatment

A blood transfusion may be necessary if bleeding is excessive. The mother-to-be may be advised to rest and also to avoid sexual intercourse. A placenta that is very close to the cervix will prevent a normal delivery, so a caesarean section will be advised.

placental abruption

Abruption occurs when the placenta becomes detached from the wall of the uterus. This occurs in about 1 per cent of pregnancies and results in maternal bleeding, which may or may not be apparent, depending on how close to the cervix the placenta is situated.

Risk factors for placental abruption include:
• Previous placental abruption
• Hypertension
• Abdominal injury
• Smoking
• Use of cocaine
• Pregnancy later in life
• Several previous pregnancies

symptoms

The classic symptoms of placental abruption include severe abdominal pain and bleeding. With a severe abruption the uterus will be tender and rigid. The amount of blood lost through the vagina may not accurately reflect the true amount of bleeding, because much of the blood can remain concealed within the uterus. This is a risk not only to the baby, because of the placenta becoming detached, but also to the mother, who may develop major problems with blood clotting.

treatment

Treatment depends on the severity of the abruption. A mild abruption may only require a period of observation in hospital to check that both the baby and mother are doing fine. More severe cases may require resuscitation of the mother and early delivery.

retained placenta

The third stage of labour covers the birth of the baby to the delivery of the placenta. In 1–2 per cent of pregnancies the placenta fails to come out, despite carefully pulling on the umbilical cord. In these circumstances, the mother is at risk of bleeding because the uterus is unable to contract properly.

treatment

Sometimes a short wait (up to 30 minutes or so) resolves the problem. If not, it may be necessary to remove the placenta manually. This is carried out under anaesthetic (usually an epidural or a spinal) and the obstetrician gently inserts his fingers into the vagina and can then separate the placenta from the wall of the uterus. Once the placenta has been removed, the mother will be given oxytocin intravenously to help the uterus contract and thus reduce further blood loss. Antibiotics will usually be recommended because of the increased risk of infection.

blood clotting

Any major haemorrhage can disturb the blood-clotting system. These disturbances are more common after a placental abruption because the amount of bleeding may be very much greater than that revealed. Other conditions, such as pre-eclampsia (in which abruption can occur), can also directly affect the mother's blood-clotting system.

placental problems

placenta in normal position

placenta

placental abruption

placenta

blood

placenta praevia

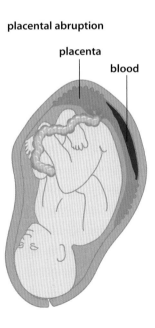

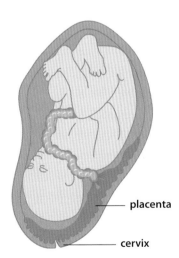

placenta

cervix

Placenta in normal position
Normally the placenta is located in the upper part of the uterus, firmly attached to the uterine wall until after the delivery of the baby.

Placental abruption
The placenta detaches prematurely from the uterine wall, causing bleeding and reducing the supply of oxygen and nutrients to the fetus.

Placenta praevia
The placenta is located over or near the cervix, in the lower part of the uterus.

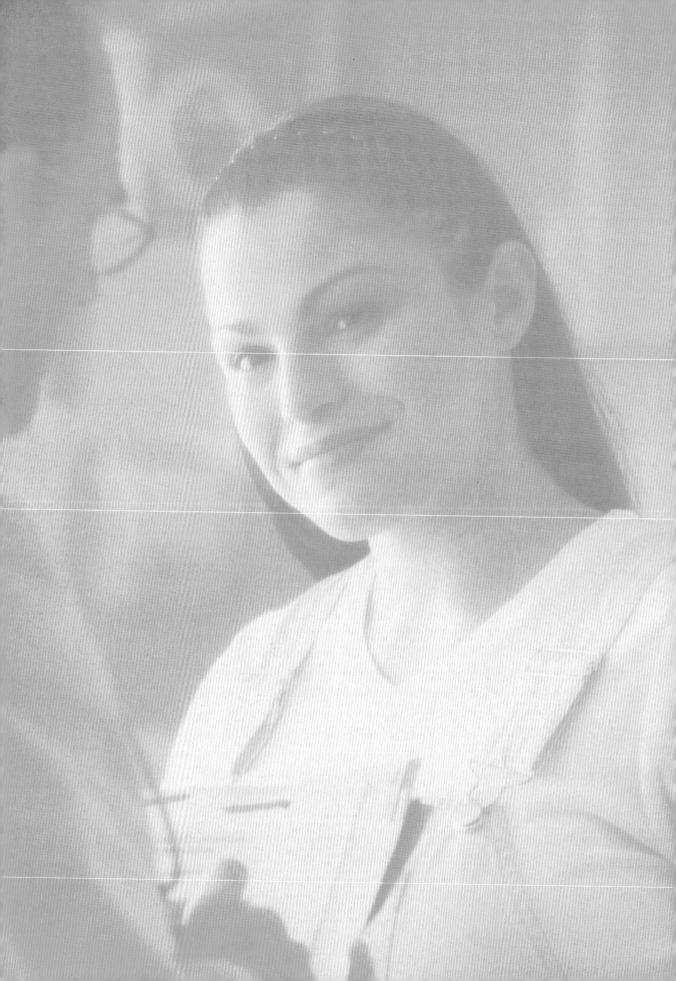

antenatal
care

A whole schedule of routine tests and assessments awaits you during pregnancy – from the initial ultrasound scan through to routine checks in the last few weeks before your baby is born. You may have some choice about your antenatal care but if your pregnancy turns out to be high risk you will be monitored more closely. There is no reason to be anxious about any of these procedures as they are designed to check that you and your baby are healthy.

choice of
antenatal care

There are options when it comes to choosing where to have your baby. These include not only home and hospital but also which hospital. There may be several hospitals in the area where you live, and different types of care, ranging from birthing centres to consultant-led units, may be available. The choice is about where to have your baby and who is to be the main provider of your antenatal care.

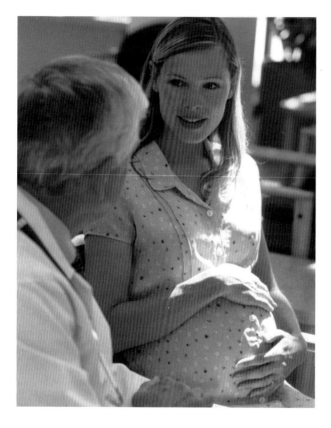

Getting as much information as you can will help you to choose the care that is right for you when it comes to having your baby.

Whatever you decide, circumstances may change during your pregnancy which influence your decision. However, there is no contract to sign, so do not worry about changing your mind.

midwife-led care

Where care is midwife-led, midwives provide all your antenatal care and, as long as your pregnancy continues to be straightforward, a midwife will also provide your labour and postnatal care. How this care is provided depends on where you live and what is available in the area.

Your community midwife can provide your antenatal checks, either in a clinic or in your home. You may see various midwives who are part of a team, or you may have one named midwife throughout your pregnancy. There may be a domino scheme, where your midwife accompanies you to hospital when you are in labour and discharges you home soon after the birth. Some doctors like to see women from their practice at some time during their pregnancy but, if you prefer, or are more comfortable, just to see a midwife, that should be quite acceptable. It is your choice.

shared care

In this case, antenatal care is shared between the midwife, doctor and a consultant obstetrician at the hospital or maternity unit. This is usually recommended if your pregnancy falls into a 'higher risk' category, for example, if you have a complicated obstetric or medical history, are pregnant with twins or have diabetes. Your midwife will explain why this recommendation is being made but, again, ultimately it is your choice.

private care

Some women choose to employ an independent midwife to provide all of their care. They like to feel that there is a guarantee that they will have the same midwife providing continuity of care throughout their pregnancy, birth and also postnatally. Statistically, independent midwives have a high proportion of homebirths.

You could also pay to see an obstetrician privately for your antenatal care, or choose to give birth in a private maternity unit.

home birth

Some women would prefer to give birth at home, where they feel comfortable and with their family close at hand, rather than in the unfamiliar, more clinical surroundings of a hospital. If your pregnancy is uncomplicated then statistically it appears to be just as safe to give birth at home as in hospital. The reality is that women who give birth at home need less pain relief, experience less intervention, are more likely to know the midwife who looks after them, and feel more in control throughout the birth.

hospital (consultant unit)

These units have obstetricians on their staff, as well as the facilities to deal with any complications during the birth. If your labour is straightforward you will have a midwife caring for you in labour and during the birth. However, if there are any problems, an obstetrician will be available to carry out an instrumental delivery (forceps or ventouse) or a caesarean section.

You will also have the option of a full range of pain relief, including an epidural, which is administered by an anaesthetist.

midwife unit

This is usually a much smaller, often stand-alone, unit, or birthing centre, where midwives, and healthcare assistants, provide the care. Women are encouraged to have an active birth and a birthing pool is usually available.

This type of unit is more suitable for women with uncomplicated pregnancies who do not anticipate any problems in labour as there are no facilities for administering epidurals and no special-care baby unit.

birth plans

Drawing up a birth plan makes you consider the options available and what is important to you and your partner. It acts as a communication tool between you and your midwife and helps to set the 'tone' of the sort of labour and delivery that you are hoping for.

To make choices you need to have information, and it is never too early to start finding out what is available. Reading, talking to other women who have had babies, attending antenatal classes and chatting with your midwife should give you some idea of the sort of birth that you would prefer.

The best way of presenting a birth plan is in the form of a letter. This is far more personal than a form printed off a website, and will give the midwife caring for you some idea of your personality. Rather than just completing boxes, put something of yourself into the plan and explain what you and your partner feel is important and why. Some antenatal notes have a space for you to write a birth plan, but you can always write one up separately. Just remember to hand it over when you find out who will be caring for you during labour.

some points to consider:
- Do you prefer to be cared for by women?
- Do you have any preferences about pain relief?
- What are your views on induced labour?
- Do you want your waters broken only if necessary?
- Do you want to avoid continual fetal monitoring which would stop you moving about during labour?
- Do you want to be encouraged to move in labour?
- Do you want the midwife to encourage you to push or leave you to push spontaneously?
- Do you want to see the sex of your baby for yourselves rather than be told?
- Under what circumstances would you be prepared to have an episiotomy?
- Does your partner want to cut the cord?
- Do you want to put your baby straight to the breast?

birth
partners

The greatest influence on your ability to cope in labour is the support that you receive. This will come not only from your midwife, but also from the person or people you choose as your birth partner or partners. You need to feel confident that they will be able to give you the emotional support and practical care that you will need during the birth.

doulas

Some women decide to employ a doula, if only to be sure of having continuity of care. The word 'doula' comes from a Greek word meaning 'a woman care-giver'. It has come to mean a woman, experienced in childbirth, who provides emotional and practical support to another woman during and after birth. A doula is well informed, understands the physiology of birth, and can help you and your partner to make informed decisions on the choices that are available to you. Her aim is to make the experience of labour and childbirth more positive. During labour, she will help you with breathing and relaxation and encourage you to change positions as your labour progresses.

Research shows that having continuous support from another woman is associated with:
• Less pain relief
• A slightly shorter labour
• Fewer forceps and ventouse deliveries
• Fewer caesarean sections

Most maternity units are happy for you to have two people with you during labour because research shows that continual support benefits mothers in a number of ways, such as:
• Feeling more in control of labour
• Feeling more positive about the birth experience
• Suffering less depression at 6 weeks after the birth
• Being more confident about motherhood.

choosing your birth partner

Although most fathers want to be at the birth, this is not right for everyone. The most important thing is to have good support in labour, regardless of who provides it. In some cultures, men are discouraged

Q **My partner hates the sight of blood and is really worried in case he cannot cope with being at the birth. Should I just insist that he is there?**

A Although most fathers attend the birth, some do worry about how they will cope with seeing their partner in pain, what their emotional response will be or how they will react to the sight of blood. It can be a good idea to have a second birth partner around, someone with whom you would both feel comfortable. The chances are that, when the baby is born, your partner will be too involved with the intense experience to notice any blood loss. The only thing that tends to make partners feel faint is the heat in the delivery room, so make sure that he does not wear warm clothes. Good support in labour is essential so you must be able to rely on whoever you decide to be with you on the day.

from attending a birth and two female relatives attend instead. You must trust the people you choose to stay with you and be honest about what you expect from them during your labour – but essentially they should want to be there.

Consider who would be best able to provide this support. It may be your baby's father, a friend, a sister or your mother. Women who have had children before will not worry about seeing you in pain and are more able to reassure you that everything is completely normal.

If your partner is anxious about how he will feel during labour, encourage him to go to antenatal classes with you. The opportunity to talk with other men in the group and discovering that he is not alone in his fears may make him more confident about being there. Many men have fears about delivery – the most common being concerns about seeing their partner in pain and not being able to 'cure' them of it. By going to classes, feeling prepared, and chatting with the midwife, he will feel more confident about being with you on the day.

involving your birth partner

Try to involve your birth partner during your pregnancy as much as possible, for example, by sharing visits to the midwife, scans and antenatal classes. A basic understanding of the process of labour will help to remove some of the anxiety. It is essential that your birth partner is there to help you cope with the contractions. Most importantly he, or she, needs to listen to you and provide comfort and emotional support.

how your birth partner can help

It is essential that you stay relaxed during labour and this is where your birth partner can have a huge influence. Your birth partner can:

- Time your contractions, keep a record and phone the midwife to let her know that you're on the way.
- Get drinks and snacks for you while you are at home waiting for your contractions to get close enough together.
- Give you a supporting arm if you want to go for a walk and need the reassurance.
- Encourage you to keep moving around, change positions and keep off the bed.
- Provide you with drinks.
- Offer verbal encouragement and reassurance.
- Help you find a pattern of breathing during your contractions.
- Talk to your midwife about aspects of your labour if you do not feel up to it.
- Keep you cool by placing a cold flannel on your brow.
- Massage your back and shoulders if you want him or her to.
- Support you if you want to sit up or lean forward during the second stage of labour.
- Encourage you during the last few pushes by telling you the progress of the baby's head.

'Mike was not sure how he would cope with the birth as he is pretty squeamish, but having my sister there as well took the pressure off him. Because he could keep disappearing for 5 minutes it actually helped him to feel more in control of what was going on. Needless to say, he stayed with me during the birth and I could not believe it when he even asked to cut the cord!'

Eve, mother of
Erin, 6 weeks

shared
experience

tests during
pregnancy

Pregnancy involves a lot of tests, not only to find out right at the start whether you are really pregnant or not but also to check your health, and your baby's health, throughout your pregnancy. The results are entered on your antenatal notes, which you will probably be asked to carry with you. It can therefore be helpful to know what the results mean.

pregnancy tests

Pregnancy test kits are readily available in supermarkets or chemists. They often come in a double pack so that you can do a repeat test a few days later if the result is negative but your period is overdue. Tests nowadays are more than 99 per cent accurate if used correctly.

Some tests can be used from the day your period is due; these detect human chorionic gonadotrophin (HCG) in your urine; this hormone is produced by the embryo. However, you need to be sure when your period is due. If you have conceived a few days later than you thought, this will affect the point at which the test will show positive, which will be 2 weeks following conception. A positive result is nearly always correct, whereas a negative result may need checking.

It is also possible to go to your family planning clinic, doctor or midwife for a pregnancy test. HCG in a urine or blood sample will indicate that you are pregnant.

routine checks

Throughout your pregnancy your midwife or doctor, who will be monitoring the wellbeing of you and your baby, will see you regularly. The first check will usually be the longest because your midwife will need to take details of your medical, obstetric and family history and current circumstances. At the first visit you will be weighed and you will be given a series of checks during later visits.

You will also get the opportunity to ask questions, for example, about the availability of antenatal classes or how to get comfortable at night. The midwife or doctor will give you general advice on health, for example, diet and exercise, and take blood tests as necessary.

understanding antenatal notes

At each visit, the details of your check-up will be recorded in your notes. You may be given many of these to carry with you, so that you can present them at other check-ups. You will obviously read them so it is useful to understand what the tests are for, what they involve and how to interpret the results.

blood test

You will be advised to have blood tests that check what blood group you are, and if any antibodies are present in your blood. They will also check whether you're immune to rubella, and will check for hepatitis and syphillis. Your haemoglobin will be checked to see whether you have anaemia. Some screening tests will also be offered to you (see page 126) as well as an HIV test.

blood pressure

High blood pressure (hypertension) can affect the growth of your baby and can also develop into a life-threatening condition called eclampsia (see page 110), which is one of the reasons for checking your blood pressure at every visit. Approximately 10 per cent of women develop pre-eclampsia during their pregnancy but, with careful monitoring, it does not become a problem.

urine

You should take a urine sample to every check-up, where it will be tested for:

Sugar which can show up if you have recently consumed a lot of sugary foods or drinks. It can also be a sign of diabetes.

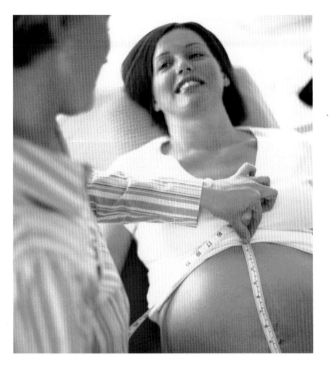

Measuring your expanding bump – what midwives and doctors call your fundus – checks that your baby is growing normally as your pregnancy progresses.

engagement of the head

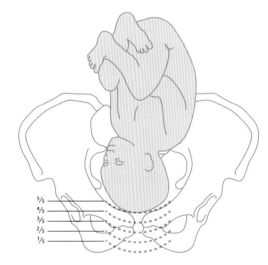

If the midwife can feel all of your baby's head above the pelvic brim, she will record his position as 5/5 palpable. If your baby's head has engaged into the pelvis, she will only be able to feel two-fifths of it, which she will record it as 2/5 palpable (see also page 208).

Protein which can be a sign of pre eclampsia (see page 110) when accompanied by a rise in blood pressure or oedema (swelling, see page 102). It can also sometimes be a sign of an infection.

Ketones which indicate that your body is short of sugar. These are often found in women who have severe pregnancy sickness.

The results may be entered on your notes as NAD (nothing abnormal detected), or trace or + (meaning that small amounts of the substance are present).

swelling (oedema)

Your midwife will ask if you have any swelling, although a certain amount of swelling around the feet and hands is normal, particularly towards the end of your pregnancy. If you have no other signs of pre-eclampsia, such as high blood pressure or protein in your urine, there is no need to worry.

position and presentation

This refers to the way your baby is lying in the uterus and which way up he is. Results are shown as Ceph. (or VX), meaning head down; Br., meaning breech; or Tr., meaning transverse, or lying sideways across the uterus. (see also page 218).

Fundus refers to the height of your uterus. If you are 28 weeks pregnant and the midwife feels that the growth of your baby is right for the gestation, she will write: = dates, or = 28 weeks. 'Weeks' refers to the duration of your pregnancy on the day of your check.

fetal heart

The midwife will examine you and listen to the fetal heart using a hand-held Doppler or a pinnard, which looks like an ear trumpet. She will record the results as FMF (meaning fetal movements felt) and FHHR (meaning fetal heart heard and regular).

relation to the brim

Towards the end of your pregnancy the midwife will record how much of your baby's head can still be felt above the brim of the pelvis and how much has descended into the pelvis. This is expressed in terms of fifths (see left). With a first baby, the head usually engages before labour starts, and this can happen at any time from six weeks beforehand. With subsequent pregnancies this often doesn't happen until the contractions are established.

ultrasound scans

In the late 1950s, using the knowledge of sonar and radar that he acquired in the Royal Air Force, Professor Ian Donald in Glasgow, Scotland, pioneered the use of ultrasound in pregnant mothers. In those days it was only possible to take very basic measurements of the fetal head. Now ultrasound can provide the detailed examination of almost all fetal structures, and has become a useful diagnostic tool.

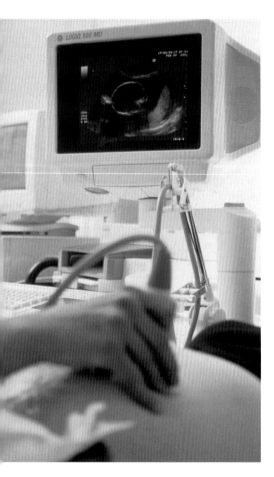

During an ultrasound scan the transducer is moved over the abdomen. It emits high frequency sound waves and detects the echoes. The results build up an image of the unborn child in the womb, as can be seen on the monitor.

what an ultrasound scan involves

To start with, the person doing the scan will rub a special gel onto your abdomen to reduce signal loss. He or she will then place a probe (a transducer) onto your abdomen. The transducer both emits and receives ultrasound waves. These reflected ultrasound waves are continuously assembled into a picture on a screen. This shows solid structures as white and liquid structures as black. Moving structures, such as the fetal heart, can be assessed, and freezing the picture enables accurate measurements of the fetus to be taken. In the first 3 months of pregnancy, you will need to have a full bladder before a scan in order to improve image quality. An internal scan using a transvaginal probe can be helpful in early pregnancy.

uses of ultrasound scans

Ultrasound has been shown to be safe, it has become widely acceptable to mothers and an indispensable part of antenatal care. Ultrasound scans are used for a number of purposes, as well as those described below.

monitoring fetal growth and wellbeing

Until 14 weeks, the size of your baby is measured by his crown-rump length. After this, fetal weight can be estimated by measuring the head circumference (HC), biparietal diameter (BPD – the width of the head), abdominal circumference (AC), and femur length (FL – length of the thigh bone). If necessary, growth measurements will be taken every 2 weeks. The amount of amniotic fluid (see page 118) is also important. A low amount may indicate that your baby is not getting enough nutrients.

locating the placenta

Ultrasound is used to locate the placenta. If the placenta is too low down and remains that way in late pregnancy (see placenta praevia, page 114), you may need a caesarean section.

guiding invasive procedures

Procedures such as chorionic villus sampling and amniocentesis (see pages 129 and 130) are best performed under continuous ultrasound control. In this way the needle can be safely guided to the sampling site without harming you or your baby.

ultrasound scans in early pregnancy (5–14 weeks)

It is possible to diagnose pregnancy from about 4–5 weeks after your last menstrual period using ultrasound. Detection of a fetal heart beat at 5–6 weeks will confirm the viability of your pregnancy. Ultrasound is therefore extremely useful if you experience vaginal bleeding during early pregnancy (see page 99) because it often makes it possible to determine the site and viability of your pregnancy.

If you are unsure of your dates, an ultrasound scan in early pregnancy is particularly useful. Later in pregnancy, dating becomes progressively less accurate. An early scan can confirm a multiple pregnancy and determine the number of placentas (see page 24). Also, between 11 and 14 weeks, it can screen the fetus for chromosomal abnormalities, such as trisomy 21 (Down's syndrome, see page 127), by measuring the thickness of the fat pad at the back of the neck (nuchal translucency, see page 126).

detailed scan at 18–20 weeks

You may be offered a scan to look for any abnormalities in your baby. This scan carefully examines each part of your baby in turn and any problems are noted. The scan will detect even small abnormalities, such as a cleft lip or tiny holes in your baby's heart. Sometimes a scan shows an abnormality which, by itself, is of little significance but which may be associated with an underlying problem, such as an abnormal number of chromosomes (for example, Down's syndrome).

Such findings are called 'soft markers' and include: too much fluid on the kidney (hydronephrosis), short femurs, bright areas within the heart (echogenic foci) and a bright appearance of the fetal bowel (echogenic bowel). Although the presence of a soft marker may indicate an increased risk of chromosome abnormality, this is not as common as previously thought.

colour doppler ultrasound

The use of a colour Doppler converts the movement of structures (for example, blood moving around the fetus) into different colours on the screen. This allows particular blood vessels to be examined to see how much blood is flowing through them.

For example, both the umbilical cord (see page 113) and the uterine arteries can be visualized and blood flow can be measured. A high resistance flow in the umbilical arteries may indicate a problem with the baby, while a similar measurement in the uterine arteries suggests an increased risk of the mother developing pre-eclampsia (see page 110).

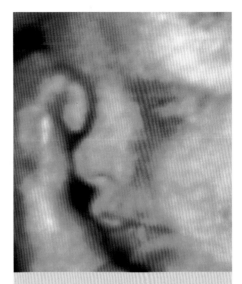

the future – 3D ultrasound

Recently, 3D ultrasound has become more available. This technique provides beautifully clear pictures of the surface of the baby, particularly the face. Clinically, this can be useful in the assessment of cleft lip and palate. Its full role has yet to be established, but as technology improves, and more uses are found for it, 3D ultrasound may well become the standard technique for examining the fetus.

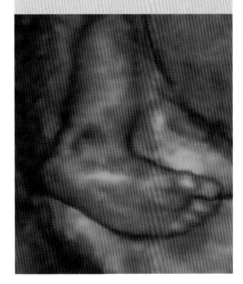

screening tests

The series of tests that you are given throughout your pregnancy helps to ascertain whether you or your baby have any problems. Some of these tests are given routinely to every pregnant woman. Others may only be offered to women whose babies are considered to be in 'at-risk groups' of having or developing a particular condition that might require special care or intervention.

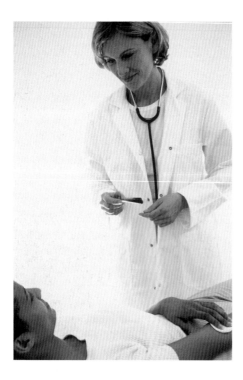

Routine blood tests are simply done and virtually painless these days – they are especially important in mid-pregnancy when your blood becomes very diluted.

at-risk groups

Several factors are taken into account when determining whether you fall into an at-risk group:

- Medical history, for example, previous pregnancies.
- Family history, for example, if there are inherited conditions such as cystic fibrosis among members of your family or your partner's family.
- Ethnic group (and that of your partner) and where your family comes from. (Higher rates of thalassaemia are found in people of Mediterranean origin; sickle-cell anaemia is mainly found among people of African descent, and cystic fibrosis occurs in white people of western European origin.)

the purpose of screening tests

Screening tests are designed to ascertain the level of risk and include blood tests, urine tests and ultrasound scans. If a screening test indicates an increased risk for a condition, it will usually be followed by a diagnostic test (see page 128), which will determine whether or not the condition is present.

Some hospitals offer certain screening tests routinely to all women, while others offer them only to women in at-risk groups. For example, some hospitals offer all pregnant women blood tests to check for the possibility of Down's syndrome, but others offer them only to older women.

ultrasound scans

At different stages during pregnancy, you will be given ultrasound scans (see page 124) to check on your baby's development.

nuchal scan

This may form part of the routine ultrasound scan at 11–14 weeks. The fold of skin at the back of your baby's neck (the nuchal fold) is checked to see whether excess fluid is present, which is a possible sign of Down's syndrome.

anomaly scan

Given at 18–20 weeks, this scan provides a check of the baby's growth and development and an opportunity to check for signs of spina bifida, changes that might be associated with Down's syndrome, and conditions that might require antenatal monitoring and neonatal care.

blood tests

As well as the blood test given to all women at their first appointment (see page 122), you may be offered blood tests (also referred to as serum screening) to check for specific conditions if you are at risk.

serum screening at around 10 weeks

If you are at risk of having a baby with Down's syndrome, you will have a blood test to establish the levels of the fetal hormones plasma protein A and human chorionic gonadotrophin (HCG) in your blood.

serum screening at around 16 weeks

You will be given further tests to check the levels of fetal hormones in your blood at about 16 weeks. Depending on the hospital, this will be an AFP test (to check for alphafetoprotein, or AFP), a triple test (which also checks for HCG and oestriol), or a triple-plus test, or quadruple test (which checks for inhibin A, too). Abnormal levels of these hormones may be an indication of spina bifida or Down's syndrome.

genetic screening

Your blood can also be tested for inherited conditions, for example, sickle-cell anaemia, haemophilia, thalassaemia and cystic fibrosis, according to your ethnic, family or geographical background. For conditions such as sickle-cell, if you test positive, your partner will also be screened. It is important to remember that these tests only indicate the possibility of a baby inheriting a condition. If the results are positive, you will be offered diagnostic tests (see page 128) in order to investigate further.

to test or not to test?

There are a number of things to consider when deciding whether or not to have any screening test. It can be very reassuring to find that the results indicate a low risk, but what if they indicate a high risk?

Even if you are sure you will love your baby whatever, and would never consider a termination, you may wish to consider screening. A low-risk assessment will be reassuring, while a higher-risk assessment will give you the opportunity to decide whether to have follow-up diagnostic tests, so you can be fully prepared for your baby's arrival.

Many women find the stress of screening very disturbing and they prefer not to have it done. Your midwife and doctor have your best interests at heart and should talk through the options of further tests with you. However, the decision rests with you. At this stage, it may be wise to start thinking about what you will do if the result is positive.

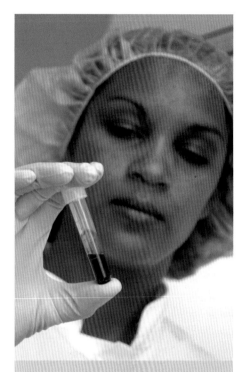

false positive or false negative?

You should remember that, although the accuracy of detection rates has improved, no screening method is perfect. For example, raised levels of alphafetoprotein (AFP) in your blood may have other causes, such as a twin pregnancy. On average, only 1 in 20 women is assessed as being at high risk of carrying a baby with Down's syndrome and offered diagnostic testing. However, of these assessments, only 1 in 60 will be correct. Similarly, screening misses about 30 per cent of all cases of Down's syndrome.

diagnostic
tests

If the result of a screening test (see page 126) indicates that your baby is at high risk of abnormality, you will be offered a follow-up diagnostic test, for example, chorionic villus sampling (CVS) or amniocentesis. These tests are not routinely available or performed because they are invasive, and there is a risk of provoking a miscarriage in 1–2 per cent of cases.

The decision to undergo diagnostic testing is therefore often difficult and causes a huge amount of anxiety. The midwife or obstetrician is there to ensure that you fully understand the benefits and risks of any test. Remember that no one has to have a diagnostic test. The final decision has to be made by the parents.

who is offered a diagnostic test?

A diagnostic test is offered to women who have an increased risk of having a baby with a chromosomal abnormality. The risk factors include:

- Late age (that is, late 30s and 40s)
- A history of a chromosome abnormality (for example, a previous child with Down's syndrome)
- A family history of a genetic disorder like cystic fibrosis
- A problem seen on the ultrasound sound scan
- An increased serum screening risk or a raised nuchal translucency (see page 126).

after a diagnostic test

If the test result is abnormal, you will be invited to discuss the available options with your obstetrician. It is

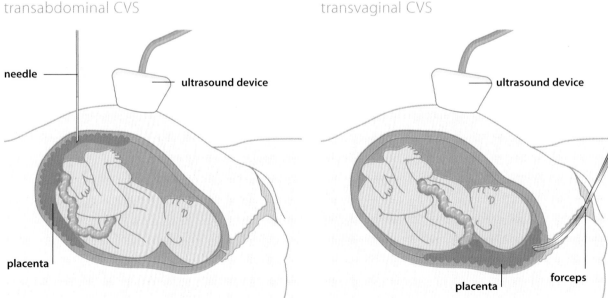

transabdominal CVS

needle — **ultrasound device**

placenta

Ultrasound is used to locate the placenta and a needle is guided into the placenta to take a small sample of cells to look for genetic defects and chromosomal abnormalities.

transvaginal CVS

ultrasound device

placenta **forceps**

Ultrasound is used to locate the placenta. A catheter or biopsy forceps are passed through the cervix to take a sample of placental tissue.

important to remember that a normal result, although reassuring, does not rule out the possibility of there being other problems.

chorionic villus sampling (CVS)

CVS is the removal and examination of a small amount of placental tissue (afterbirth), known as chorionic villi. Because the placenta and fetus are made up of the same cells, an analysis of the cells of the placental tissue provides information about the fetus itself. Analysis of the chromosomes in these cells will detect any abnormalities, while analysis of the individual genes will reveal any genetic defects.

when can it be performed?

CVS is only performed after 11 weeks because some evidence suggests that CVS performed before 10 weeks can result in limb deformities.

how is it performed?

Before performing the procedure, your doctor will discuss it with you fully and will usually obtain your written consent. CVS involves injecting a local anaesthetic and then, under ultrasound guidance, passing a needle through the skin and layers of your abdomen into the placenta. A sample of the placenta is then taken and sent for analysis. Occasionally the procedure is performed through the cervix, for example, if the placenta is very low or the uterus is tilted back (retroverted). If you are Rhesus negative, you will be given an injection of Anti-D (see page 82).

what is it used for?

CVS detects chromosome abnormalities (for example, Down's syndrome) and genetic disorders (for example, muscular dystrophy, Huntingdon's chorea, sickle-cell anaemia and cystic fibrosis). The sex of the baby can also be determined in this test.

how quickly are the results available?

An initial result is usually available within 2–3 days. The full culture result (obtained from a culture of the cells) takes about 2 weeks.

does it hurt?

Most women who have had a CVS describe the procedure as uncomfortable but not too painful. Afterwards, it is normal to experience some abdominal discomfort, which can be relieved by mild painkillers, such as paracetamol. If the symptoms worsen or any bleeding occurs after this test, you should contact your doctor urgently.

amniocentesis

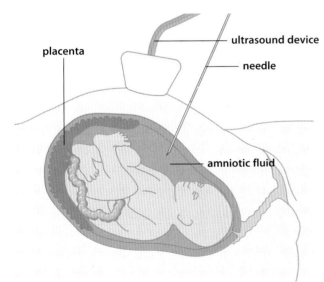

Ultrasound is used to guide a fine needle into the amniotic sac to take a sample of fluid to look for chromosomal abnormalities and genetic defects.

fetal blood sampling

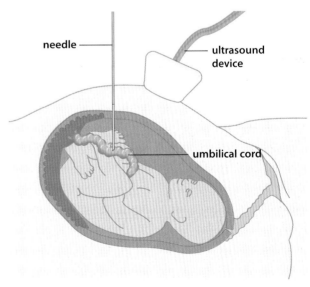

Under ultrasound guidance a very fine needle is passed into the umbilical cord to obtain a sample of the fetus's blood to perform a full chromosomal analysis.

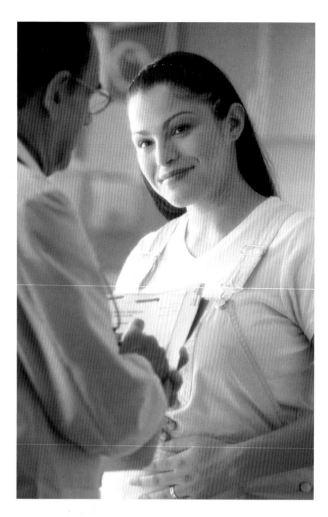

Even if you have exhausted the local bookshop and library of pregnancy books and leaflets, be sure to ask your midwife or doctor if you have any worries or unanswered questions.

what are the risks?

The risk of miscarriage from CVS is about 1–2 per cent. If miscarriage does occur, it usually takes place within a week of the test. In rare cases (about 1 in 100), an abnormality is seen in the placenta cells that is not found in the fetus. In this case, it may be necessary to perform another amniocentesis in order to confirm that the fetus is normal. In about 1 in 200 cases, no full culture result is obtained.

amniocentesis

Amniocentesis is the removal of a small amount of the amniotic fluid that surrounds the fetus. Amniotic fluid contains skin cells from the baby that can be tested for chromosomal defects, for example, Down's syndrome.

when can it be performed?

The procedure is only performed after 15 weeks. Before 14 weeks, there is evidence of an increased risk of club feet (talipes) and the chances of causing a miscarriage are raised.

how is it performed?

As with CVS, the doctor performing the procedure will make sure that you fully understand the procedure and will obtain your written consent. You may not require an anaesthetic because the needle used for amniocentesis is finer than that used for CVS.

The procedure is conducted under ultrasound guidance and involves passing a needle through the skin and layers of your abdominal wall into the uterus, avoiding the fetus and, if possible, avoiding the placenta. A small sample of fluid (for example, 15 ml at 15 weeks) is then removed. If you are Rhesus negative, you will be given an injection of Anti-D (see page 82).

what is it used for?

Amniocentesis is mainly used to detect chromosome abnormalities (for example, Down's syndrome, or trisomy 21), genetic disorders (such as cystic fibrosis) and fetal infection. Amniocentesis is occasionally used late in pregnancy to assess whether your baby's lungs are mature enough for him to breathe on his own. Like CVS, the sex of the fetus can also be determined.

how quickly are the results available?

Some hospitals offer rapid tests in addition to the full culture test. These are usually known by their initials – FISH or PCR (fluorescence in situ hybridization or polymerase chain reaction). These results are available with 2–3 days of the procedure and provide specific information, for example, whether or not the fetus has Down's syndrome. The full culture results take longer (usually about 2 weeks).

is it painful?

As with CVS, many women find the procedure uncomfortable but not too painful. Amniocentesis usually takes only about 10 minutes and is thus well tolerated by most women who have it.

what are the risks?

The risk of miscarriage after amniocentesis is about 1 per cent and it usually occurs within a week of the procedure. In about 1 in 200 cases, no full culture result is obtained, in which case the FISH and PCR results are usually reliable. Otherwise, it may be necessary to repeat the test.

fetal blood sampling

Another method of diagnostic testing is sampling the fetal blood, either from the cord (cordocentesis) or from a vein in the fetal liver (intrahepatic vein). The technique is similar to amniocentesis and CVS except that the aim is to obtain a small sample of fetal blood rather than amniotic fluid or placental tissue.

when can it be performed?
Fetal blood sampling is usually performed after 18–20 weeks of pregnancy.

how is it performed?
For cordocentesis, ultrasound is used to locate the point where the umbilical cord inserts into the placenta. The procedure then involves inserting a fine needle through the abdomen and uterine walls into the umbilical cord, using ultrasound as a guide. Once the fetal blood sample has been obtained, it is sent to the laboratory for analysis. A full chromosome result is usually available within 72 hours.

Blood samples from the intrahepatic vein are taken in a similar way, except that the needle is guided into the fetal liver.

what is it used for?
Fetal blood sampling was formerly used to obtain a full chromosome analysis of the fetus, which took just a few days. However, since the advent of rapid testing of amniotic fluid (by PCR or FISH, see above), it has been used less often for this purpose because amniocentesis is technically less demanding.

Instead, fetal blood sampling is now mainly reserved for conditions such as fetal anaemia (for example as a result of Rhesus disease), fetal infection (for example toxoplasmosis or rubella) or fetal blood disorders (such as sickle-cell disease). If fetal anaemia is diagnosed, the fetus can be given a blood transfusion using the same needle.

what are the risks?
The major risk of fetal blood sampling is a 1–2 per cent risk of miscarriage.

the future: non-invasive diagnostic tests

In the not-too-distant future, the use of CVS and amniocentesis may largely be replaced by a blood test on the mother. The main advantage of this method of testing is that it is non-invasive and carries no risk of miscarriage.

Research has shown that it is possible to identify fetal cells as well as the fetal DNA that normally circulates in the mother's blood. The challenge is to accurately distinguish between the components derived from the fetus and those of the mother. It is already possible to determine fetal gender and blood group in this way.

'I had CVS with both of my boys. As I was an "older mother", I needed to know they were healthy. The risk of a possible miscarriage for either of my much-wanted babies was difficult to bear, but thankfully it was fine. I didn't feel a thing during the CVS, but for the next couple of days I felt like I'd been kicked in the stomach, although this gradually eased. Waiting for the final results was horrendous, but the initial results come through within a few days now and that was reassuring. And the wonderful news that all was well with my babies meant I could relax and get on with the rest of my pregnancy.'

Paula, mother of 6-year-old Charlie and 1-year-old Edward

shared experience

twin
pregnancies

The number of twin pregnancies has steadily increased over the last decade. In Europe approximately 1 in 80 pregnancies are twins and multiple births are more common nowadays. This is partly due to the increase in fertility treatment and also because women are delaying getting pregnant, thus increasing their chances of multiple pregnancy. Whatever the reason, having twins is something special.

Twin and multiple pregnancies are considered high-risk for both mother and baby. For the mother, there is an increased risk of complications, for example, gestational diabetes (see page 81), pre-eclampsia (see page 110) and anaemia. For the babies, the risk of growth restriction and pre-term labour are of particular concern. Therefore, you will be offered close antenatal care and regular scans to monitor the growth of your babies.

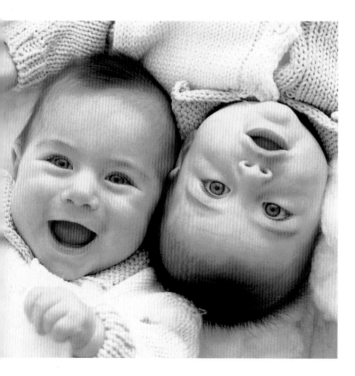

Double the trouble or twice the fun? However you look at it, having twins can be challenging but is ultimately worthwhile.

the first few months

In early pregnancy, an increase in common symptoms, such as pregnancy sickness or excessive tiredness, or simply an unusually large uterus, may suggest that you are carrying twins. However, the obstetrician needs to know not just how many babies there are but also the number of placentas.

In the majority of twin pregnancies, there are separate placentas (dichorionic twins). In about 20 per cent of these pregnancies, the placenta is shared (monochorionic twins). Monochorionic twins have much higher complication rates and therefore need closer monitoring.

ultrasound monitoring

As with one baby, twins can be screened for Down's syndrome at 11–14 weeks by looking at the nuchal translucency (see page 126). A detailed scan is also performed at 18–20 weeks. Twins are more likely to have certain structural abnormalities, for example congenital heart disease and neural tube defects (such as spina bifida).

All twins are monitored at least every 4 weeks by ultrasound to look for growth restriction. This affects about 25 per cent of dichorionic twins and almost 50 per cent of monochorionic twins. The major risk to monochorionic twins, however, is the development of twin-twin transfusion syndrome.

twin-twin transfusion syndrome

About 15 per cent of twins who share a placenta develop a condition known as twin-twin transfusion syndrome (TTTS, see page 79).

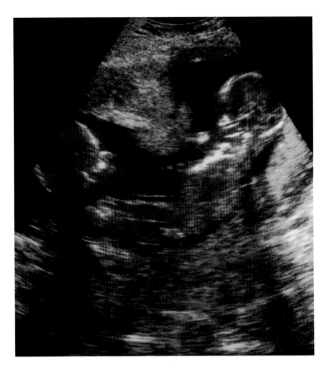

Two precious little packages – your pregnancy will be monitored more closely when you are having twins, and it is a good idea to take it easy whenever you get the chance.

coping with twins

Having two babies is especially exciting, and even a little awesome, for both you and the people around you. It can also be overwhelming at times. If you are carrying twins, it is important to have regular antenatal checks in order to identify any potential complications. Many obstetricians recommend iron and folate supplements to prevent anaemia.

Pregnancy symptoms are often more pronounced with twins and multiple pregnancies – for example, you may experience more sickness, fatigue, heartburn, haemorrhoids – because your body is working harder and carrying more weight than during a singleton pregnancy. You are also more likely to develop high blood pressure (hypertension) and you may need to give up work earlier – many women stop work at around 26 weeks of pregnancy. Do not worry – both you and your babies will be monitored closely throughout your pregnancy.

Since early delivery is much more common in twins and multiple pregnancies, you should visit the hospital to be checked over if you notice any hint of labour occurring. You are more likely to deliver early if you have a short cervix, and some hospitals offer a scan at 24 weeks to measure the length of this. Almost all twins are delivered in hospital and both of them are monitored continually throughout labour.

during pregnancy

Take any opportunity to talk to others with twins for practical tips and advice. You could start attending a support group for the parents of twins, if there is one in your area, in order to build up a support network ready for when your babies are born.

It is even more important to maintain your energy levels by eating a healthy, balanced diet. It is often easier to digest small, frequent snacks than three main meals a day. Small meals, such as pasta or a jacket potato, based on slow-release carbohydrates will keep your energy levels higher for longer than a biscuit or doughnut, which will only give you a short 'sugar high'.

did you know?

The average length of a twin pregnancy is 36 weeks, and 34 weeks for triplets.

Tall women are more likely to conceive twins.

Women over 35 are more likely to have twins.

The highest rate of twins are born to Nigerian women.

Up to 22 per cent of twins are left-handed while for non-twins the rate is just under 10 per cent.

The United States has one of the highest rates for multiple births, while Japan has one of the lowest.

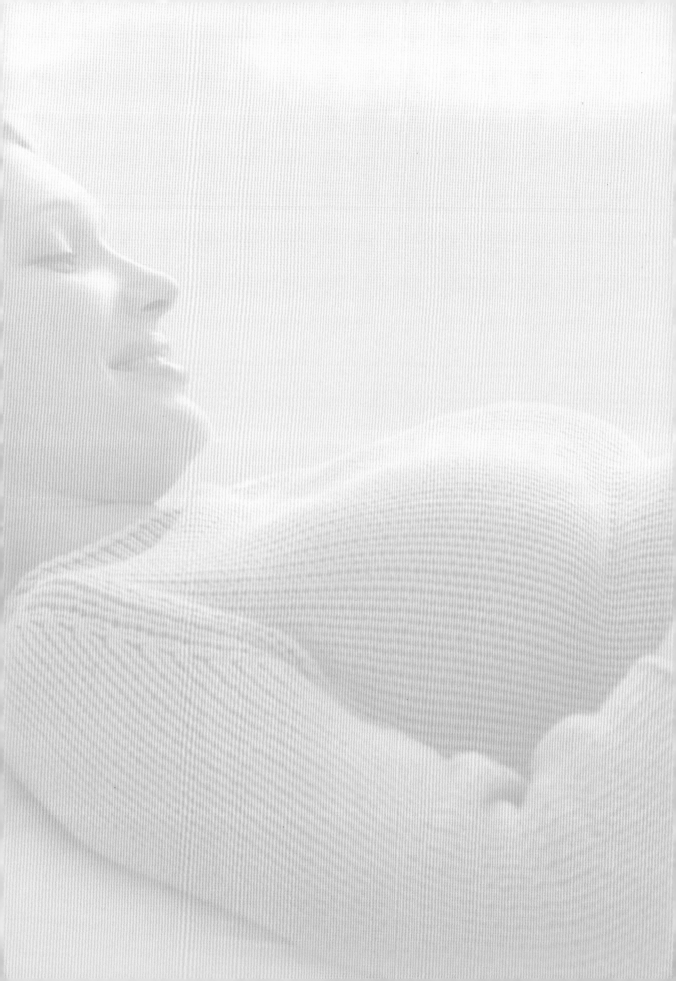

early
pregnancy

You have found out that you are pregnant and already you are noticing oddities, such as a strange taste in your mouth and sore breasts. Although your body will still look the same, amazing events are going on inside you. A rapid and startling transformation is underway in your uterus, and by the end of 12 weeks a tiny bundle of cells has grown and developed into a baby with a beating heart, fingers and toes, and a functioning brain.

your body at
1–8 weeks

For many women the first sign that they are pregnant is a missed period, although women who have an irregular menstrual cycle may only decide to do a pregnancy test when they get other symptoms, for example, tiredness, tender breasts or a need to pass urine more frequently. Some women just instinctively feel 'different' and know that they are pregnant, particularly if they have been pregnant before.

' I did not believe the first pregnancy test when it showed positive so I made my partner buy another test kit. In the end I took four positive pregnancy tests before I actually believed the result! '

Mandy, 5 weeks pregnant

shared experiences

' We have decided not to tell anyone that we are having a baby until after the first scan but it is so hard. I feel as if I am carrying around the most enormous secret and wonder if people can tell by looking at me! '

Jemma, 8 weeks pregnant

The beginning of your pregnancy is dated from the first day of your last period. Therefore, when you are 4 weeks pregnant, this is actually only 2 weeks after the conception of your baby.

how you may feel

You may have very mixed emotions when you discover that you are pregnant. Even if you have planned to have a baby, the reality of being pregnant may be overwhelming. Like many women, you may wonder if you are mistaken and insist on repeating the test. However, it is extremely rare for a test to give a false positive result.

The knowledge that you are pregnant can make you feel very special, and many women want to shout the news to everyone. Others prefer to wait until after they are 12 weeks pregnant, when there is less risk of a miscarriage.

You will probably have started to feel very tired – not helped by the frequent need to pass urine during the night – and you may well be suffering from nausea or vomiting. Feeling continually sick is almost as bad as being sick, but there are steps you can take to help the symptoms (see page 90). Try to see these as positive signs of pregnancy and not an illness, because attitude can have a huge effect on the way you feel during your pregnancy.

your changing body

Your body may feel different but it will not look very different, so others will not be able to tell that you are pregnant. Early symptoms of pregnancy can be very similar to the signs that you get when your period is due, for example, your lower abdomen and pelvis may feel congested. You may even get a small amount of breakthrough bleeding (an implantation bleed) 6–10 days after conception, when the fertilized egg implants in the lining of the uterus.

It is not surprising that you feel tired because, although you will have no obvious bump at this stage, your body is working very hard as the embryo rapidly develops and grows. Your cervix will be softer and your

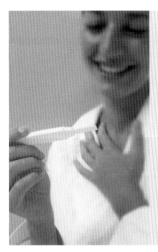

signs of pregnancy

- Missed period
- Tender breasts
- Tiredness
- Irritability
- Frequent urination
- Nausea or vomiting
- Metallic taste in mouth
- Pelvic congestion
- Positive pregnancy test

week reminders

what you should be eating

Start taking folic acid supplements (0.4 mg daily) if you have not done so already. Folic acid is known to reduce the risk of your baby having spina bifida, other neural tube defects and cleft palate.

jobs to do

Make an appointment to see the midwife at around 8 weeks of pregnancy.

uterus will swell as it stretches to make room for the embryo. You may notice the area around your nipples (areola) becoming darker and the tiny glands around the nipples becoming more prominent.

your health

Headaches are very common, especially when you are tired (see page 95).
Constipation is common because the muscles of your intestine are relaxing, making it sluggish (see page 89).

your weight gain
None.

fundal height
Your body shape will not have changed, although by 7 weeks your uterus will be the size of a small tangerine and will be squashed against your bladder.

your baby at
1–3 weeks

Your pregnancy is dated from the start of your last period, although conception usually occurs 2 weeks later. Thus, by the time you miss a period, you will probably be 5 weeks pregnant. A full-term pregnancy lasts 40 weeks so your estimated date of delivery (EDD) will be 40 weeks from your last menstrual period (LMP). Making a note of this date helps the midwife when it comes to working out your due date.

development

Approximately 14 days before your period is due, your body releases an egg (ovum) and the lining of your uterus starts to thicken. It only takes one sperm – out of the millions that are released and the hundreds that make the long journey up the Fallopian tube – to fertilize the egg and for the process of growth and development to begin. The tail separates from the head of the sperm as soon as it penetrates the egg, and cell division begins. Within hours, the fertilized egg becomes two cells, then four, then eight and so on, and is called a zygote. Approximately 4 days after fertilization it is a solid cluster of cells, called a morula.

About a week after fertilization, the ball of cells – now hollow in the centre and called a blastocyst – reaches the uterus. The blastocyst will attach itself to the wall of your uterus and begin to embed deep into its lining. This process is called implantation. The cluster of cells very quickly produces an outer layer, which will develop into the placenta and amniotic sac, and an inner layer, which will develop into the embryo. The outer layer has root-like structures that bury into the lining of the uterus. These become the route by which nutrients and oxygen are transported from your circulation to what will soon be the developing placenta and embryo.

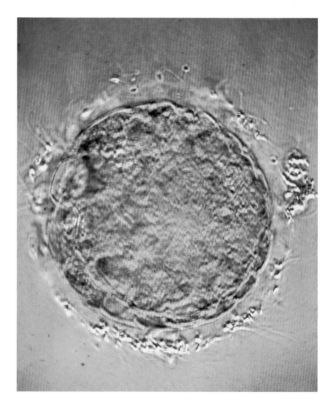

In this false-colour image, 6 days after fertilization, the morula is surrounded by a ring of sperm that failed to penetrate and fertilize the ovum.

appearance

The morula is microscopic in size and resembles a mulberry. By the time it implants in the uterus, at around day 10, it resembles a greyish blackberry and is called a blastocyst. This hollow cluster of cells will grow and develop into the embryo.

your baby at
4 weeks

Your body is producing high levels of human chorionic gonadotrophin (HCG), especially in the morning. This happens after successful conception, that is, once a fertilized egg is implanted in the lining of the uterus. High levels of HCG, which makes pregnancy tests read positive, are necessary to sustain pregnancy. A plug of mucus develops at the entrance of the uterus to protect the embryo from infection.

development

At 4 weeks the cells are dividing and multiplying rapidly, and three layers of cells have now formed:
- The outer layer (the ectoderm) will develop into your baby's brain, nervous system, skin, hair, nails and teeth.
- The middle layer (the mesoderm) will become her heart and blood vessels, bones, muscles and reproductive organs.
- The inner layer (the endoderm) will develop into her lungs, liver, bladder and digestive system.

appearance

The cells of the embryo grow lengthwise, so that the initially round cluster of cells assumes a leaner shape.

The outer cells extend tiny finger-like projections (villi), which link up with your circulation.

Within each of the embryo's body cells are 46 chromosomes in 23 pairs (see page 22) with one of each pair inherited from each parent. As cell division takes places, so long as the chromosomes have been copied correctly, each new cell will have the same number of chromosomes and the same genetic information.

Q **I accidentally got pregnant while taking the pill. I stopped taking it as soon as I found out. Will this have harmed my baby?**

A   It is very unlikely that this will have caused any damage at all to your developing baby because the amounts of hormones that are contained in the contraceptive pill are relatively small. The synthetic hormones from the pill will have cleared from your body by now and you will be making your own natural pregnancy hormones. If you are still worried, talk to your doctor or midwife, who can provide information to reassure you about this.

Q **Does it really matter what I eat and drink so early in pregnancy?**

A   By 12 weeks of pregnancy the embryo will be almost fully developed, which means that the majority of development happens at the start of your pregnancy. Sometimes, things go wrong for no apparent reason, but you can take steps to improve the chances of a successful pregnancy. Avoiding certain foods (see pages 40–43) and taking folic acid will give the tiny embryo extra protection.

You should also avoid drugs, smoking and alcohol, all of which can affect development. It is also best to avoid close contact with certain chemicals and and toxic substances around this time. If you have a problem with dependency or addiction, confide in your midwife who can help to refer you for additional support.

your baby at
5 weeks

Your period is now overdue, so your pregnancy may just have been confirmed. You may not feel any different, but a tremendous amount of activity is going on inside your uterus. At first the hormone progesterone is produced by the discarded follicle to prevent womb lining from shedding. Later the placenta will produce progesterone in order to sustain the pregnancy.

For a small number of women (about 1 in 200 in the UK), the fertilized egg starts to develop outside the uterus, usually in a Fallopian tube. This is known as an ectopic pregnancy (see page 108). It is often detected around this stage but may still become apparent up until 10 weeks.

development

The tiny embryo that will become your baby has a head end and a tail end. By this time all the building blocks for your baby's vital organs are in place. The central nervous system (brain and spinal cord) has already started to form. A basic circulation has begun to work, from you to your baby, and tiny blood vessels are now forming.

The embryo is taking oxygen via the developing placenta, and the bag of membranes (the amniotic sac) is also developing. This will contain the water (amniotic fluid) in which your baby will be protected and continue to grow.

Even at this early stage, the developing heart can be seen as a bulge, no bigger than a poppy seed, at the front of the embryo.

appearance

Under a microscope, the embryo would look rather like a prawn in shape – but no bigger than a grain of rice. At this stage, the head can already be distinguished clearly from the body.

The embryo has a curved back, like the letter C, with a stripe down it, which marks the beginning of the central nervous system. The embryo is attached by a stalk to the developing placenta.

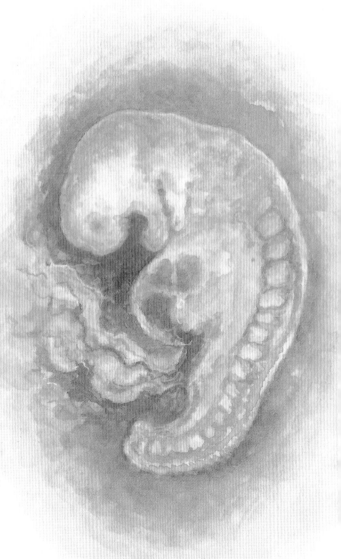

At this stage the embryo that will become your baby is curled up in a C-shape, like a tiny comma.

your baby at
6 weeks

In certain cases where it is necessary to confirm a pregnancy very early on, an ultrasound scan may be given, but it may not be able to detect the embryo at less than 8 weeks. Alternatively, you may be offered a trans-vaginal ultrasound scan – where a probe is placed into the vagina. This may just be able to show the 'flickering' of your baby's heart at 6 weeks of pregnancy.

Babies, up to 14 weeks, are measured in terms of crown to rump length, that is from the top of the head to the end of the bottom, measured as if they were sitting down. This measurement can be used to determine how many weeks pregnant you are and so give you an estimated delivery date (EDD). These scans are most accurate when they are done at around 10 weeks because there is more variation in fetus size later in pregnancy.

development

Your baby's embryonic heart is now beating, but it only has two chambers (not four), because the circulation is not yet completely developed.

The most advanced system at this stage is the central nervous system: the neural tube has now closed over and the brain is developing at one end. The liver begins to develop before the rest of the digestive system.

appearance

Your developing baby now resembles a tiny seahorse. This is because the tissue at the tail end grows faster than that at the front end, giving this distinctive shape. She is floating in a bubble of fluid, which will eventually develop into the amniotic sac. At this stage it is known as the yolk sac, and it provides your baby with oxygen and nutrients until the placenta is fully formed.

The large head seems out of proportion to the body, but the growth of the brain and head is particularly rapid at this early stage of development. Limb buds have appeared and, at the base of the head, there are folds that will develop into facial features, such as the eyes and ears.

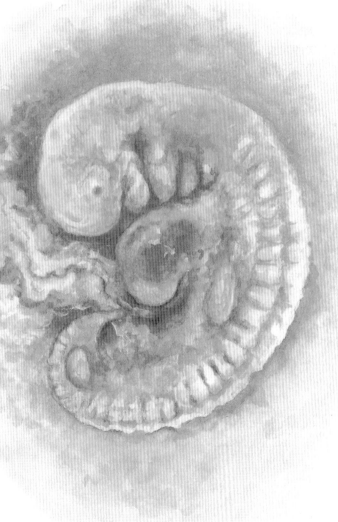

At 6 weeks your baby looks like a minute seahorse, with a large head and tail.

141

your baby at
7 weeks

By now you will probably be more aware of being pregnant because of the hormones rushing around your body, in particular progesterone, oestrogen, HPL and HCG. Your body is still working incredibly hard, and you will feel tired. It is during this week and the next that the tiny embryo that is your baby will be transformed into a human-looking fetus.

development

The heart now has four clearly defined chambers and, although it is still simple, it has a regular beat. The lungs are developing, the muscles and bones are forming, and the limbs are beginning to take shape. The head and brain are growing rapidly, with ridges defining the three areas of the brain. These areas will develop into:

- The forebrain, which controls memory and thinking.
- The midbrain, which is responsible for co-ordinating messages.
- The hindbrain, which regulates the heart, breathing and movements of muscles in the body.

Nasal and oral cavities are developing, which will rapidly become facial features, such as the eyes, ears and mouth. Amazingly, your baby already has an appendix!

appearance

The limb buds are now developing into more recognizable, paddle-shaped arms and legs. A neck is starting to separate the relatively large head from the body. There is a dark tinge where the eyes are forming, and eyelids are also developing. In profile, the tip of the nose is present. Your baby even has lips and a tongue, even though it is only the size of a baked bean!

movement

Your baby will start to make tiny 'twitching' movements that may be detected by sensitive ultrasound equipment. However, you will not be able to feel any movements until approximately 18 weeks of pregnancy.

The sex glands are now developing, although, at this stage, it is impossible to tell the sex by ultrasound scan.

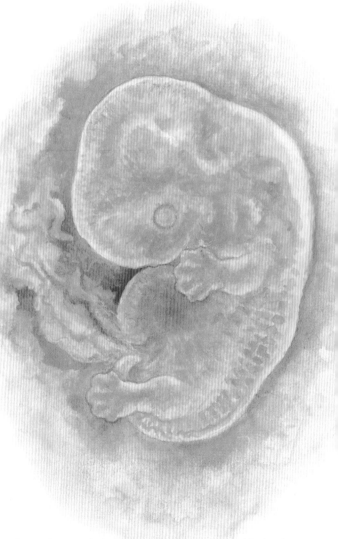

By week 7 your baby has a regular heartbeat and limbs that are just recognizable as arms and legs.

your baby at
8 weeks

Medically speaking, the embryo is now officially called a fetus (meaning 'young' or 'little one'), although you have probably referred to it as 'your baby' from the very beginning. Over the next 4 weeks development will be almost completed – with all major organs and systems working and features present, there will be rapid growth over the following months.

development

The bones start to harden and lengthen, with distinguishable joints, such as wrists, shoulders and elbows. The pituitary gland, which is responsible for the production of hormones and growth, is developing. The kidneys now start to produce urine for the first time. The major organs are still developing but all of them are now in place. The intestines are long and some of them protrude into the umbilical cord. Your baby is living in warm amniotic fluid that consists mainly of water. This keeps her at a constant temperature, and protects and cushions her from any knocks or pressure, encouraging movement.

appearance

Your baby is now recognizably human, with much more distinct features. Her body is losing its curved appearance and becoming straighter, and her limbs are more in proportion. Her skin is transparent, and blood vessels are visible beneath it. Eyelids continue to develop over her eyes, which are wide apart, on the sides of the head, rather like those of a bird. They will move to a more central position as her head and face develop further. The outer parts of her ears are developing on the side of her neck. Her fingers and toes are distinguishable, despite the webbing between them.

movement

Messages are passing along the nerves to your baby's muscles, enabling her to make spontaneous movements, such as gentle kicking, rather than the previous 'twitches'. At this stage, the messages are coming from the spinal cord rather than the brain.

amniotic fluid

Amniotic fluid is the straw-coloured, watery substance that surrounds your baby, protecting her and enabling her to move freely, and keeps the temperature in the uterus constant.

- At 37.5 °C, the temperature of amniotic fluid is higher than that of your body.
- Until 14 weeks, amniotic fluid is absorbed by your baby's skin. Once her kidneys start to function and she develops a sucking reflex, she swallows the fluid and excretes it back into the amniotic sac. However, all her nutrients come from the placenta via the umbilical cord.
- Amniotic fluid contains a range of substances, for example, glucose, fructose, salt, proteins, amino acids, citric acid, urea, lactic acids and fatty acids. However, most of the fluid in the amniotic sac is actually sterile urine.
- Amniotic fluid is a good conductor of sound, although most of what your baby hears in the womb will be muffled.

how your baby has grown

your baby (actual size)

Length 14–25 mm from crown to rump
Weight 4 g

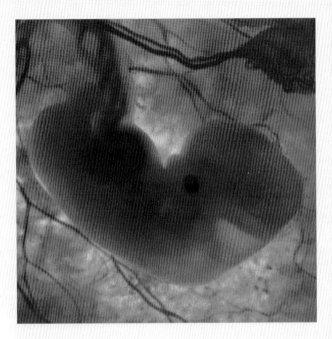

Your baby is surrounded and protected by amniotic fluid.

8

your baby's development

skin
Skin is translucent. Fingers and toes are webbed.

muscles
Muscles are developing and tiny movements begin.

bones
The soft, pliable cartilage is starting to harden and lengthen. Joints are distinguishable and there are tiny movements of the spine.

organs
All major internal organs are in place and developing.

circulatory system
The four chambers of the heart are forming and the heart is beating approximately 170 times per minute.

digestive system
Stomach and intestines have developed. The muscles of the digestive tract are already functioning.

nervous system
The brain and spinal cord are now in place.

urinary system
Kidneys are preparing to produce urine.

respiratory system
Lungs have formed and will continue to develop.

ears
Outer ear structures are developing on each side of the neck.

eyes
Eyes are wide apart on the sides of the head. Eyelids are starting to form over them.

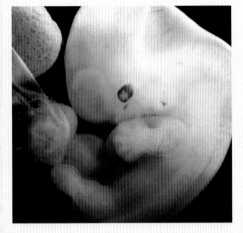

Your baby's limbs are more in proportion to her body.

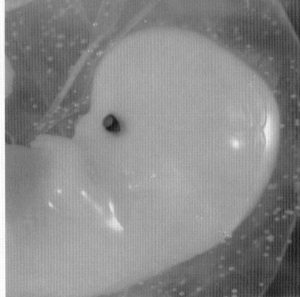

The eyes are set far apart, on each side of her head.

your body at
9–12 weeks

By now, you have probably got used to the idea that you are pregnant. You are likely to have had your first antenatal appointment with your midwife or doctor, you may have seen an image of your baby on an ultrasound scan, and even brought home a copy of the scan to show to everyone, once you decide to let on that you are pregnant.

You may not experience some of the more unpleasant symptoms of early pregnancy, however, even if you have had more than your fair share, you may not mind because they are all signs that indicate that you really are pregnant!

how you may feel

The reality of pregnancy may now be hitting home. Many women choose to tell friends and family about their pregnancy as they approach the twelfth week because the risk of miscarriage is much less. Other people's reactions – surprise from friends, concern from your family, who may be worried that you are too old or too young – can affect how you feel. By the end of this period, the tiredness and nausea should lessen although, for a small minority of women, it will continue. You may also feel very hungry at this stage.

your changing body

Your breasts will now be bigger and you may find that your veins become more prominent. From 9 weeks of pregnancy, you might notice that your waist is getting thicker and that your clothes feel tighter, but this has nothing to do with the size of your baby. It is more likely to be the result of general congestion: your circulation is now more sluggish and you may also be suffering from constipation and wind.

You may notice an increase in vaginal discharge, which is normal during pregnancy. Meanwhile, your uterus has been expanding to accommodate your growing baby and, by 12 weeks, you should be able to feel it through the wall of your abdomen, just above your pubic bone.

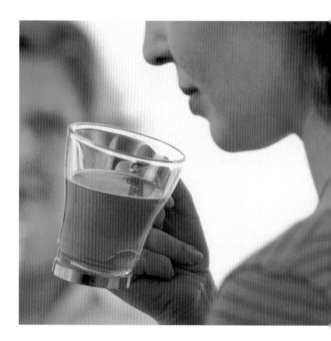

An aversion to coffee is common in the early weeks of pregnancy – many women switch to herbal teas instead.

your health

Sinusitis You may be particularly 'snuffly' as a result of nasal congestion (see page 93).

Gum problems Your gums become softer as a result of the pregnancy hormones and they may bleed (see page 89).

Candida (thrush) An increased vaginal discharge is normal, but women are also more prone to this yeast infection, which produces a white itchy discharge and soreness (see page 99).

Q **I am 10 weeks pregnant and I am being sick every day. It is really getting me down. Is there anything I can do?**

A This is thought to be caused by the pregnancy hormone human chorionic gonadotrophin (HCG) and is sometimes made worse if your blood sugar levels fall. Try to eat little and often throughout the day. Ginger or peppermint is also thought to help nausea, and some women swear by travel bands. These apply pressure to the acupuncture points in the wrist that control sickness. Try sucking ice cubes if you cannot face drinking anything and see your doctor if you find yourself becoming dehydrated. In the majority of cases the sickness is a normal, if unpleasant, part of pregnancy and generally passes by 14 weeks. (See also page 90.)

what you should be eating

Continue to take your folic acid supplements and make sure that you are eating enough iron-rich foods, for example, red meat, dried apricots, raisins, pulses, green leafy vegetables and dark oily fish.

jobs to do

Make an appointment to see your midwife or doctor if you have not done so already. They will need to take blood tests and may arrange a dating scan.

If you decide to have a chorionic villus sampling (CVS), a prenatal screening test to detect genetic defects (see page 129), it would be done around now.

Ask your midwife or doctor for the appropriate certificate if you can claim free prescriptions and dental care.

your weight gain

Up to 1 kg
Some women lose weight due to sickness.

fundal height

The top of your uterus should be just above your pubic bone.

your baby's position

Your baby will be changing position all the time.

your baby at 9 weeks

During the last 3 weeks, your baby has increased more than three times in size and now looks far more human. The 'tail' has disappeared and the growth of the limbs is more in proportion to the body. As your baby goes through this major growth phase, so the placenta is also busy enlarging and building for its important life-supporting role.

development

Your baby's heart is almost fully developed and is beating approximately 170 times per minute, more than twice as fast as that of an adult. An important band of muscle, which will become the diaphragm, now separates the cavity of the chest and the abdomen. The placental tissue is becoming concentrated in one area of the uterine wall but is not yet fully functional.

appearance

Your baby's development and appearance is becoming more 'refined'. This week, growth of his hands and feet and his arms and legs is particularly rapid. His fingers have separated and his feet have lengthened. His upper lip is fully formed and his ears are more recognizable. His head is growing rapidly and is almost half the size of his body, appearing out of proportion. Growth is fast and, during the next 3 weeks, his body will more than double in length.

movement

Your baby is now starting to make more definite movements, exercising his muscles, which will encourage their growth. As well as kicking his feet, he can also move his arms and spine, although you will not be aware of these movements for several weeks yet. Movements are one indication of a healthy baby and if you choose to have an ultrasound scan you will be amazed to see how much movement your baby does make, even though you do not feel it.

Q I did not realize that I was pregnant and I had too much to drink one night at a party. Will it have affected my baby?

A Many women worry about what they ate or drank before they realized that they were pregnant. However, now that you do know, there is a lot that you can do to give your baby the best chance possible. Even if you have never drunk alcohol, there is no guarantee that your baby will be free from problems, so adopt the healthiest lifestyle you can. Binge-drinking can be dangerous for the baby but the chance of one evening's overindulgence causing a problem is very small.

'I was unsure of my dates so the midwife arranged an ultrasound scan. The sonographer pointed out a tiny shape, like a seahorse, with a flickering heartbeat. Although I'd had a positive pregnancy test, it only felt real when I could see it with my own eyes!'

Liz, 9 weeks pregnant

shared experience

your baby at
10 weeks

Your baby is floating in approximately 50 ml of amniotic fluid and as she continues to grow, the amount of fluid will also increase, as it is largely made up of the urine she excretes! Your baby is developing rapidly, with changes taking place daily. Muscles in your baby's face are developing that will eventually enable her to suck and chew. By this stage, she even has distinctive fingerprints.

development

The structure of your baby's brain is complete, although the cells continue to multiply. The palate of her mouth is forming and tooth sockets have formed in her gums. The umbilical cord is fully formed and blood is beginning to circulate through it, although the placenta is not yet formed. Her stomach and intestines are developed, and the muscles of her digestive tract are functional and starting to contract. Your baby's sex is still unclear because the genitals are not fully formed, but male and female characteristics are beginning to show.

One of this baby's eyes is clearly visible as the dark spot above her hands. Her head is large in proportion to her body.

appearance

The most dramatic change is in your baby's face, which is really taking shape and now looks distinctly human. Her head is still large in relation to her body. Her eyes are moving from the sides of the head to the front, and are now covered by the eyelids. Her ears and mouth are forming. Her fingers and toes are no longer webbed.

movement

As your baby's nervous system becomes more developed, her movements increase. You can detect even tiny movements of her toes. It has been observed on ultrasound scan that, if your abdomen is prodded, your baby will move in response.

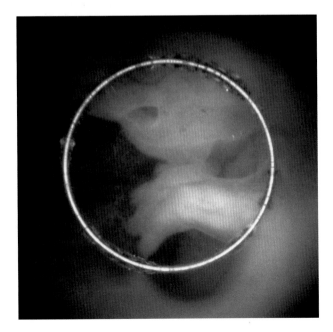

did you know?

If you are having a dating scan, it will usually be around week 10. Drink plenty beforehand because, when your bladder is full, it helps the sonographer to get a clearer picture of your baby. It will be at this point that the number of babies you are carrying will be confirmed – although, if you are pregnant with twins, you might already have a suspicion because early pregnancy symptoms tend to be much worse.

The sonographer will take measurements of your baby, from which he or she will work out when your baby is due. It is a good idea to take some change with you because you might be able to buy a picture of your baby!

your baby at
11 weeks

By this point of your pregnancy your baby has grown to approximately the size of a small lime. By the end of this week his organs are not only formed but are also working. As a result of this, your pregnancy is stronger, your baby's development is not so vulnerable to environmental risks and the danger of you suffering a miscarriage is reduced.

development

Your baby's heart is working hard, pumping blood around his body and through the umbilical cord to the area that is developing into the placenta. His outer ears are moving from the neck to the sides of the head, and the middle and inner ears are completely formed. The ovaries and testicles have developed inside the body but your baby's sex is not obvious from the outside because the genitals have not developed.

appearance

Most of the time your baby will be in the fetal position, with chin bent down and knees curled up, but, despite that, he is very active. His limbs remain quite short but they are undeveloped because he has not as yet been moving them.

The more he moves, the stronger his muscles will become, and this will encourage their growth. His head appears large and out of proportion to his body, but his face is more rounded with discernable features.

movement

Your baby is making more definite movements, moving his spine and stretching his arms and legs. He can even open and close his mouth!

old wives' tales
According to folklore, if you suffer from heartburn in pregnancy, your baby will be born with a good head of hair!

the umbilical cord
- At full term, the cord is about 50 cm long and 1–1.5 cm thick.
- Your baby does not feel anything when the cord is cut after the birth.
- After the birth, when your baby breathes, the cord has no further function though it provides him with extra blood and oxygen until it is clamped.

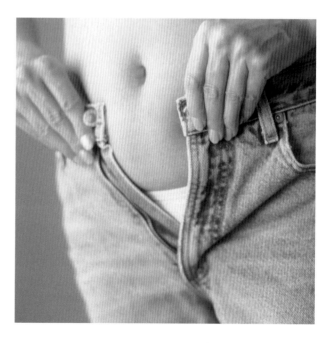

Even though your baby is quite small (about 6.5 cm long), his presence means that your clothes start to feel tight.

your baby at
12 weeks

Your baby has grown to about the size of a lemon. This stage of pregnancy, which marks the end of the first 3 months, often feels like a milestone for many women because the risk of miscarriage is reduced after week 12. The major development of your baby is complete and the emphasis is now on growth. Although the placenta is small, it is now complete.

development

Your baby's ears have moved to the sides of her head and the remainder of her face is now formed. Her jaws have tooth buds in place, and she can suck and swallow. She has an unmistakable chin and her nose is more obvious. Her eyelids are fused shut over her eyes. Her circulation is fully functioning, her kidneys are working, and her bones are becoming harder.

The muscles of your baby's intestine are moving, practising peristalsis, the contractions used to move food through the bowels.

appearance

Her skin remains very thin and translucent and the blood vessels are visible through it. Her limbs are growing in length and are more in proportion to the rest of her body.

Tiny nails are growing on her fully formed fingers and toes. Her external genitals are forming, although it would still be very difficult to determine the sex of your baby on an ultrasound scan.

movement

The movements of your baby will increase as the muscles in her limbs develop, although you will not be aware of them. She can even move her fingers, clenching and unclenching her hands. Researchers have described a baby's movements, seen on an ultrasound scan at this stage, as 'graceful'.

'She became absorbed in her own body and obsessed with her pregnancy, I felt pushed out. After the scan it seemed far more real to me than it had previously!'

Michael, partner of
Cheryl, 14 weeks pregnant

shared experiences

'I held back from telling people I was pregnant until after my 12-week scan. It wasn't just the relief of knowing that the risk of miscarriage was less; in a funny way it didn't feel like I was really pregnant until I actually saw my baby on the scan and saw it move. At last I felt I could tell my family, friends and people at work that I was going to have a baby, although I think that some of them had already guessed and were just waiting for me to say something!'

Kate, 19
weeks pregnant

how your baby
has grown

your baby (actual size)

Length approximately 6.5 cm from crown to rump
Weight 14 g

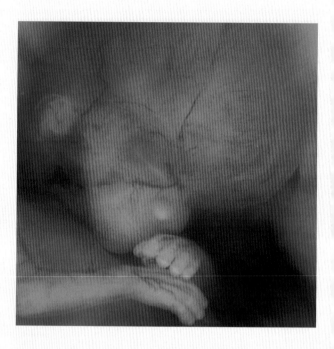

Nails are starting to appear on fingers and toes.

12
weeks

your baby's development

skin and hair
Skin is translucent. Fingers and toes are no longer webbed and nails are beginning to develop.

muscles
Developing muscles are linked with the nervous system. The diaphragm has formed.

bones
All bones are in place. Bones continue to harden.

organs
All major internal organs are formed, but still maturing.

circulatory system
This is fully functioning. The heart is pumping blood.

digestive system
Fully formed and fuctional.

endocrine system
This is starting to manufacture growth hormone and produce alphafetoprotein (AFP, see page 127).

nervous system
The brain is now complete but still developing. Messages pass between the spinal cord and muscles.

renal system
Kidneys are functioning.

respiratory system
Your baby is practising breathing movements.

ears
Outer ears have moved from the neck to the side of the head. The outer ear continues to develop but the middle and inner ears are fully formed.

eyes
Eyes, although still wide apart, have moved from the sides of the head to the front. Eyelids are fused shut.

This 3-D scan shows how the shape of your baby's body has altered.

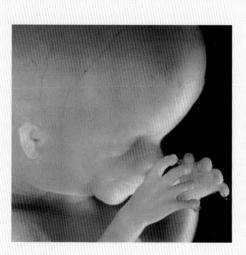

Your baby's eyes are sealed closed.

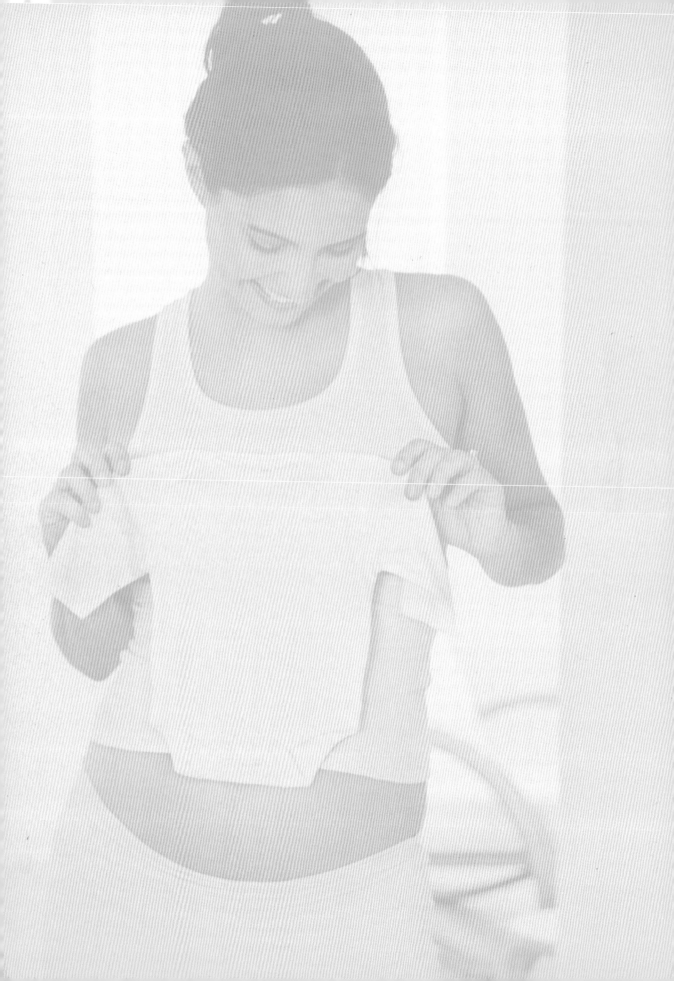

mid-pregnancy

Like many women at this stage of pregnancy, you will probably be blooming and full of energy. What is more, the first obvious sign of your new status is making itself known in the form of your ever-expanding bump. Your baby is growing fast and taking up more room but your bump is not yet big enough to feel heavy or wear you down. Any day now, too, you'll feel those amazing and longed-for first flickering movements – your baby somersaulting inside you.

your body at
13–16 weeks

As you enter the second 3 months of pregnancy, you will probably start to 'bloom'. This is when many women feel at their best. Your tiredness and nausea should improve and your energy levels should pick up, and you will also become aware of your changing shape and find that your usual clothes are too tight. But look in the mirror – you are at last starting to look pregnant!

five reasons to go to antenatal classes

1 It is a good way of meeting other pregnant women and building a support network for after the birth. Years later, many women keep in touch with the people they met through these classes.

2 Most classes encourage partners to come along, which is a good way of making them feel involved, in both the birth and the pregnancy.

3 You will be given information on everything to do with childbirth, for example, pain relief, positions in labour, signs of labour, types of delivery, feeding and baby care. Research shows that, the more information you have, the more likely you are to stay in control throughout your labour.

4 You will get the opportunity to tour the maternity unit. You can see how to get there, where to park and the ward you will go to, as well as the options that are available. Even if you are planning a home birth, it is still a good idea to have the tour in case you need to be transferred to the unit.

5 You will be able to ask questions in an informal setting. Some subjects that you are keen to ask will probably be covered by the midwife or childbirth educator during the classes.

how you may feel

Many women feel at their most feminine during pregnancy, because their breasts become larger, their abdomen rounds and the condition of their skin and hair improves. By this stage, you will have accepted and become more confident in your pregnancy, and you have probably shared the news with others.

It is quite normal to be preoccupied with your pregnancy and you may find that your short-term memory is poor: you may forget what you need in the supermarket or keep mislaying things. You should also be feeling more energetic because your sleep is being less disrupted by nightly visits to the toilet.

Your midwife or doctor will have used a Doppler (see page 159) to listen to your baby's heartbeat. Listening to this for the first time is an emotional moment, and it may make you feel much closer to your baby. Many women say that they wish they could simply lie down and listen to their baby's heartbeat until it is time for the birth!

your changing body

Changes in your skin are common at this stage (see page 84). Your uterus has now risen out of your pubic cavity and is the size of a grapefruit. If you have had a baby before, your bump is often more obvious because your muscles have been stretched and are not as toned. Your veins expand during pregnancy and therefore become more prominent: you might notice them as blue lines not only on your breasts, but also on your legs and abdomen. Although many women delight in the changes others find it difficult to make the adjustment.

your health

Heartburn You may experience an unpleasant burning sensation when stomach acids leak into your oesophagus. This is because the valve that normally stops this from happening relaxes during pregnancy (see page 90).

Varicose veins are common during pregnancy and are due to the sluggish circulation caused by pregnancy hormones (see page 102).

Q Can my baby get cold in the uterus?

A It is highly unlikely that your baby could get cold. Your body temperature and the warm amniotic fluid maintain her temperature. She also has a light covering of hair (lanugo) as well as the waxy vernix, both of which give her some protection.

week 13–16 reminders

what you should be eating

Increase your intake of calcium by eating plenty of dairy foods (particularly milk, yoghurt and hard cheese), tinned fish, white bread, spinach, baked beans, kidney beans, almonds and oranges. Calcium is necessary for the growth of your baby's teeth, bones and muscles and also helps your blood to clot and may protect against hypertension (high blood pressure).

Do not take any vitamin supplements other than folic acid unless advised to do so by your midwife or doctor. Vitamin A supplements and foods high in animal-source vitamin A – such as liver – can harm your unborn baby.

jobs to do

Make sure that you have had all the blood tests that you need by the end of this period. It is important to establish your blood group during pregnancy in case of any bleeding. You should have an injection of Anti-D (see page 82) if you are Rhesus negative and have any bleeding.

Ask your midwife about antenatal exercise classes in your area, such as aqua-natal or yoga.

your weight gain
0–2 kg

fundal height
If you lie down you can feel the top of your uterus about 3 fingers depth above your pubic bone.

your baby's position
Your baby has plenty of room and is constantly exercising by moving and changing position.

your baby at
13 weeks

Your baby is about the size of a peach, which is incredible when you think that he was only the size of a baked bean 6 weeks ago. He will grow rapidly over the next few months and, if you feel your lower abdomen, you may just be able to feel the curve of your expanding uterus. External genitalia is now just about developed enough for an ultrasound to detect gender.

development

Although your baby's organs are formed they still need to mature over the following weeks. His hands and feet are fully developed and making lots of movements as messages pass from the spinal cord to the muscles. His joints and bones continue to get harder (ossify), a process that will continue even after he is born.

appearance

Your baby's head is still relatively large but his neck is more defined. His arms and legs are growing longer, which makes them more in proportion with the rest of his body. He is sprouting fine hair (lanugo) over his body and at last, although tiny, he looks like a baby.

movement

Because your baby's neck is now developed he can move his head freely. If you see your baby on ultrasound scan at this stage you would be amazed at how active he is. Because he can make movements with his mouth he seems to be making facial expressions!

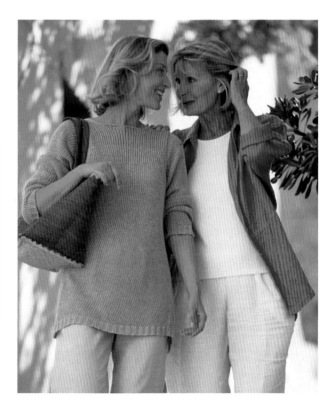

how smoking can affect your baby

- Smoking affects the growth of your baby by diminishing the supply of oxygen.
- Smoking increases the risk of miscarriage, premature birth and cot death.
- Smoking increases the risk of stillbirth or of death within the first week of life.
- Babies of smokers generally have a lower birth weight.
- Babies of smokers are more likely to have breathing difficulties.
- Babies of smokers are more likely to smoke as adults.

Your baby is already a big part of your life and you will probably want to share your feelings with someone else.

your baby at
14 weeks

Your baby is able to make facial expressions now and she will exercise her face muscles by frowning and pulling a variety of expressions. She weighs around 70 g and is the size of a pear, and would fit into the palm of your hand. Her face and body are far more defined than a few weeks ago – she is tiny and fragile, but very obviously a baby.

development

Around this time your baby's thyroid gland starts to produce hormones. The external genitals are developing further and, in most cases, can be seen on an ultrasound scan. In girls, the ovaries descend into the pelvis and, in boys, the prostate gland appears. The skeleton is getting harder and becoming stronger and she even has tiny taste buds, which look like those of an adult but are not yet functioning.

appearance

Your baby's neck is longer and her chin is now more defined, refining the shape of her head and face. Her eyes have become closer, although they will be sealed closed by the eyelids until 28 weeks of pregnancy. The bridge of her nose appears and her ears are higher on her head. Her face is now well developed and she even has very faint eyebrows appearing.

doppler scanning

Your midwife or doctor can use an ultrasound device, called a Doppler, to listen to your baby's heartbeat. The heartbeat will be amplified so that you can hear it too. It will sound very fast and will be about 150 beats per minute at this stage. The Doppler works by bouncing sound waves off red blood cells, which shows how fast they are moving, and how fast the blood is flowing. This checks the baby's growth rate and how well the placenta is functioning.

movement

Your baby can easily move around in the amniotic fluid and has plenty of space to do so. She is strengthening and encouraging the development of her muscles by exercising them more and more. She is kicking and twisting, her fists can grasp and clench, and she can even put her thumb into her mouth. She has periods of being awake and asleep, although, at the moment, you will not be aware of this.

Q **My partner does not seem to be bonding with my unborn baby in the same way that I am. How can I encourage him to feel differently?**

A Bonding can be difficult for a partner because he is not the one experiencing the signs and symptoms of pregnancy and it is easier for him to feel removed from it. At this stage of pregnancy the bones in your baby's ears are hardening so you can encourage your partner to talk to your baby, while gently laying his head on your bump. In a few weeks he will be able to feel the baby move when he places a hand on your bump. Involve him as much as you can by encouraging him to come to your antenatal checks and ultrasound scans. When he sees the baby on the screen, or hears the baby's heartbeat, your pregnancy will probably seem more real to him.

your baby at
15 weeks

Talk to your baby because the amniotic fluid that surrounds him will conduct sound. As well as your voice, he will be able to hear your heart beating and your stomach rumbling. Research shows that a newborn baby is very attuned to his mother's voice, presumably because he has got used to hearing it, even though it is muffled, from within the uterus.

development

Although his eyes are fused shut, he is becoming sensitive to light and will appear to squint. If he has genes for dark hair, the cells of his hair follicles will be producing a dark pigment. He is opening his mouth and regularly swallowing amniotic fluid. He will turn towards the direction of any stimulus of his mouth.

appearance

Overall, your baby's body is generally in proportion now and his legs are longer than his arms. As well, as the soft coating of hair over his body (lanugo) he is growing fluffy hair on his head. Very faint eyebrows and eyelashes are starting to appear, although his eyes are still closed. His skin is still very thin and translucent, and the complicated network of developing blood vessels can be seen beneath it.

movement

Your baby is moving freely in the uterus as he still has plenty of room to do so. Although he may be laying head down one minute, he can easily be bottom down (breech) the next, as he twists and turns unhampered in the amniotic fluid.

Q **Why does the size of babies vary so much?**

A There are many things that determine a baby's size, some of which you have influence over and some of which you do not. Your baby inherits genes from two biological parents so, if both parents are small, he will probably be small as well. Lifestyle also has an effect on your baby's size. For example, your baby is more likely to be smaller if you smoke because he is receiving less oxygen and nutrients than he should. Your diet can affect the size of the baby, and if you eat a healthy balanced diet your baby is less likely to have a low birth weight. Medical conditions, such as diabetes or high blood pressure, can affect a baby's size but these are things that your midwife and doctor assess when they feel your abdomen. If they had any cause for concern they would refer you for a scan to assess the growth. The size of your baby at birth is not necessarily related to his eventual size as an adult.

---

think about your baby

It is important to make time to think about your baby and to prepare yourself emotionally. If it is your first baby, you will probably know exactly how many weeks and days pregnant you are. However, if you have already had children, the weeks seem to fly by, often without a thought for the new baby inside you. This is where it can be beneficial to make time to attend aqua-natal or parent-craft classes because you can set aside time when you can think about your baby and chat to others about the pregnancy.

your baby at
16 weeks

Your baby is fully formed and is continuing to grow rapidly. When you see an ultrasound image of her you might even feel that you can discern familiar facial features, such has her father's chin, or your mother's nose! You may also be surprised by her athletic prowess as you see her turns and squirms in the uterus, playing and exploring her environment.

development

If your baby is a girl, more than 4 million eggs will have formed in her ovaries, although this number will reduce by the time she is born.

Nails are appearing on her fingers and toes, and her skeleton has developed to such an extent that it would be visible on an X-ray. Although she is receiving oxygen from blood, via the umbilical cord, she is practising breathing movements, encouraging her lungs to develop.

appearance

Your baby's face looks human in appearance, particularly now she can produce different expressions. She can hold her head up straighter, yawn and may even suck her thumb.

movement

This is the earliest stage at which you can feel your baby move, especially if this is not your first child. She is making a lot of movements, but they will be very subtle. At first, you may not be sure whether she is moving at all. Imagine the fluttering of a miniature butterfly or the popping of bubbles in a fizzy drink – a tiny movement – that is barely discernable and can sometimes be mistaken for wind! If you have any anxiety about not being able to tell if she is moving or not, do not worry. Her movements will get stronger each week, until you are in absolutely no doubt at all when she moves.

six facts about your baby's movements

1 Although you will not have been aware of it, your baby started moving shortly after you were 8 weeks pregnant.

2 The first movements that you feel are referred to as 'quickening'. If this is your first baby, you usually notice these at around 18–22 weeks. Otherwise you may recognize them earlier – closer to 16 weeks.

3 After 28 weeks of pregnancy you should feel your baby move approximately ten times a day.

4 Babies should not move any less as you get closer to your delivery date. If you feel that the movements are reducing or are less than ten a day, contact your midwife or the maternity unit so that you and your baby can be checked over.

5 Some women feel fewer movements than others, possibly because of the position of their baby. However, even if this is the case, you should still have close monitoring on a regular basis.

6 If a bright light is shone onto your abdomen at 16 weeks of pregnancy, your baby may raise an arm to shield her eyes.

how your baby has grown

your baby (actual size)

Length Approximately 11 cm from crown to rump
Weight 85 g

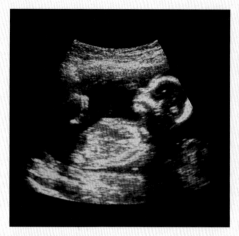

This colour ultrasound scan shows that your baby looks completely human.

16

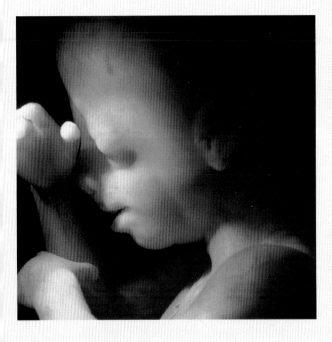

His external ears have moved up from the neck area to the sides of his head.

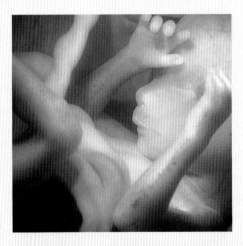

Your baby appears to make different facial expressions at this age.

your baby's development

skin and hair
Skin is thin and translucent. Body is covered in lanugo. Head hair, eyebrows and eyelashes are starting to grow and hair colour is developing. Nails are forming.

muscles
Muscles become stronger with increasing movement.

bones
Calcium is being laid down so the bones continue to harden. Skeleton is now visible on an X-ray.

circulatory system
Oxygen and nutrition are acquired via the umbilical cord. The heart beats at about 160 times per minute.

digestive system
Organs are formed but still maturing.

endocrine system
Thyroid gland starts to produce hormones.

nervous system
Brain and nervous system continue to develop. Messages are sent from the spinal cord to the muscles.

reproductive system
External genitals are obvious. Female babies have eggs.

respiratory system
Lungs are still developing but baby is practising breathing movements.

urinary system
Your baby is gulping amniotic fluid and urinating small amounts, maintaining the volume of fluid.

ears
Bones of the inner ear formed. Can hear some sounds.

eyes
Eyes can respond to bright lights. Eyelids are still fused.

your body at
17–20 weeks

Many women enjoy the middle 3 months of pregnancy because they have the fun of looking pregnant without feeling cumbersome. Once your baby starts to move you will feel reassured that everything is alright, and have even more confidence in your pregnancy. The early weeks may have passed slowly but time will seem to fly by from now on.

'I felt more feminine than ever before when I was pregnant. It gave me an excuse to experiment with clothes, change my hairstyle and I loved having a decent cleavage!'

Cilla, mother of 3-week-old Callum

shared experiences

'I didn't realize that being pregnant involves more than just an ever-growing bump. I've put on weight all over my body and feel fat and cumbersome. My partner has been wonderful: he's always reassuring me that my bump is perfect and that I look beautiful.'

Debbie, 20 weeks pregnant

how you may feel

Many women bloom at this stage: nausea decreases, energy levels increase and they begin to look noticeably pregnant. Learning about the options for birth, antenatal classes and talking with other women who have children all make pregnancy more enjoyable. You may enjoy looking for maternity clothes to show off your bump. You might have felt your baby move, and you will certainly have heard his heart beat, so you will probably be feeling very protective of your baby.

your changing body

You will now look pregnant, with a noticeable bump and a vanishing waistline. Many women feel happier once they look pregnant, but others find it difficult to adjust to their changing body image. You may notice some changes in the pigmentation of your skins, such as a dark line on your stomach, or a discolouration on your face (see page 84). These usually fade after the baby is born.

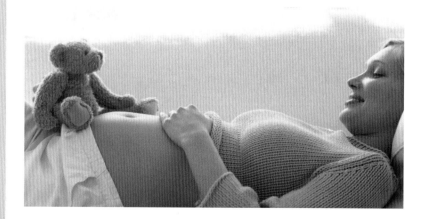

Chances are, you're now feeling full of energy but take time out occasionally to put your feet up during the day and relax. Although you cannot feel him move yet, you can enjoy visualizing your baby inside you.

Q **My last baby was born by caesarean section 18 months ago. I am now 17 weeks pregnant; will I need a caesarean section again?**

A It depends on the reason for the operation. If your pelvis was too narrow for the baby then you would be advised to have another caesarean. In most circumstances, however, there is no reason for you to have another caesarean unless you want one. Recovery from a vaginal delivery is quicker and, as this is your second baby, you probably won't want to stay in hospital longer than totally necessary. Your obstetrician and midwife will discuss the delivery with you and you can make the decision.

your health

Nosebleeds can be more frequent during pregnancy because of increases in blood supply and nasal congestion (see page 101).

what you should be eating
Include plenty of iron-rich foods to avoid getting anaemia and be sure that you are getting enough vitamin C to help your body absorb the iron.

jobs to do
Think about enrolling in an antenatal class. Although it is probably too early to begin them, you might need to go on a waiting list to avoid disappointment.

Pay attention to your posture. During pregnancy, your ligaments stretch and your joints separate slightly, making you more prone to back problems, so avoid unnecessary bending and lifting. Good posture will help reduce heartburn.

your weight gain
2–3 kg

fundal height
The top of your uterus will be about 4 finger-widths beneath your navel.

your baby's position
Your baby will be changing position frequently. She still has plenty of room and can even somersault.

your baby at
17 weeks

If the baby you are expecting is a boy, his testosterone levels will have peaked between 12 and 16 weeks gestation, not only affecting the development of his sexual organs but also that of his brain. Scientists have found that regular ultrasound scans beginning a few weeks after this can distinguish a male from a female brain.

development

Your baby now begins to lay down brown fat, which will play an important part in generating heat when he is born. The placenta is also growing quickly, providing a huge surface area that will provide him with nutrients and remove his waste products. No new structures are forming now, but existing ones are growing in size, developing further and becoming stronger. These are essential if your baby is to lead an independent existence outside of the uterus. By this stage he will weigh about 100 g and would still be able to fit into the palm of your hand.

appearance

The soft downy lanugo makes swirly patterns, similar to those of fingerprints, all over your baby's body. His skin is still thin and very fragile because there is very little fat on his body.

movement

His chest is making breathing movements like those he will make when he is born. However, he is not actually breathing yet because oxygen is being supplied via the umbilical cord. Rapid eye movements have been detected at this stage, suggesting that your baby dreams!

Q **I'm 17 weeks pregnant and feel really low and miserable, and the slightest thing has me in tears. Will it affect my baby?**

A Mood swings and tearfulness are common in pregnancy because of the increased hormones in your body and because of sheer tiredness. Normal mood swings are unlikely to harm your baby. However, 10–15 per cent of women do get antenatal depression (in varying degrees). Talk to your midwife about how you are feeling as soon as possible. It is important to address this and to explore the cause, as there is an increased risk of developing postnatal depression, which, it is thought, can potentially affect the emotional development of your baby.

the placenta

- By 17 weeks, the placenta is almost the same size as your baby.
- After the first 3 months of pregnancy, when your placenta is fully functioning, it takes over the production of your pregnancy hormones.
- At full term the placenta is round and flat, about 23 cm in diameter and 2 cm thick in the middle, getting thinner towards the edges.
- In the last few weeks of pregnancy the placenta is normally situated n the top half of the uterus.
- Nicotine, drugs and alcohol can pass through the placenta to your baby.
- The placenta transmits some of your antibodies to your baby, helping to protect him against diseases to which you are immune.

your baby at
18 weeks

No new structures will be formed now. Your baby has everything she needs, but she is not mature enough to survive if she was born at this stage. You will probably start to feel her moving around this time. Babies appear to move more when their mothers are still so it may be movement that lulls them to sleep. It seems that babies continue to find being 'on the move' comforting after they are born.

development
The last organ to develop is the lungs, and will take many weeks. This is why premature babies often need help with their breathing. At this stage, tiny air sacs (alveoli) are beginning to form in the lungs. Her muscles are strengthening. Her kidneys are working and she is swallowing amniotic fluid and also urinating, thus maintaining the volume of amniotic fluid.

appearance
Your baby's head and body are more in proportion now, and the facial features are very clear. Her skin looks red and her body is still very thin because the majority of fat will not be laid down until the final weeks.

movement
There is plenty of room for your baby to move around. This movement is vital for the proper development of the muscles, joints and bones. Ultrasound scans have shown babies crossing their legs, somersaulting, or resting while sucking their thumb. She might already have a pattern of activity and rest time.

anomaly scan

This ultrasound scan at 18–20 weeks of pregnancy checks for obvious abnormalities with your baby and for the position of the placenta (see page 124). Some sonographers will tell you the sex of your baby at this point.

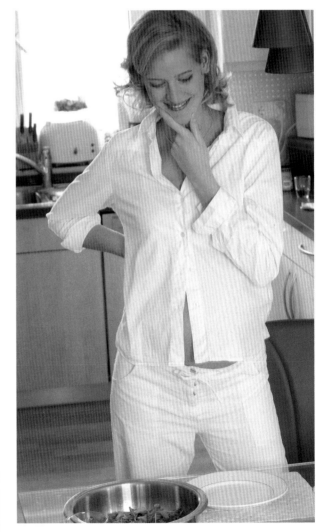

It is important to eat a good variety of food, so that your baby grows well.

your baby at
19 weeks

Your baby is responding to sound, movement, touch and light by this time and is much more aware of the outside world than he was earlier in your pregnancy. If he hears a loud noise outside your body, especially if it is sudden, he may jump or move around vigorously in reaction to it, although you may not always be aware of these movements.

development

Millions of cells are growing in your baby's brain, and nerves are now connecting the brain to the muscles, so that he has more control of his movements. He has the same number of nerve cells as an adult but the nerves have yet to receive a protective layer of myelin. His system of temperature regulation continues to develop, and small amounts of a substance called 'brown fat' are being deposited around his neck, chest and groin. At this stage the placenta is fully formed and will continue to grow in size. It is almost the same size as your baby, who is moving around in just a cupful of amniotic fluid.

appearance

Your baby's ears now stand out from the sides of his head, whereas previously they were flat. Permanent tooth buds are appearing behind the buds of his milk teeth. His skin is wrinkled and is covered in a waxy substance called vernix, which is secreted from the sebaceous glands and provides a waterproof coating, as well as giving him some protection from infection.

movement

You may be aware of some movement, although some women do not notice anything until 22 weeks. Your baby is still relatively small so there may be days when you do not feel very much – the foot that kicks you is only around 2 cm long! He has far more control over his movements and is using his joints to kick and punch, making fists with his hands and curling his toes.

If you could see him, you would see his tongue when he opens his mouth and see the expressions on his face changing.

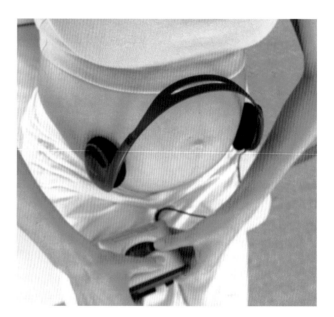

Your baby can hear from about week 12, so by the time your bump is well and truly showing, why not play him some music?

noise

Your baby's life in the uterus is so noisy that he gets used to constant noise. After he is born he may be comforted by sounds such as running water, the vacuum cleaner or a hairdryer. Some parents record the sound of a washing machine to play at bedtime! As far back as the 5th century BC, Hippocrates told pregnant women to listen to beautiful music.

your baby at
20 weeks

Your baby's growth starts to slow down now and she is approximately half the length of a full-term baby. Her fat is not yet laid down and she weighs about 340 g. She is about the size of a small mango. From this point on she will start to put on weight at a rate of approximately 50 g per week. If she is to arrive on her due date, she's half way there.

development

Your baby's development is focused on the lungs and digestive and immune systems. Her kidneys are passing approximately 7–17 ml of urine every 24 hours. Areas of her brain are developing that are specific to the senses of taste, smell, hearing, sight and touch. Her heartbeat is stronger and can be heard using a stethoscope.

appearance

Your baby is thin and looks very delicate. Her eyes seem large because her face has not yet rounded out, and her eyes can move from side to side, although her eyelids are closed. She has more hair on her head, and her eyelashes and eyebrows are taking shape. Her legs are almost in proportion with the rest of her body.

movement

Your baby's nervous system is more developed so she can co-ordinate her movements and is very active. She can grasp firmly, and can roll and turn.

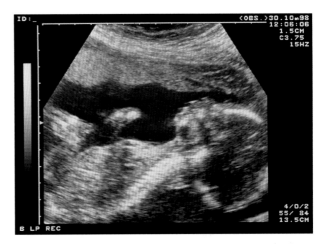

This ultrasound of a baby at 20 weeks clearly shows how her skeleton is developing; the line of hardening vertebrae in her spine (centre) and her skull (right) are visible. She has one arm raised and one of her legs (of which the bones are visible in this scan) is bent. At this stage she has plenty of room to move within the uterus.

vernix

This greasy white coating is produced by oil glands in your baby's skin. It keeps her skin supple and protects it from immersion in the amniotic fluid. It is very thick around the eyebrows and is anchored in place by the lanugo. It lubricates and protects the skin during delivery. In some hospitals, it is cleaned off but it rubs off naturally after a couple of days.

listening to your baby

Get your partner to place a cardboard tube from an empty kitchen roll low down on your abdomen. If he listens through it, he may be able to hear the baby's heartbeat. It will be a very subtle sound – like a very light pulsation. However, you should not worry if he cannot hear it – it takes practice to get the technique right.

how your baby
has grown

your baby (actual size)

Length Approximately 16 cm from crown to rump
Weight 340 g

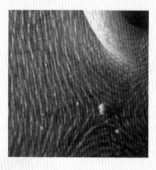

Your baby's skin is covered in fine hair called lanugo.

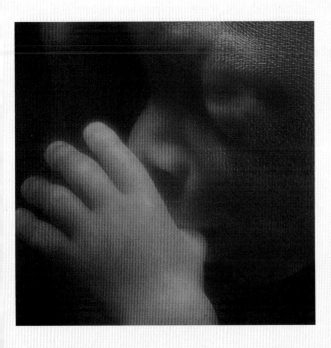

Scans have shown babies sucking their thumbs and grasping the umbilical cord.

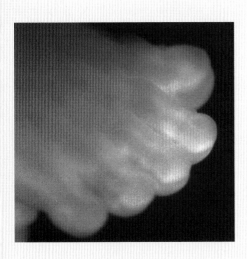

The feet and toes are not as fully developed as the hands and fingers.

20 weeks

your baby's development

skin and hair
Skin is red, thin and wrinkled. Hair is appearing on the head. Fine eyebrows and eyelashes are taking shape.

muscles
Muscles are becoming stronger and moving more frequently. The baby still has room for exercise.

bones
Bones are still soft but continue to harden each week.

organs
Organs are growing and developing.

circulatory system
This is now completely functional. A strong heartbeat can be heard through a stethoscope.

digestive system
Your baby is absorbing small amounts of water and sugar from the amniotic fluid and passing a tiny amount of meconium into the bowel.

nervous system
Nerve cells of the brain are developing and the brain can now send messages to parts of the body.

respiratory system
Lungs take many weeks to develop but air sacs are starting to form.

urinary system
Kidneys are working well and the baby is drinking amniotic fluid and passing 7–17 ml urine per day.

ears
Ears are in the final position and stand out. Your baby can hear sounds inside and outside the uterus.

eyes
Closed but respond to light and dark, and move from side to side.

your body at 21–24 weeks

This can be an exhilarating stage of pregnancy. You will have a rounded bump, which is growing week by week. Your baby's movements will also be reassuring: you may even feel him jumping in response to a loud noise. You will have also seen your baby's image when you had your ultrasound scan, so you have seen the incredible development of the tiny life inside you.

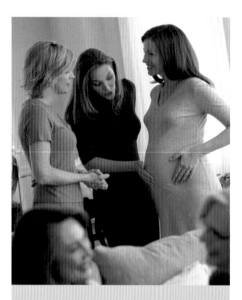

'I do not mind people asking me when the baby's due, but I cannot believe the way in which people I do not know comment on my size. I would not dream of passing comment on the size of their non-pregnant stomach – maybe I should!'

Jessica, 24 weeks pregnant

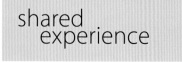

shared experience

how you may feel

As your pregnancy becomes obvious, you may sometimes feel that you have become public property. It is normal to be very sensitive to other people's comments, and remarks about the size of your bump do not help.

Many women get very excited about their pregnancy at this stage but, equally, they can be gripped by fear in the middle of the night about potential problems with the baby or the birth. Tell your midwife or doctor if you have any worries because they can help to reassure you and put things into perspective.

You may want to find out more about labour and you may have ideas of what sort of birth you would like. However, it is also normal for women to avoid these concerns and just concentrate on enjoying their pregnancy.

your changing body

Your body will now look very different and you may no longer be able to wear your normal clothes. This is when many women choose to move into their maternity clothes – these will probably emphasize your changing shape. Towards the end of the day, you may notice that your ankles are swollen (oedema). This is due to the accumulation of fluid caused by sluggish circulation. Sit with your feet up during the evening and put them on a pillow when you are in bed.

your health

Urinary tract infection Commonly known as cystitis, this causes a stinging, burning sensation when passing urine (see page 98). It is common in pregnancy as the blood vessels in the pelvic region become engorged.

Haemorrhoids (piles) can cause a great deal of discomfort during pregnancy. These varicose veins of the rectum are caused by sluggish circulation, constipation and the weight of the baby on the pelvic floor (see page 101).

Q **My baby is very active. I am worried that she could damage me. Is this possible?**

A A baby's kicks can certainly feel uncomfortable but she is unable to harm you because the uterus in which she is confined is made out of thick muscle. Also she is surrounded by amniotic fluid, which acts as a 'shock absorber', cushioning her movements. It is good for babies to be active.

what you should be eating
Continue to eat iron-rich foods because the volume of your blood has increased and is more dilute than previously. Also eat foods rich in vitamin D, for example, oily fish, eggs, milk, fortified margarine and breakfast cereals. This vitamin is essential for the development of your baby's bones and teeth. It also helps your body to absorb calcium and is made in the body as a result of exposure of the skin to sunlight.

jobs to do
Make time to rest, however you feel. Also set aside time each day to think about your baby because it is important to be prepared emotionally and practically, as well as physically.

Ask for a blood test to check your haemoglobin levels if you are feeling particularly tired.

Check your situation at work. Has your employer carried out a risk assessment? Do you spend too long standing or carrying heavy weights? Start to think about when you would like to give up work and how practical it will be to continue working until close to your due date.

your weight gain
Approximately 5 kg

fundal height
You should be able to feel the top of your uterus at around the same level as your navel.

Your baby's position
Your baby still has plenty of room and is changing position all the time. Your midwife or doctor will not pay much attention to your baby's position until 36 weeks of pregnancy.

your baby at
21 weeks

Your baby is now a smaller, thinner version of how he will look at full term. He may already have recognizable family features! The next few weeks are crucial as his lungs mature, which is essential for his survival outside of the uterus. Even though he won't take his first breath of air for another 19 weeks, he still 'practises' breathing movements.

development

The growth of your baby's brain is very rapid. It is at around this time that he is thought to develop memory, so play soothing pieces of music – they may also calm him after he is born. His tongue, complete with taste buds, is fully developed. He already has a high number of red blood cells and it is now that white blood cells are produced. These cells are essential for helping him to fight infection. If your baby is a girl, her uterus and vagina will have developed. If your baby is a boy, his testes will probably have started to descend towards the scrotum.

appearance

Lanugo now covers your baby's entire body, but the hair growing on his head is far more visible, with eyebrows and eyelashes becoming more defined. His skin is growing, and he will soon start to lay down some fat. Over the next few weeks he will become less thin but will still be red and wrinkled.

movement

Your baby is very active and you will probably be aware of his movements. Babies appear to use the umbilical cord as a toy, trying to grab it and even squeeze it.

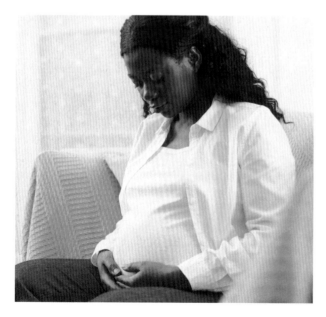

Becoming aware of your baby's somersaults and acrobatics is a longed-for and welcome time in most pregnancies.

Q I've been told that I'm definitely carrying a boy because of the shape of my bump. Is this true or not?

A Among all of the myths associated with pregnancy one of the most common is that the shape of your bump – to the front or all round, is dictated by the sex of the baby that you are expecting. The reality is that the shape of your bump depends on a number of factors related more to you than to your baby, including which way the baby is lying in your uterus, how much weight you have put on during your pregnancy, your height, if your muscles have been stretched during previous pregnancies and the shape of your pelvis.

your baby at
22 weeks

Your baby is now the length of a large banana and would be too big to hold in the palm of one hand. By feeling (palpating) your abdomen, your midwife can now work out her position. However, there is plenty of time for this to change, and it may do so frequently. Knowing which position she is in can help you to visualize how she looks inside your uterus.

development

Your baby's sense of touch is maturing, and she will frequently stroke her face and suck her thumb. She is learning that she can move her limbs and make them touch each other. She can 'play' at crossing and uncrossing her legs, reaching out and bending her head to touch her hand. She is developing an awareness of herself and how the parts of her body are related and will use her hands to grasp other parts of her body.

Twins have been seen on ultrasound scans reaching out, touching and responding to each other.

appearance

Your baby's skin looks too loose for her, like that of a newborn puppy, because there is only very little fat underneath it. Her fingernails and toenails are growing and the lines and creases on the palms of her hands are becoming obvious.

movement

By now you will be aware of your baby's movements, especially when she 'startles' in response to a loud noise. Even at this stage she will jump or kick if she hears the crash of a dustbin lid or loud music!

Do not worry if she has a quiet day and does not seem to move very much. She is still only small and she may be awake while you are asleep. Your baby will be awake and asleep as much now as when she is born at full term.

However, by 28 weeks of pregnancy you should feel her moving at least ten times a day. If you have any worries about your baby's movement, get in touch with your midwife.

did you know?
Of the average weight gain in pregnancy, 38 per cent is the weight of the baby. The rest is made up of the placenta, fluid and blood, and the increased weight of the breasts and uterus.

Q **I am 22 weeks pregnant and am worried about getting chickenpox as a couple of my friends' children have it at the moment. Is there anything I can do to avoid it? Can it damage my unborn baby?**

A Most adults are immune to chickenpox, but if you cannot remember whether or not you had it as a child you can have your blood tested for antibodies. Developing chickenpox during pregnancy is rare, but it could affect a baby's development if the virus was contracted before 20 weeks or after 36 weeks of pregnancy. If you develop chickenpox, your baby could contract the virus (varicella infection of the newborn). If you think that you have contracted chickenpox during your pregnancy, you can be given an injection of immunoglobulin containing chickenpox antibodies, which will lessen the effect on your baby.

your baby at
23 weeks

If your partner lays his head on your abdomen, he may be aware of your baby's heartbeat as well as feeling some small ripples of movement. This will be a very special moment for him as it could be his first real opportunity to bond. Also, if the baby has older siblings, it is a good idea to let them enjoy this moment too, as it can help them feel that the new baby is already part of their family.

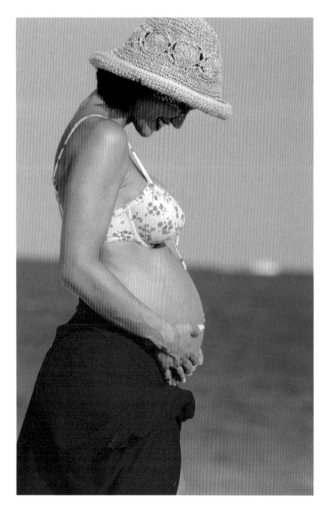

Your baby's eyes are formed by week 12 but his eyelids stay shut until about week 28. It is now that he will see sunlight as a reddish haze if you expose your ever-expanding bulge to bright sunlight.

development

Your baby's bones, muscles and organs are steadily growing and his lungs continue to develop. There is also a lot of activity in his brain. Babies at this stage appear to prefer the taste of sweet to bitter!

appearance

Your baby's skin still looks 'too big' for him – so he looks as if he is wearing an over-sized baby-grow suit – but it will fill out once the fat develops beneath it. The lanugo covering him darkens and the amount of sticky vernix increases, some of which may still be there when he is born. His eyes are still closed, but their colour is starting to develop.

movement

You may notice that your baby is developing a pattern of waking and sleeping. Many babies are active at night, when their mothers are still, but are rocked to sleep during the day when their mothers are moving around. This is probably why it is soothing for them to be held and walked around when they are newborn.

did you know?

Researchers in California have found that, the happier the mother during pregnancy, the healthier the baby will be when it is born. Apparently, the babies of women who have plenty of support from friends and family during their pregnancy grow better in the uterus.

your baby at
24 weeks

Depending upon the country in which you live, it is usually around 24 weeks of pregnancy that your baby is considered 'viable', which means she is capable of a separate existence. If she were born prematurely at 24 weeks, she might be able to survive in a special-care baby unit with the help of medical expertise and a ventilator to assist with breathing.

development

Her lungs continue to develop daily, forming more air sacs. She is getting plenty of practice at breathing, by taking small amounts of fluid in and out of the lungs, her chest moving up and down. The centres of her bones are getting harder, and she has a normal amount of muscle. Her brainwaves show that she is almost as active as a newborn baby – increases in her pulse rate show that she reacts to sounds, such as loud noises.

appearance

Your baby's face looks much as it will do when she is born, only not as well rounded. Her eyes are still closed, with distinctive eyebrows and eyelashes. More hair is growing on her head, and at this stage, you can even tell what colour it is. The vernix being produced sticks to her eyebrows and other hair on her body.

movement

You may feel a tiny rhythmic movement in your lower abdomen that means your baby has hiccoughs! She is also responding much more to touch and sound.

Q **I am 24 weeks pregnant and have just started antenatal classes. I am convinced that my bump is much smaller than everyone else's in the group and now I am worried that my baby is not growing properly.**

A   Tell your midwife about your worries. She can reassure you and explain what she is doing at your antenatal check. One of these checks includes feeling the top of the uterus to make sure that it is growing at the right rate and noting the size of your bump. If there is any cause for concern, your midwife will closely monitor you and refer you to the hospital for growth scans. Obviously some babies are bigger or smaller than average and the size of women's bumps always vary. Comparing fully clothed bumps is not an accurate way of judging the size of a baby because size varies depending on how many babies a woman has had before, the amount of fluid around the baby, the height of the woman and her baby's position.

Q **Why does my baby get fits of hiccoughs in the uterus?**

A   These are probably a result of your baby moving her chest in practice 'breathing'. These movements are thought to help babies to expand their lungs in preparation for their first real breath after they are born. Hiccoughs will be felt as a series of rhythmical movements and can last for up to 30 minutes. Don't worry about them, there are certainly not doing her any harm – many women find the sensation amusing.

how your baby has grown

your baby (actual size)

Length Approximately 21 cm from crown to rump
Weight 530 g

24 weeks

your baby's development

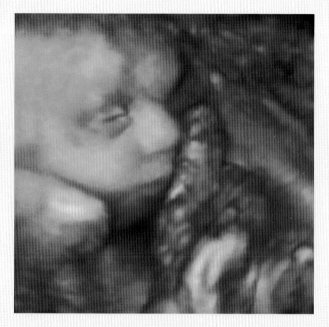

By this age, your baby may have recognizable family features.

skin and hair
Skin is thin and wrinkled. Body is covered in fine hair known as lanugo and a greasy substance called vernix. More hair is developing on the head and eyelashes and eyebrows protect the eyes.

muscles
There is a normal amount of muscle, built up from the vigorous movements.

bones
The backbone has 150 joints. The centres of the bones are getting harder.

organs
All internal organs are formed and are growing and maturing.

circulatory system
White blood cells are being produced to help combat infection. The heart is beating approximately 160 times per minute.

nervous system
There is a lot of brain activity.

respiratory system
Air sacs are still developing in the lungs. Your baby takes small amounts of amniotic fluid in and out of her lungs. His chest rises and falls, practising her breathing movements.

ears
Ears are formed and in their final position. Your baby is hearing sounds, including music and voices.

eyes
Eyes are closed but are developing colour. Your baby reacts to light and starts to develop a waking/sleeping pattern.

your body at
25–28 weeks

You will probably be relieved to have made it to the last 3 months, taking comfort from the fact that, if your baby were to be born at 28 weeks, he would have about an 85 per cent chance of surviving. However, the realization that the birth is not very far away can bring a whole new set of anxieties: suddenly there is a great deal to do and very little time!

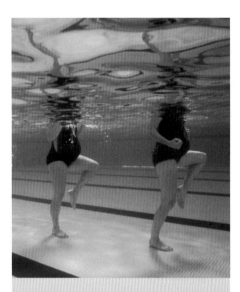

'I love aqua-natal classes, as we all go out afterwards and talk about our pregnancies. It is great being able to indulge in pregnancy and baby talk, with people who have the same hopes and fears as I do.'

Maggie, 27 weeks pregnant

shared experience

how you may feel

You may find yourself worrying about your health or your baby's health and the impending labour. You may also be experiencing stress associated with work, particularly if you have a demanding job. If your baby is active, or pressing on your bladder, you may find yourself waking at night to visit the toilet.

All this can leave you feeling very tired, and you may be short-tempered with family and colleagues – or tearful as you try to cope with everything. If you have other children you may feel guilty about being too tired to take them to their usual activities. It is a good idea to get toddlers used to having a 'quiet time' in the afternoon when you can both rest – and to continue this once the baby arrives.

your changing body

Women vary in the amount of weight that they put on and the size of their bumps. You will probably find yourself comparing your shape to other pregnant women and worry about being too big or too small. You will notice that your centre of gravity is changing and may sometimes lose your balance or become clumsy.

By this stage your baby is curled up inside you and, although he no longer has much room to move freely, he will still kick (often hard), roll and wriggle. If he is in a head-down position, you may notice more jabbing at the top of your bump or kicking in the ribs.

Your breasts are getting ready for your baby's first feed and may start leaking a few drops of colostrum (the first milk, rich in antibodies) as your body prepares for breast-feeding.

your health

Stress incontinence The pressure of your uterus and baby may make you leak a little urine when you cough, sneeze or laugh (see page 98).
Sciatica The weight of your uterus may press on the sciatic nerve, producing a sharp pain in the lower back, buttock or hip and radiating down one leg (see page 97).

Q **I am only 28 weeks pregnant but already I am worrying in case there will be students at the birth. Is there any way I can make sure that this does not happen?**

A Women often imagine that there will be a crowd of medical students in white coats gathered in the delivery room but this does not happen any more. At most there might be a student midwife, student nurse or medical student who needs to spend a certain number of hours on a labour ward as part of his or her training. He or she would be supervised by a midwife or doctor, who is responsible for them. The midwife looking after you should ask your permission before a student joins in with your care, so you can say how you feel early in labour or put it into your birth plan (see page 119).

what you should be eating

Drink plenty of water and eat fibre-rich foods, such as wholegrain cereals, fruit and vegetables, to avoid getting constipated.

Eat foods containing essential fatty acids, which are found in seeds (including sunflower and linseed, and oily fish (such as sardines). Your baby's brain is growing rapidly and these are important 'brain foods'.

jobs to do

Make a note of your next antenatal appointment, as your short-term memory can be poor during pregnancy and your antenatal checks will be more frequent.

Have a blood test to check for anaemia, which is common at this stage of pregnancy.

You may be offered an injection of Anti-D at 28 weeks (see page 82) if your blood group is Rhesus negative.

your weight gain

Approximately 8 kg

fundal height

The top of your bump should have reached a point about 4 finger-widths above your navel and 3 or 4 finger-widths below the top of your ribcage – hence the discomfort.

your baby's position

Your baby may be head down. If not, there is still plenty of time for him to turn, even though he now has less room to somersault.

your baby at
25 weeks

From 6 months, try singing the same songs or nursery rhymes to your baby on a regular basis. Singing combines a right (music) with a left (words) brain activity and will encourage the connections between the two halves of your baby's brain to grow. A fetus generally seems to react to his mother's voice best, and then to deep male voices.

development

Your baby now weighs about 680–850 g. The lungs, which were originally spongy-solid, are now filling with air sacs, each wrapped in a network of blood vessels. There is no air inside them at the moment, just fluid from the amniotic sac. This passes in and out as your baby practises breathing, his chest rising and falling as he does so.

appearance

Your baby is looking more like a proper baby, although his head is still relatively large in comparison to the rest of his body – even a newborn baby's head takes up one quarter of his length and is wider than his shoulders. His arms and legs are still quite thin, as the fat stores at this stage of his development make up just 1 per cent of his total body weight.

movement

Floating in the amniotic fluid, your baby is able to move vigorously and to stretch his arms and legs in a more deliberate way. He is reaching out and touching whatever he encounters around him, like the umbilical cord, grabbing his feet, and even sucking his thumb or fingers.

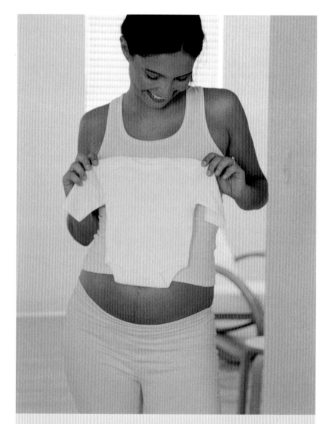

did you know?
Nerve cells (or, properly, neurons) are produced in the fetus at a (mind-boggling) average rate of 250,000 per minute!

preparing yourself

Mentally preparing yourself is part of adjusting to life with a baby, particularly if you have a busy life. Try to make time every day when you can think about your baby. Imagine how he looks now, and what position he is in and what he will be like when he arrives. Talk to him as you stroke your bump.

your baby at
26 weeks

It is encouraging to think that your baby would have a good chance of survival if she was born now, although she would still need a great deal of highly skilled medical attention to help her survive. From 7 months, play classical music to your baby. This will help to speed the development of right-brain spatial skills and increase the likelihood that your child will excel in sports!

development

Your baby's nervous system is maturing, including the cells in the cortex of her brain that are used for conscious thought. Her brain is increasing in size, and the nerve circuits are linked up with the brain cells. The nerve fibres are now encased in myelin, a fatty substance that enables messages to travel faster along the nerves, thus boosting her ability to learn, remember and move. Meanwhile the smooth surface of her brain develops the ridges and valleys that vastly increase its surface area. At this point, she can feel pain. This week, she will partly open her eyes, which are almost fully formed. A few babies are born with brown eyes, but most babies' eyes are blue and remain blue until the colouring develops, often several weeks after they are born.

appearance

Your baby's skin is not as red as it was in earlier weeks, and it is no longer translucent. A thin layer of fat has already started to accumulate under her skin, which makes her look paler, less wrinkled and generally less fragile overall.

movement

You will be very aware of your baby's movements as she still has room to turn around and will prod against the wall of your uterus with her sharp fists and knees. You may start to recognize the parts of her body as she kicks and prods you, making odd shapes on your abdomen. Some mothers-to-be say that they can even feel the 'scratching' of their baby's minute fingers against the wall of the uterus.

Q **I'm 26 weeks pregnant and I'm having real problems sleeping and feel so exhausted the whole time. Can I ask my doctor for some sleeping pills or would they harm my baby?**

A Like all medicines, sleeping tablets are best avoided during pregnancy. It is better to try to get to sleep naturally if you can. The best means of doing this is to make sure that you are relaxed and comfortable. Try to get some light exercise during the day. Avoid eating heavy meals late in the evening or you will not have time to digest them, but if you are peckish, have a light snack or a glass of warm milk.

Make sure that the bedroom is at a comfortable temperature: being too hot or too cold will make sleeping difficult.

Although it sounds easy, try not to worry about being unable to sleep, this will just make it more difficult. Distract yourself by getting up to watch the television for a while, or read a book or magazine. When you feel sleepy, try again.

If no commonsense ideas seem to work, talk to your doctor who may prescribe something for you.

your baby at
27 weeks

Your baby now weighs approximately 1 kg, about the same as half a honeydew melon! He may be lying in a bottom-down position at this stage or even across the womb (transverse), but he is quite likely to turn into the more usual head-down position any time from now, in preparation for birth. This may not happen until quite close to full term, however, and you may still feel quite sharp movements.

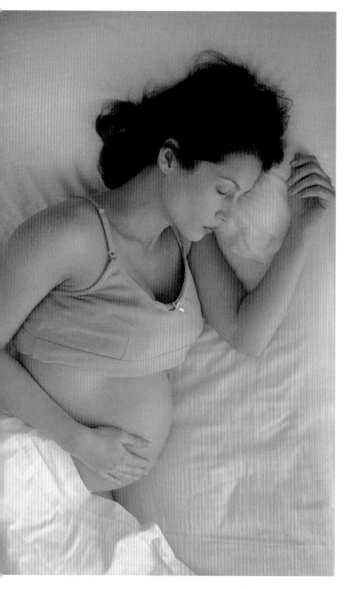

development

Your baby's bones, muscles and organs continue to grow, and he is becoming stronger with every passing week. If he was born now, and given the right specialist care, he would have about an 85 per cent chance of survival. However, he would still be unable to keep his lungs inflated and would have a problem keeping himself warm because there is not enough fat on his body yet. He would also be more susceptible to infection because his immune system is immature. Although he could probably survive in an incubator, the best incubator by far over the next few weeks, providing him with everything he needs to thrive, is your uterus.

appearance

Your baby's eyelids are open and he will start to blink. He looks much the same as he will at full term, only smaller and thinner.

movement

It would be convenient if your baby's sleep–wake phases coincided with yours, but they rarely do. Perhaps this is nature's way of preparing you for disturbed sleep after the birth!

A more likely theory is that your baby is rocked to sleep by your daytime activities, which takes up about four-fifths of his time, then wakes up and starts his own stretch-and-exercise routine just as you settle down for the evening.

By now, you will probably have got to know your baby's pattern of wakefulness and sleep – usually opposite to yours!

your baby at
28 weeks

You may feel more in touch with your baby now, recognizing her wakeful times and the sort of sounds that she likes. You may feel that she is responding to your moods. Indeed there is evidence to show that the mother's hormones (for example the stress hormone, cortisol) do actually cross the placenta so your baby may be relaxed or agitated according to how you feel.

development

Most of the smaller airways and tiny air sacs (alveoli) in your baby's lungs have developed. The amount of fat on her body is increasing, making it easier for your midwife or doctor to identify the position that she is in when they feel your abdomen. However, she still needs to develop substantially more subcutaneous fat in order to be able to regulate her own temperature when she is outside of the uterus.

In baby boys, the testicles may have descended into the scrotum by now, although, in some cases, this will not happen until after they are born.

appearance

Your baby's head is more in proportion with the rest of her body. Her hair, although still fine, is growing longer. The lanugo gradually starts to disappear, remaining only in a few patches around her neck and shoulders. Her skin is damp and shiny, well covered now with white vernix, and is generally looks less wrinkled, becoming plumper every day.

movement

Your baby may move around, making your bump heave and bulge, to show you that she is uncomfortable with the way you are sitting and lying. At other times a loud noise might startle her.

She may respond to chemicals and hormones from your body, which enter her bloodstream via the placenta and umbilical cord.

Many women enjoy tracing the development of their growing bump for themselves by measuring it every couple of weeks.

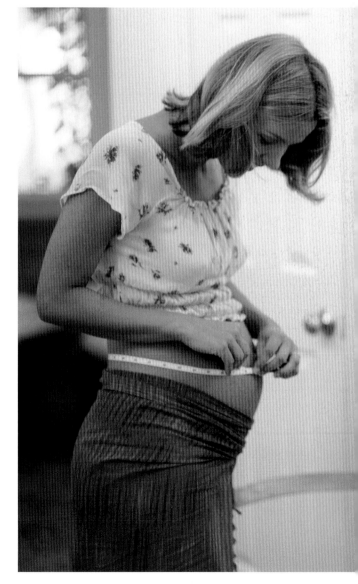

how your baby has grown

your baby (actual size)

Length Approximately 25 cm from crown to rump
Weight 1.1 kg

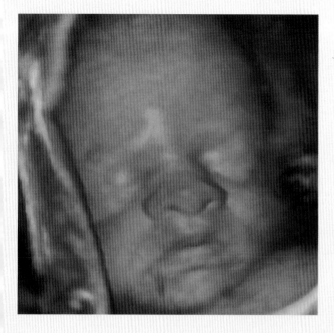

By now, your baby is developing her own sleep–wake pattern.

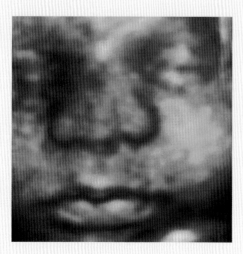

Your baby is now laying down layers of fat under the skin, so appears less wrinkly.

28 weeks

your baby's development

skin and hair
Skin appears paler, as fat is laid down, and is no longer translucent. Hair continues to grow on the head and eyelashes and eyebrows are clearly defined. Lanugo starts to disappear.

muscles
Muscles are now well developed, strong from the vigorous movement. Your baby can make a fist and punch against the uterine wall.

circulatory system
Heart is beating approximately 150–160 times per minute – about twice as fast as an adult.

digestive system
Meconium (the baby's first bowel movement) is collecting in the colon. Drinks and excretes amniotic fluid.

nervous system
Brain cells are multiplying rapidly and folds and grooves are appearing on the brain's surface. More links are being made between the brain and the rest of the nervous system. Your baby can respond to pain, touch, sound, taste and light, and also has a memory.

respiratory system
The tiny air sacs (alveoli) and air ways are developing.

ears
Your baby can recognize your voice and may respond to loud noises and music.

eyes
Eyes have now opened. Your baby can look around and follow the light of a torch shone across your abdomen.

187

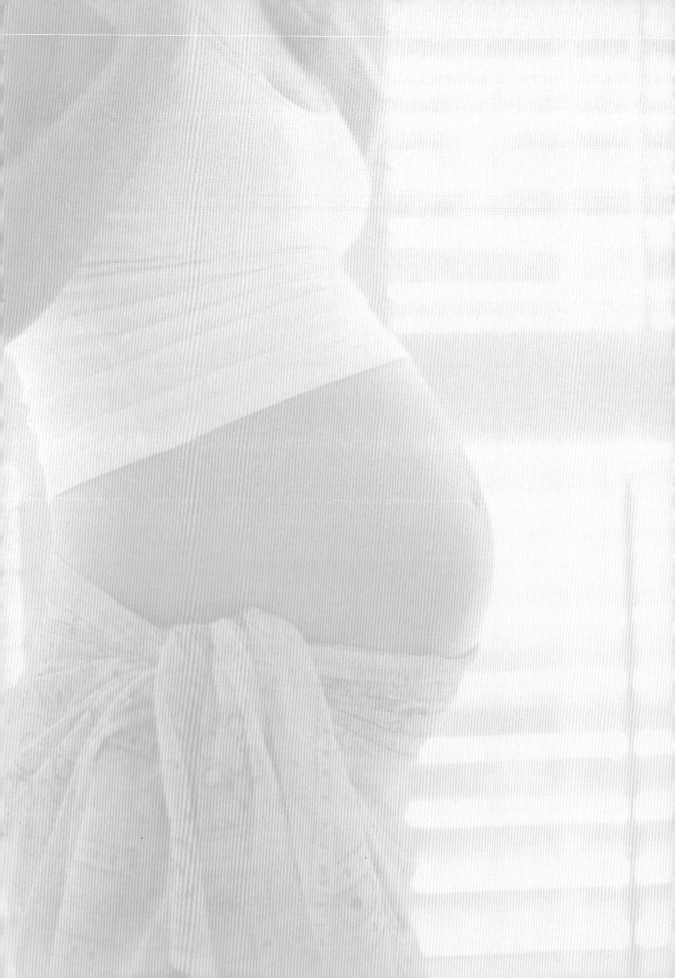

late
pregnancy

This can be an exciting, but also, apprehensive time. Your baby is coming soon – just a matter of weeks now – but you might not feel quite ready. This is completely normal. You will also probably be starting to feel a bit weary now as your baby's weight has rocketed up and she is piling on the fat, ready for her arrival into the outside world. So, take it easy and enjoy the final weeks of growing your baby.

your body at
29–32 weeks

The period of 'blooming' may now seem a long way in the past. By now, you are starting to feel the weight of your baby and to experience discomfort as your stomach gets squashed by your expanding uterus. Other organs are pushed aside as well, and you may start to feel breathless as you move about. You may not always feel it, but pregnancy is beautiful and others will think you look incredibly special.

'I love going for my antenatal checks. When I hear my baby's heartbeat, I could happily stay in the room and carry on listening, until I go into labour!'

Kristina, 31 weeks pregnant

shared experience

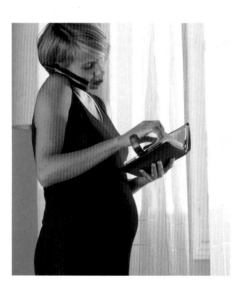

Get organized. If you've not sorted out any antenatal classes, now is the time to do so.

how you may feel

This period can be one of mixed emotions as the birth becomes more imminent. At times you may be excited and impatient to meet your baby, while at others you may be fearful of the prospect of labour and becoming a mother. Originally, you may have intended to work until late into your pregnancy, but you now find that being heavily pregnant is making you tired and breathless.

Many women have difficulty sleeping around now, because of waking frequently to pass water, the baby's activity, not being able to get comfortable in bed and their mind becoming active in the middle of the night. Try to take a nap during the day, even if for only 15 minutes; otherwise you will feel increasingly tired over the final weeks.

your changing body

Your expanding uterus is squashing against your internal organs and pushing your stomach higher, making you prone to heartburn because the valve between your stomach and oesophagus allows acid to leak into the latter. You may find that eating little and often suits you better than having fewer larger meals.

Your centre of gravity changes and you may find yourself developing the familiar pregnancy 'waddle'. Be aware of your posture, however, because it is easy to slouch when your shape changes and this can cause back problems.

You may start to retain fluid (oedema), so that your fingers and feet become swollen – particularly at the end of the day. It is a good idea to remove any rings while you still can.

your health

Breathlessness The pressure of your baby on your diaphragm, and your expanding uterus, changes your breathing pattern and you may become short of breath (see page 93).
Vulval varicose veins You may develop varicose veins in your vulva, particularly as your baby becomes heavier (see page 103).

Q What happens in an antenatal class?

A Despite the word 'class', this is not held in a classroom environment and there is no test at the end. It usually takes the form of a small informal group, led by a midwife or childbirth educator, in which all aspects of pregnancy, childbirth and parenting are discussed. The subjects are often dictated by what the members want to know most about, which is usually pain relief, signs of labour, birth plans, how to cope with labour, and feeding the baby. Classes provide a great opportunity for pregnant women to meet each other and talk about any worries. Many classes encourage you to bring a birth partner along but others are specifically for women.

week 29–32
reminders

what you should be eating and drinking
Drink cranberry juice, to reduce the risk of getting a urinary tract infection.

Eat brown rice, strawberries, eggs, spinach, onions and green beans, which are all good sources of manganese – essential for the healthy development of your baby's bones and joints.

jobs to do
You should have started to attend antenatal classes by now.

If you are not familiar with the maternity unit, arrange a visit and ask a member of staff to show you around. Find out about car-parking arrangements and which entrance is open in the middle of the night. It is better know these things in advance.

Buy a 'sleep bra' to wear at night if your breasts are feeling heavy. At 32 weeks, start to massage the perineum (the area between the vagina and the anus) with sweet almond or wheat germ oil. This may help the area to stretch and become more supple, reducing the risk of tearing.

your weight gain
Approximately 8 kg

fundal height
If you place your hand on your abdomen, with your little finger just above your navel, the top of your uterus will be close to your thumb.

your baby's position
Your baby is still active but is now not as quick to turn. By now she will be drawing up her knees into the fetal position because she no longer has much room. She may be head down, ready for birth. If not, there is still time for her to turn.

191

your baby at
29 weeks

You may start to feel impatient, imagining what your baby looks like, and wish that labour would come early. However these next few weeks in the womb are absolutely crucial to your baby's development, as he lays down fat stores that will keep him warm in the outside world and his lungs mature preparing him for independent breathing.

development

Your baby's eyes can now focus and he can also blink. He may be able to see shadows and silhouettes of shapes of the outside world. Beneath his skin, a layer of fat is building up that he will use for warmth and energy when he is born. His lungs are continuing to develop and he is growing at a rate of approximately 1 cm each week.

appearance

Your baby's head is now in proportion to his arms and legs. The fatty deposits under his skin give him a less wrinkled appearance. He has not yet acquired the plump appearance of a full-term newborn baby but he is looking far less 'prune-like' than before. Because his skin is thicker, you can no longer see the network of tiny blood vessels beneath it.

movement

There is still plenty of space for your baby to move, and you should be feeling at least ten movements a day. He may not be somersaulting as often as before, but he can still turn in your uterus and will be very active, often when you want to sleep.

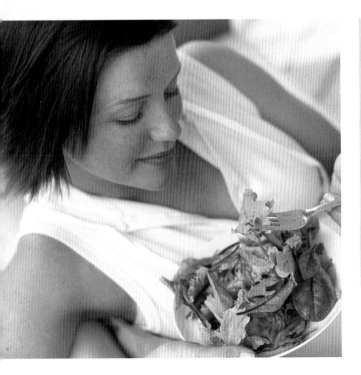

small babies

'Small for dates' babies (also known as fetal growth retardation, small for gestational age or intrauterine growth restriction) are often detected at around this time.

If your baby is suspected to be smaller than expected for his gestation then you may be offered some ultrasound scans to monitor his growth. You will also need more frequent antenatal checks. You may also be offered a scan that looks at the blood flow through the placenta to the baby, to check that it is working efficiently.

'Eating little and often' is coming into its own now as our baby squashes your stomach, making you feel full much sooner. Eating smaller amounts can also help with heartburn.

your baby at
30 weeks

Although you are probably counting the days to the birth now, you may also become anxious as the date becomes closer and more of a reality. Many women worry that they may go into premature labour, especially if they have particularly strong Braxton Hicks tightenings (see page 95). These can be uncomfortable but should never be painful.

development

If your baby was born at this stage, she would have an excellent chance of survival, although her immune system and lungs are still immature and will continue to develop. Your placenta has been transmitting your antibodies to your baby, providing her with some immunity against infections and diseases. By breast-feeding, you will continue to provide her with antibodies after she is born.

appearance

Your baby will probably be lying head down, with her knees curled up into her chest. She is becoming plumper now, so her skin is looking smooth, but she is still covered in greasy, white vernix.

movement

Your baby will still be able to stretch out and kick you or punch against the wall of your uterus. You may be able to recognize which way she is lying and the different parts of her body as she moves. You may even feel a 'scratching' sensation as she moves her fingers against the wall of your uterus. Do not worry about any possible injury to either you or the baby. She is surrounded by fluid, which protects you both and lessens the impact of any strong movements.

Introduce your bump to your other children – she will already have been listening to their voices and so will recognize them when she arrives in the outside world. Interest your older child in your bump and explain that there is a new younger brother or sister on the way, so that he or she can be looking forward to the event, too.

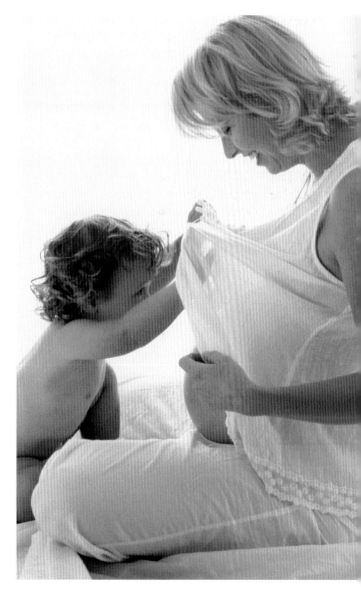

your baby at
31 weeks

Your baby is now at least as long as a stick of celery! He is very aware of the noises and movements inside your uterus as well as influences from the outside. He will be aware of you exercising, talking, singing and playing music, and of changes in light. He will even be able to feel you massaging your abdomen, so talk to him as you do it so that he can also hear your voice.

development

The main developments at this stage are in your baby's lungs. The cells lining the air sacs of the lungs secrete a substance that is known as surfactant. This is a lubricant that prevents the tissues of the lungs sticking together. This is a major milestone in your baby's development, because without surfactant, he will be unable to breathe outside the uterus.

appearance

Now the layers of subcutaneous fat are getting thicker and the blood vessels no longer show through, your baby's skin looks much healthier and is not as dark or reddish as it was earlier in his development. The skin on his face, in particular, is smoother and his face looks round and chubby. His body fat now accounts for 3.5 per cent of his bodyweight but, by birth, this will rise to 15 per cent.

movement

Your baby is becoming more aware of stimuli so will be very active, responding to sounds and movements. He can even feel when you have a Braxton Hicks contraction – which is no cause for alarm as they do not hurt him although you may find them uncomfortable. Since his 'living conditions' are now rather cramped, due to his size, for most of the time he will have his chin on his chest, his arms across his chest and his knees curled up. Even though he has less space than earlier, you should still be feeling at least 10 movements a day.

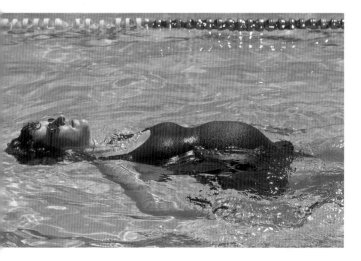

Give your baby some space while doing some swimming. He will welcome any chance to move about.

Q **I am 31 weeks pregnant and worried about having a premature baby. If I go into early labour can anything be done to stop it?**

A This will depend on whether or not your cervix has started to dilate. A drug can be administered via a drip to relax the uterus and stop the contractions but, if your cervix is opening, then labour will probably continue. Women who show signs of premature labour are often advised to have two steroid injections that will help with the development of the baby's lungs.

your baby at
32 weeks

As your baby grows, she no longer 'floats' in the amniotic fluid but rests in the uterus, most often in the head-down position. If your midwife confirms that your baby has not yet turned head down, you can encourage her to do so by adopting an all-fours position (see page 231). Do not worry, though. There is still plenty of time for her to get into her final position.

development

Your baby's hearing is becoming more finely attuned. Her environment is constantly filled with noise – the sounds of your stomach, your heartbeat and the blood rushing through the umbilical cord. It is not surprising that newborn babies do not need quiet to sleep when they have become used to such constant sounds. The lining in the air sacs of your baby's lungs continue to secrete surfactant. Unless her breathing system is mature, she will not be able to breathe unaided when she is born.

appearance

Your baby looks like a smaller version of a full-term baby but is still very delicate. A few creases are developing where she is laying down fat, at the top of her thighs and on her arms. The hair on her head continues to grow and there may still be a light covering of soft lanugo across the back of her shoulders and along the tops of her arms.

movement

Your baby may still be looking for a position in which to settle when it comes to the birth. By now most babies are head down, but there are many who will still turn around. She no longer has as much room to somersault but mothers often notice when their baby changes position and can tell the difference between a hard head and a bony bottom, or a rounded fist and a pointed elbow!

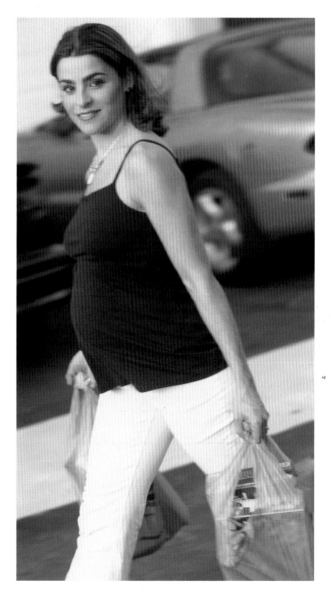

When you are shopping, don't carry anything too heavy and make sure your load is evenly balanced.

how your baby has grown

your baby (actual size)

Length Approximately 29 cm from crown to rump
Weight 1.6 kg

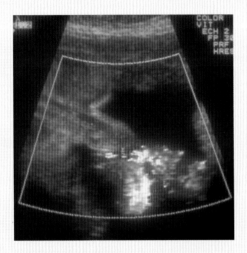

This Doppler scan shows the genital area of a baby boy, with scrotal sac (left) and penis (centre). The blue, red and white areas indicate that he is urinating into the amniotic fluid.

your baby's development

skin and hair
Skin is smooth and no longer transparent. Head hair has a distinct colour. Most lanugo has been shed but some may still be present across the back and shoulders.

bones
Bones continue to harden, except those of the skull.

muscles
Muscles are strong. Frequent movements mean that baby is exercising her limbs, strengthening them further.

circulatory system
Heart is beating approximately 150 times per minute.

digestive system
Water, nutrients and waste are being exchanged through the placenta. Your baby is swallowing and urinating amniotic fluid.

nervous system
Connections are still being made in the brain and nervous system.

respiratory system
Lungs continue to develop. Cells now lining the air sacs are secreting surfactant.

ears
Hearing is your baby's main link with the outside world.

eyes
Your baby may have developed a more obvious pattern of sleeping and waking. When awake the eyes will be open, turning towards the light and able to blink.

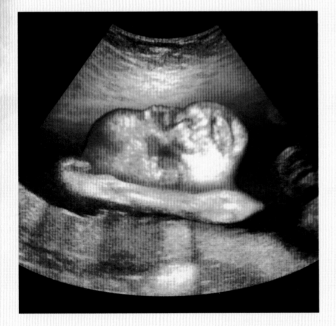

At 36 weeks, your baby is beginning to run out of space to manoeuvre.

your body at
33–36 weeks

As your due date approaches, you are probably becoming quite excited. Inevitably, there will still be days where you feel anxious about the birth or becoming a mother, but this is a very normal part of pregnancy. Your pregnancy is probably starting to take its toll physically. You are probably not feeling as energetic as in previous weeks and, if you have not done so already, will be preparing to stop work.

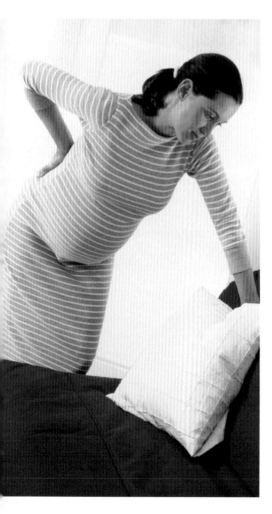

Your extra-heavy bump may put additional strain on your lower back so avoid bending over to pick things up and sit down and rest if you experience any discomfort.

how you may feel

Part of the mental process of becoming a mother is the time spent beforehand, when you can prepare for your baby in practical terms. However, if you work, or are busy with your other children, you may not have had time to get excited and really think about the arrival of your new baby. You may be curious about other babies, wanting to be with them, and comparing their size with that of baby you are carrying. You may be feeling tired, particularly if you are waking frequently during the night to pass urine, so try to rest during the day.

your changing body

If you are fortunate, you should have had a few weeks of 'blooming' and feeling energetic before these final weeks. For many women, there is a return to the discomforts of early pregnancy. As your baby is resting, probably head down, in your uterus, rather than 'floating' inside you, you will feel pressure on your bladder – which means frequent trips to the toilet. Your stomach is getting squashed, higher up, as your uterus grows, which means a return to the indigestion and heartburn that you may have experienced in the early weeks.

You may feel discomfort under your ribcage as your baby pushes against it with a foot or his bottom. Many women start to experience backache towards the end of pregnancy and it is important to be aware of your posture, standing straight, with your bottom tucked in. When you bend to pick up objects bend your knees, squat down with a straight back and then stand keeping the object close to your body. Your breasts will grow a little more and, if they have not done so already, may start to leak colostrum in preparation for breast-feeding.

your health

Raised blood pressure (hypertension) is experienced by 10 per cent of pregnant women, particularly towards full term (see page 100).
Backache As you get bigger and heavier you are more likely to get backache, especially if you are prone to back pain (see page 94).

Q **I want to breast-feed but I am 35 weeks pregnant and I have not leaked any milk. Does this mean that I will have a problem with the feeding?**

A Some women do not leak anything until after the birth, while other women leak colostrum from early on in their pregnancy. Neither has any effect on their ability to breast-feed. There will be many changes to your breasts during pregnancy: they will become more sensitive, they will get bigger, and the area around the nipple (areola) will darken. After your baby is born put her to the breast frequently to encourage the milk to come in, which will happen on about the third day after the birth. Until then she feeds on a thick creamy substance called colostrom that helps to protect your baby from infections.

what you should be eating

Eat a varied diet rich in fresh fruit and vegetables. This will not only give you energy but also help to build up your baby's immune system.

Vitamin K is essential for blood clotting and is particularly important as the birth approaches. Good sources include green leafy vegetables, cantaloupe melon, fortified cereals and wholemeal bread.

jobs to do

Get measured for a nursing bra, ideally at 36 weeks.

Your blood should be retested for antibodies and anaemia, as you get closer to the birth.

Seriously consider giving up work if you have not done so already. Remember, 37 weeks counts as a normal time for birth.

From 34 weeks, start drinking one cup of raspberry leaf tea twice a day in order to tone your uterus and prepare it for labour.

Continue to take regular gentle exercise to give you stamina to cope during labour. Women who exercise regularly are also known to recover physically more quickly from the birth.

your weight gain

Approximately 10 kg

fundal height

If you lie down, the top of your uterus will be approximately a finger-width below the bottom of your ribs.

your baby's position

Most babies have now settled into a head-down (cephalic) position ready for the birth. If your baby is still in a different position at 36 weeks, your midwife can arrange for you to see the obstetrician, who will discuss the options.

199

your baby at
33 weeks

By this stage of pregnancy you are probably communicating with your baby on a regular basis, even if you are not always aware of it. Many women inadvertently stroke their abdomen or talk to their baby, and your baby is increasingly aware of the sounds, movements and emotions that you communicate to him. Get your partner to massage your bump with gentle, sweeping, rhythmic movements.

did you know?
Your body responds to your different emotions by producing hormones, which are transmitted to your baby through the placenta. This is referred to as sympathetic communication. In this way, your baby becomes aware of whether you are frightened and upset, or happy and relaxed.

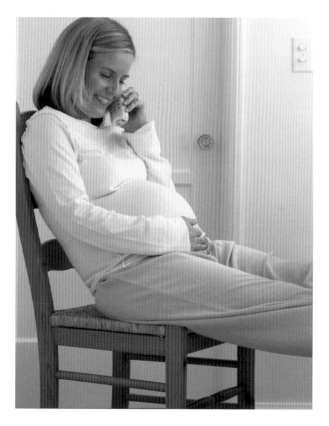

development
The main focus now is on growth. Your baby needs to become bigger, fatter and stronger in order to maintain his body temperature, feed well and fight off any infections that come his way.

His immune system is still developing and, although his major organs are complete, the extra weeks are crucial for the final stages of the development of his lungs, which are maturing fast.

appearance
Your baby looks very much the same as he will at full term, but smaller and generally more 'delicate'.

His skin appears paler because of the build-up of white fat beneath it. This fat will have a big impact on his appearance, making his skin smoother and plumper, with dimples at the elbows and knees and creases in the wrists and neck.

movement
Your baby is still quite active. You and your partner may be able to recognize the shape of a small foot or elbow pressing against your abdomen, or a little bottom pushing beneath your ribs. If this is especially uncomfortable, try changing position, which may in turn encourage your baby to shift. Getting down on all fours or going for a swim can often do the trick.

When your lively baby is on the move, you will be able to feel him pushing against your uterus. He may also respond if you press gently against your bump.

your baby at
34 weeks

As your due date comes closer there may be days when you feel positive anticipation and others when you feel very apprehensive. The best way of dealing with these fears is to gather as much information as you can about pregnancy and birth. If you haven't done so already, talk to your midwife about your concerns. It is important that you feel in control of your pregnancy as well as your baby's birth.

development

Your baby continues to lay down fat – by now fat makes up 15 per cent of her weight – which she will need to keep warm. Her lungs are almost mature and she might even be able to breathe for herself if she was born now. Although her brain and nervous system are fully developed, her sucking reflex would still be poor. Her taste buds are fully developed and there is some evidence to show that she has developed a preference for certain flavours.

appearance

Most of the soft downy lanugo has disappeared from your baby's body, but the hair on her head is becoming thicker. Her skin will be soft and smooth, and her body is covered with a layer of waxy vernix. Her gums have a 'ridged' appearance that is sometimes mistaken as being teeth.

movement

Sometimes your baby will press part of herself so hard against the wall of your uterus that you feel compelled to push back. This vigorous movement will probably be from a foot or a knee. A more gentle 'flickering' type of movement is more likely to be a hand. Although your midwife will tell you which way your baby is lying, you will probably have a good idea yourself from identifying the position of her limbs as they move.

did you know?
The placenta reaches maturity by 34 weeks. It will continue to provide your baby with oxygen and nutrition until she is born.

Ultrasound scans can detect rapid eye movements (REM) in sleeping babies before they are born. This suggests that babies spend as much as 60 per cent of their sleeping time in the last 3 months of pregnancy dreaming. For the rest of it they will be in deep, dreamless sleep.

When your baby is born, she will sleep for approximately 16–17 hours out of 24. Roughly half of this is REM sleep.

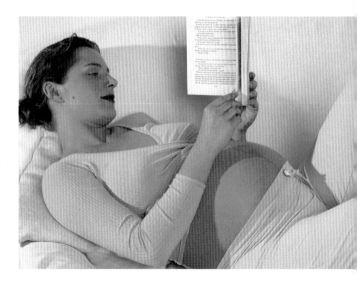

If you rest your book on your bump while reading, do not be surprised to find your baby pushing against it.

your baby at 35 weeks

You do not have much longer to wait now. After all the preparations, labour and the birth will soon be a reality. However, even if your pregnancy was twice as long, you would still never feel completely prepared for labour and your role as a mother. The years ahead will be a learning curve, with the first few months presenting the greatest challenge as you get to grips with all that needs doing.

development

Although your baby is still growing in length, his rate of growth has slowed down. He is becoming plumper, laying down fat cells, mostly around his shoulders. All his organs are fully mature, apart from the lungs. These final weeks are very important as far as his lungs are concerned. Their development needs to be complete so that he can breathe without assistance.

appearance

Your baby looks very much like the one that you will soon meet. His skin is smooth, with a few dimples, and by now he may even have a good head of hair! Dark-skinned babies normally have more hair than light-skinned ones, and it can reach up to 4 cm. He will still be covered in vernix, although some of it will have been shed into the amniotic fluid.

movement

He is reacting now, with movements and facial expressions, in a similar way as he will when he is born. Your baby will frequently respond to sounds. You will feel him 'jump' at a loud noise, or move when he recognizes a piece of music or your voice. He can hear sounds outside of the uterus at about half the volume that you can.

Q **I sometimes notice my bump tightening. Does this mean I'll go into labour early?**

A What you're describing are Braxton Hicks tightenings. These mild, irregular tightenings have, in fact, been there throughout your pregnancy but you just haven't been able to feel them until now. Braxton Hicks tightenings get more frequent and intense towards the end of pregnancy, and some women notice them from about week 25. They are in fact practice tightenings, getting your uterus ready for labour. Unlike the contractions that happen in labour, they are not painful and are irregular.

'I always took my little boy to all my antenatal checks. My midwife used to ask him to guess where she would be able to hear the heartbeat and then he would help put the gel on my tummy. He was very accepting when Amy was born and I feel sure it is because he was so involved from the start.'

Ngaio, mother of 12-week-old Amy and 3-year-old Adam

shared experience

your baby at
36 weeks

The Braxton Hicks tightenings will probably feel quite uncomfortable at times, as your uterus gets ready for labour. Practise breathing through them when you feel your abdomen tighten. Your life is probably revolving around waiting for your labour to start and confirming that all your arrangements for the birth and for the first few weeks afterwards are in place.

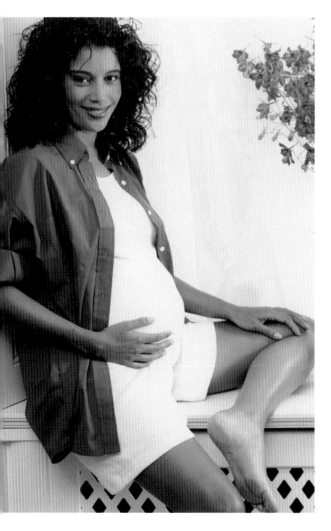

It is now that you have the time to devote solely to your baby and yourself as you have probably given up work. Make the most of this special period, you will not have time later on!

development

Your baby's development is almost complete, although she would still be considered premature if she was born at this time. Her lungs continue to develop and, every day, more fat cells are being laid down in a layer underneath her skin.

appearance

Your midwife should have a good idea of your baby's size when she palpates your uterus to check that it is still expanding at the right rate and also to feel your baby's position. Even if she is not a large baby, her cheeks will be plump. By now, her nails will reach her fingertips. When she is born they will probably be long enough for her to scratch herself – although they are very soft, almost like paper.

movement

Your baby has less room to move around but you should still feel at least ten movements a day. These will feel more like a large 'shifting' movement rather than arms and legs waving around. If she is in the breech position, you will probably be aware of an uncomfortable bump right under your ribs where her head is pressing.

did you know?
Your uterus normally weighs about 50 g, but by week 36, it weighs more than 1 kg – that is more than 20 times heavier than normal!

how your baby has grown

your baby (actual size)

Length Approximately 33 cm from crown to rump
Weight 2.75 kg

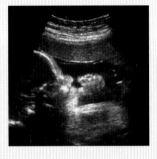

Babies appear to find sucking their thumb as comforting before birth as they do after.

your baby's development

skin and hair
Skin is smooth, as fat is now laid beneath it. Vernix may still be present. Cheeks now look plump. Lanugo is disappearing. Your baby has a good covering of hair on her head, and perfectly formed eyebrows and eyelashes.

bones
The bones of the skull remain slightly soft so that they can mould to the shape of the birth canal.

muscles
Muscles are now strong after weeks of movement.

digestive system
Meconium (the first bowel movement) has collected in the intestine and will be discarded either during or after the birth.

nervous system
Your baby is capable of a whole range of reflexes. She reacts, remembers, and is practising her breathing, swallowing and sucking movements, ready for after the birth. Brain cells increase rapidly and continue to do so even after the birth.

respiratory system
Lungs continue to mature.

urinary system
Your baby is passing approximately 600 ml of urine into the amniotic fluid each day.

ears
Your baby not only hears your voice and other sounds, but also responds to them.

eyes
Eyes are open when your baby is awake. She blinks and responds to light.

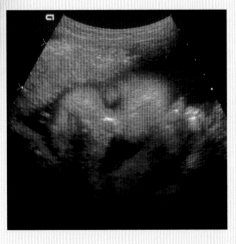

At 36 weeks, her cheeks have filled out and become chubby.

your body at
37–40 weeks

Your baby could be born at any time now and he would not be considered premature. Normal gestation is anything between 37 and 42 weeks, and not just precise 'text-book' 40-weeks pregnancy. This is the point when the telephone calls usually start – from friends and relatives wanting to know whether you have got 'any news' for them yet!

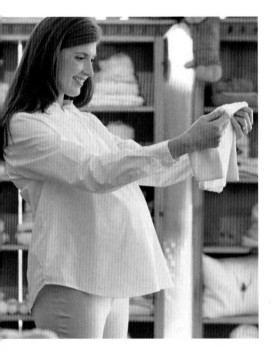

If you have the energy, indulge in some retail therapy and take your bump shopping for items to mark his arrival in a few weeks' time.

how you may feel

There will be days when you feel very excited and impatient to meet your baby and others when you feel panic-stricken at not being fully prepared. Women often find that their 'nesting instinct' kicks in around now and they start to prepare for their baby's birth. You might get a last burst of energy and find yourself cleaning out cupboards, washing baby clothes, wanting to decorate the baby's room and feeling tearful if everything is not just right.

You will probably be getting up at night, possibly several times, to empty your bladder or lying in bed awake, desperately tired, with an active baby inside your uterus. Many women feel that their baby may as well be born now, as they are getting no more rest and sleep than if he had already arrived.

your changing body

Women often get generalized swelling, including their hands and feet and, less commonly, their face and abdomen (more common if your blood pressure is rising). This is caused by fluid retention (oedema, see swelling, page 102) and occurs in up to 80 per cent of pregnant women, because the overall amount of fluid in the body increases during pregnancy. However, it is very important to get any sudden change checked by a midwife, as is could be a sign of pre-eclampsia.

When you are sitting down, put your feet up on the sofa or a footstool and do not cross your legs because this can make it worse. You will find that the swelling is less in the morning after a night's rest but it will not disappear as soon as your baby is born. In fact it sometimes gets worse for a few days before it improves.

your health

Heartburn often returns or gets worse around now, as your stomach gets pushed higher by your expanding uterus (see page 90).
Carpal tunnel syndrome is caused by swelling in the wrists causing numbness and 'pins and needles' in some fingers (see page 95).

Q **I am 35 weeks pregnant and have Group B Strep infection. Is my baby at risk?**

A Group B Streptococcus is common and often associated with a vaginal infection (typically with itchiness and excessive discoloured, smelly discharge). Up to 35 per cent of pregnant women have the infection, many without symptoms. Intravenous antibiotics in labour will help protect your baby. Various factors increase the risk of infection, including premature birth, waters not breaking for more than 18 hours, premature rupture of the membranes or the mother having a temperature in labour or an infection at the birth. Some babies become very ill if they develop this infection and may need a course of antibiotics, while others show no symptoms.

37–40
week reminders

what you should be eating

Eat plenty of iron-rich foods to stock up your iron reserves. Even if you are not anaemic, you will inevitably lose a certain amount of blood during the birth. Dried fruit such as raisins and apricots contain iron in an easily digestible form, which you can keep in your bag to snack on.

jobs to do

Attend your antenatal checks, which are probably weekly by now.

Make sure that you have a copy of your birth plan in your labour bag.

Continue to fill your diary with places to go and people to visit. If you go past your due date, time will drag if you have nothing planned.

Visit a hairdresser – this may be your last opportunity for a while!

Start attending aqua-natal classes. They are a good way of meeting other pregnant women in your locality.

Set aside some time each day to play relaxing music and concentrate on your breathing.

your weight gain
Approximately 13.5 kg

fundal height
At full term the top of your uterus will be as high as it gets – just under your breastbone. When your baby's head engages you may notice that your bump drops slightly.

Your baby's position
Most babies are now head down, ready for the birth. A few still change position, particularly if there is a lot of fluid around them or the mother has had several children before.

207

your baby at
37 weeks

If you are planning to have your baby in hospital, by now your bag should be packed. Since your baby could arrive any time, remember to take essentials (money, phone, address book) with you when you go out, and take your hospital bag with you in the car – just in case! Even if you intend to have your baby at home, you should pack a hospital bag in the event that things do not go according to plan.

development

All major development of your baby is complete. From now on he will continue to grow in size and strength and to lay down fat – up to 28 g a day! The cells in his brain will continue to multiply and develop for the first few months of life after the birth.

In boys, the testicles usually descend into the scrotum about now. However, in approximately 3 per cent of cases, this does not happen until after the birth and surgery may sometimes be necessary, usually before the age of 2 years.

appearance

Your baby's appearance will not change drastically now. He is a slightly smaller version of what he will look like when born.

movement

At about this time your baby's head will start to descend into the pelvis. Once his head is well down and engaged, you may notice that your bump has 'dropped' and looks lower.

If this is not your first baby, this dropping often does not happen until labour, because your muscles do not have the tone they had first time round and so don't hold the baby in place so well. When he does descend his movements will probably seem less vigorous, although you should still be feeling at least ten movements a day.

Your baby is nearly ready to emerge into the world and as that time approaches the big day will be on your mind. Spend plenty of time relaxing.

Q **I'm 37 weeks pregnant and last week my midwife told me that my baby is in the posterior position. What exactly does this term mean?**

A This means that, at the moment, your baby is lying with his back towards your back, although he might turn during the first stage of labour so that he is lying with his back towards your front (anterior), which is the ideal position. There are things that you can start doing now to encourage him to turn into the anterior position (see page 219).

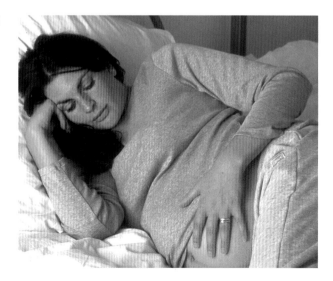

your baby at
38 weeks

Your baby is now fully formed and the birth is imminent. If her head has engaged into the pelvis, you may notice that your abdomen has changed shape. If not, do not worry – some babies, especially if this is not your first, do not engage until labour starts. Once the head has engaged you may find it more uncomfortable to walk.

development

Fat is still being laid down under your baby's skin and, as long as there are no problems with the placenta, she will continue to grow while she is inside you. The fat will be lying in folds and her cheeks will become plumper. Her heart is beating at approximately 110–160 beats per minute. She has 300 bones at the moment, whereas an adult only has 206. This is because some of her bones will later fuse together.

appearance

Most of the soft, downy lanugo covering her body has now been shed, apart from a light covering across the top of her back and shoulders and behind her ears. Her body is still covered in greasy white vernix because she will continue to need 'waterproofing' until she is born.

movement

As space becomes tight in your uterus, your baby will be tightly curled up, with her chin tucked onto her chest and her knees drawn up to her abdomen. Her movements will be less vigorous but she should still be active.

Research suggests that babies have rapid eye movement (REM) sleep from 23 weeks of pregnancy, which indicates that they are dreaming – this encourages the development of the brain. As your baby is asleep for at least 60 per cent of the time, that is a lot of time to dream!

Your baby reacts to external stimuli. If you gently prod part of your bump, she will quickly respond by poking you back with an arm or leg.

the fontanelle

The bones of your baby's skull remain soft so that bones can ride over each other and mould to the shape of the birth canal. As a result, her head may be slightly pointed when she is born and she may have some swelling on either side of the head. This is only temporary. However, there will be a soft spot on the top of her head, called the fontanelle, for about 18 months, until the bones fuse together.

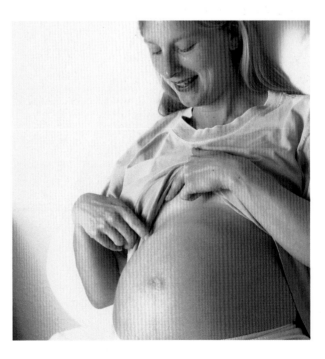

your baby at
39 weeks

You are probably feeling very uncomfortable by now and getting as much sleep, or as little, as if your baby had arrived. Your baby may also be feeling uncomfortable, squashed up with not much room to spare, and you may feel him trying to shift his position from time to time as he tries to stretch in the increasingly confined space available in your uterus.

development

Your baby's immune system continues to develop. Some of your antibodies will pass to your baby through the placenta. These will help to protect him against diseases and infections. This protection will only last a few weeks, but by breast-feeding you will boost this protection by providing him with your antibodies in the colostrum and breast milk.

appearance

Your baby's body will now be well rounded, with a healthy covering of fat. His skin is smooth, still with areas of vernix. His toenails have reached the end of his toes. The amount of hair he may have varies: he could be completely bald, have a few downy patches or have a full head of hair, although its colour may change during the first few months after he is born.

movement

If your baby has developed a pattern of waking and sleeping, this may continue after he is born. If your baby has been active at a particular time of day, this may continue even after the birth. When you go to bed, play some calming music and talk to him gently – this can soothe him if he is unsettled at a particular time of day. Many women recognize their baby's 'playtime', often during the evening and anticipate this after the birth! You should still be getting plenty of movements (at least ten a day) but they will not feel quite so vigorous now as they did in earlier weeks.

Bumps enjoy baths just as much as expectant mothers do. It is a wonderfully relaxing time to bond with your baby.

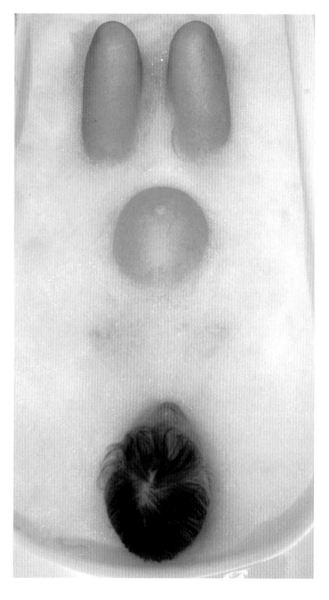

your baby at
40 weeks

This may seem like the longest week so far, particularly if you are past your due date. Some women experience a hormonal feeling, similar to premenstrual tension, just before labour begins; other women just feel 'different'. Many women experience a desperate urge to clean and tidy the house, sort through the baby's clothes, and 'nest' in preparation for their baby's arrival.

development

Your baby is fully developed. At birth, major changes will occur in the baby's heart and lungs. Up until birth the exchange of oxygen and carbon dioxide has been through the placenta. As soon as she is born and takes her first breath, the blood in her lungs will be oxygenated and she will begin to breathe normally. Her rate of respiration will be about 50 per minute, although it is often irregular for the first few days.

appearance

At this point, your baby looks the same in the uterus as she will when she is born. She will be tightly curled up so it is not surprising that babies like to be held close and made to feel secure. If she was in the breech position in the uterus, her knees may remain drawn up to her chest for a couple of days. Some babies are born with one foot or both feet turned in (positional talipes), because of their position inside the uterus, but this is only temporary.

movement

Even inside you, your baby is practising turning her head to the side to look for milk and sucking. You will probably recognize some of these squirming movements when you finally hold your baby. As he pushes out his bottom or reaches up to his face, it will seem familiar to you. Your movements and sounds will be familiar to him too.

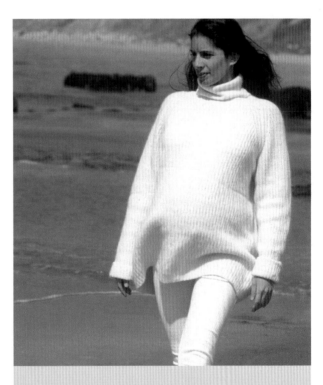

'The waiting to go into labour was unbearable. My partner and I used to sit and talk about what our baby would look like and whose colour hair he would have. I felt such a longing to see and hold him.'

Dawn, mother of 2-week-old Jack

shared
experience

how your baby
has grown

your baby (actual size)

Length 36–37 cm from crown to rump
47–51 cm from head to foot
Weight 3.5 kg

your baby's development

skin and hair
Skin is smooth, with folds of fat on the arms and top of legs. Some vernix may still be present. Most of lanugo has been shed. Your baby has a head of hair, perfectly arched eyebrows and eyelashes.

muscles
Muscles are strong from all the exercise inside the uterus. Your baby responds to sound and movement.

bones
The soft bones of the skull will overlap slightly as the baby is squeezed through the birth canal.

organs
All internal organs are fully formed. 20 per cent of your baby's fat surrounds the organs.

circulatory system
The heart is beating at 110–160 times per minute.

digestive system
Your baby may pass meconium during labour or soon after the birth.

nervous system
Now formed and sufficient for survival, although brain cells continue to multiply and will do so for some time after birth. Your baby is capable of about 70 different reflex system behaviours.

respiratory system
Now fully mature.

ears
Your baby can recognize familiar sounds: your voice and your partner's voice and music.

eyes
She does not have to see very far in the uterus, but by birth she can focus between 20 and 30 cm, the distance between your breast and face.

213

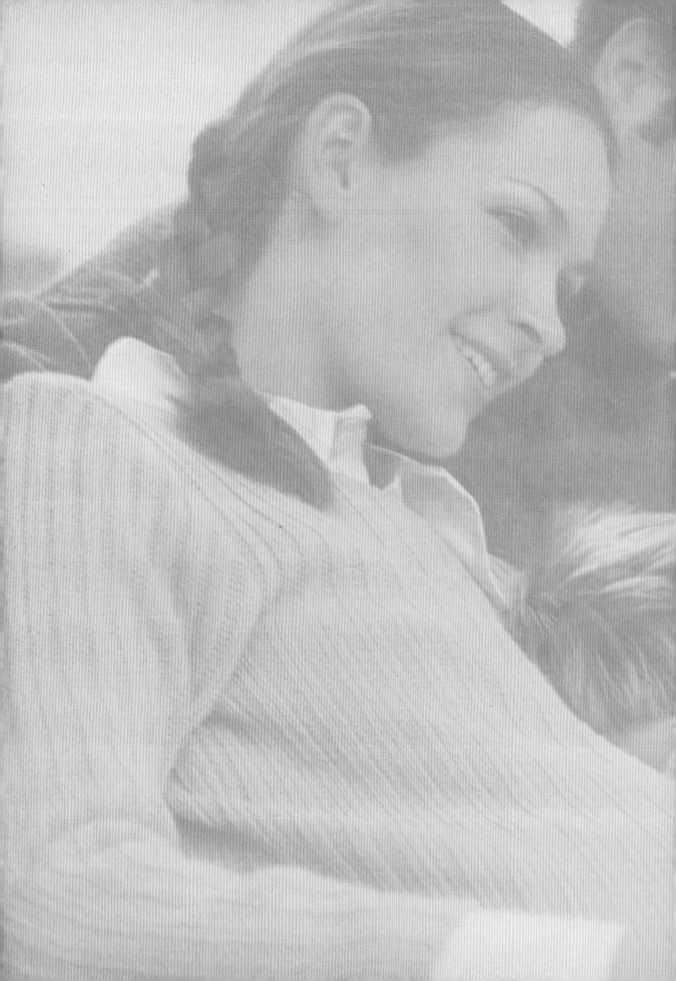

labour
and birth

The big day is fast-approaching and you need to get yourself ready, both in terms of your 'hospital' bag and in terms of your mind-set. The experience of labour and birth is highly individual, but even so it is a good idea to listen to any birth stories offered by new mothers at your antenatal classes. Soon, you will finally reap the rewards of your labour – you get to meet your precious newborn.

getting ready for
the birth

Preparing for your baby involves more than just packing your bag for the hospital and decorating the nursery. You also need time to adjust emotionally to the prospect of the alterations created in your life by having a baby. Women who continue to work late into their pregnancy may find it very difficult being at home with a baby only a week or two after giving up work.

'I was convinced I would be able to work until about 37 weeks of pregnancy. By 33 weeks I felt exhausted, I was not sleeping and I could not bear the thought of going to work. I did not need much persuading to give up and, looking back now, the time at home "nest building" was very special.'

Lou, mother of
7-week-old Gabby

shared experiences

'I loved getting ready for labour. I kept getting the baby clothes out of the drawer and gazing at them. I must have packed and unpacked my hospital bag at least every 3 days!'

Annie, mother of
3-week-old Martha

stopping work

Choosing the right time to give up work is a common problem, particularly if you intend to return to work and have a limited amount of maternity leave. Many women try to make the most of their maternity leave by working as far into their pregnancy as possible. You need to think very carefully about this.

preparations

As the birth approaches, make sure that you have everything ready, where you can access it easily.

telephone numbers

Know who to ring when you go into labour. You should have the phone number of the labour ward in your antenatal notes, as well as any other important phone numbers, for example your community midwife or ambulance control. It is always useful to have a list of phone numbers to hand – not only your partner's mobile number, but also the numbers of local taxi firms and people you will want to call with your news afterwards.

knowing where to go

Once you are in labour you need to go to the maternity unit, and it is worth calling them first to let them know that you are on your way. If you have already had a tour around the unit, you will know where to go when you arrive.

Make sure that you and your partner know how to get to the maternity unit – you would be amazed at the number of people who get lost on the way! You can even practise trying the route in rush hour, just to see how long it takes. Remember that, with a first baby, established labour lasts an average of 10–12 hours, so even if you are stuck in traffic, you will probably still have time to spare! Make sure that you can find the correct entrance, especially at night when the main doors to the hospital or maternity unit may be locked.

labour ward bag

- Comfortable clothes to wear during labour, for example, an oversized T-shirt or nightdress.
- Socks and slippers.
- Dressing gown.
- Three pairs of large disposable knickers (for when your waters break and also for immediately after the birth, when your blood loss will be quite heavy).
- Clean nightdress for afterwards.
- A sponge or flannel (to keep you cool during labour).
- Massage oils and equipment if you are using them.
- Toiletries, including mild soap, toothbrush and toothpaste, hairbrush and towel.
- Sanitary towels (maternity pads or night-time sanitary towels).
- Cartons of fruit juice and high-energy snacks (for example, dried fruit).
- Birth plan, camera.
- A hot water bottle for easing backache.
- A hand mirror – so that you can see your baby's head emerging, especially when you feel that you are not making any progress.
- A battery-operated cassette recorder or radio (sometimes electronic items from home are not allowed in the ward) and a selection of music that you can focus on through the contractions.
- Change for the telephone (you are not allowed to use mobile phones in a hospital), address book and important telephone numbers.
- For your baby: two baby-grow suits, two vests, nappies, cotton wool, hat.

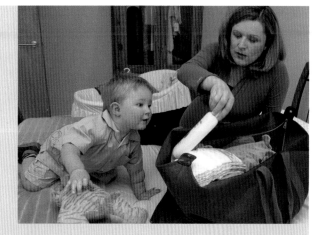

postnatal bag

- Nightdress – front-opening if you are breast-feeding.
- Several pairs of knickers.
- Nursing bra.
- A few breast pads.
- Good-quality nipple cream (ask your midwife).
- Sanitary towels (heavy-duty ones).
- Something to read – if you get time!
- For your baby: bottles, teats and formula if you are not breast-feeding and if the unit does not provide them, four baby-grow suits, four vests, a small pack of nappies, and a hat, cardigan or outdoor suit for wearing home.

If you know you are having a caesarean section, have a few more of everything, or ask your partner to bring things in as the need arises. He can also fit a baby seat or carrier to the car, ready for when you come home.

packing

Do not be over-ambitious and pack pre-pregnancy clothes for yourself – it will be a few weeks before you can get into your pre-maternity wear. Get your partner to take home any soiled clothing that you wore to the hospital or during your labour and bring you fresh comfortable replacements for when you are ready to go home. Most women opt to wear a nightdress while on the postnatal ward.

It is useful to pack two bags: one for the labour ward and one for the postnatal ward (see below).

Even if you are planning to have your baby at home, it is worthwhile packing a bag for the labour ward in case you need to be transferred to hospital part way through your labour.

your baby's
position

The position of your baby in the uterus can affect the labour and birth. Until 36 weeks of pregnancy, this is irrelevant because he may still change position. By 36 weeks of pregnancy most babies will be head down (vertex) ready for labour, but a few still move around, frequently changing their position. This is known technically as an unstable lie.

Q Can I do anything to turn my breech baby?

A If your baby is still in the breech position by 32 weeks, you could try burning Chinese moxa sticks (a tight roll of powdered herbs). When combined with acupuncture, this is believed to encourage the baby to turn head down. Be sure to consult a qualified acupuncturist and inform your midwife or doctor, because this treatment is not for women with high blood pressure.

Regular swimming, on your front may also help your baby to turn. Theoretically, the buoyancy gives your baby more room to turn around.

There are some suggestions that adopting a knee to chest position for 5–10 minutes, four times a day, can help the baby to turn.

Alternatively, kneel on the floor, knees apart, place your forehead on a cushion on the floor and raise your bottom higher up than your head.

occiput anterior

Your baby will probably be facing your back, with his back slightly to one side of your abdomen. This position is described as occiput anterior (OA; the occiput is the back of the baby's head). This is the ideal position for a baby to pass through the pelvis and the majority of babies adopt this position. If the baby's back is on the right side, his position is said to be right occipital anterior (ROA) while, if it is on the left, it is said to be left occipital anterior (LOA).

occiput posterior

If your baby is lying with his back against your back, facing your abdomen, this is called an occiput posterior (OP) position. However, only about 5 per cent of these babies fail to move into an OA position. If your baby is one of this 5 per cent, it does not mean that you cannot have a vaginal birth. However, labour may take longer, you may have backache (see page 94) and you are more likely to need an assisted delivery (see page 248).

breech

A breech position is when your baby's buttocks are facing down and his head is under your ribs. His legs may be tucked up (frank breech) or he may have one or both legs pointing down (footling breech). If your baby is breech, you may be offered an external cephalic version (ECV) at about 37 weeks. This is where the obstetrician manipulates your abdomen to try to turn the baby around.

transverse lie

If your baby has head towards your left or right side, this is known as a transverse lie. Unless he turns you will need a caesarean.

unstable lie

A baby that keeps changing position after 37 weeks is referred to as an unstable lie. Labour may be induced while he has his head down.

exercises

To encourage your baby to get into the best position for labour, try the following:

- Sit with your knees lower than your hips.
- When standing, lean over slightly as much as possible, for example, over a work surface, thus allowing more space for your baby to turn.
- Swim – breaststroke is best.
- Kneel and lean over a beanbag to watch television.

positions in late pregnancy

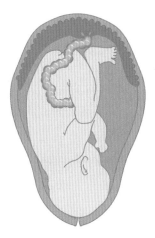
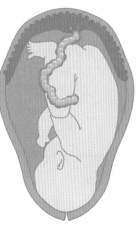
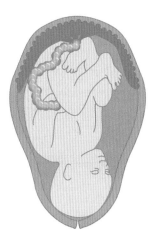
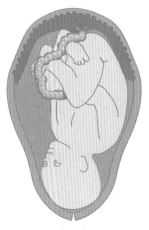

Right occiput anterior (ROA). He is head down, facing your back and to the right side of your body.

Left occiput anterior (LOA). He is head down, facing your back and to the left side of your body.

Right occiput posterior (ROP). He is head down, facing front and on the right side of your body.

Left occiput posterior (LOP). He is head down, facing front and on the left side of your body.

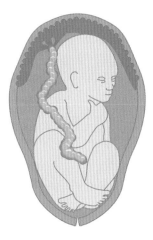
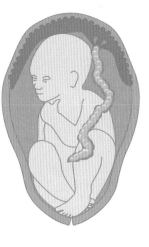
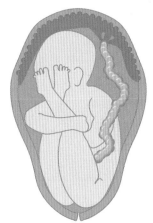
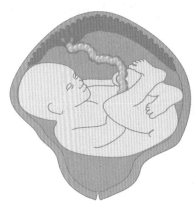

Breech. He is bottom down and has his legs and arms crossed.

Footling breech. One or both legs are pointing down and he will emerge feet first.

Frank breech. He is bottom down and his legs are completely tucked up.

Transverse lie (TR). He lies across the uterus with his head on one side and his buttocks on the other.

overdue babies

It can be depressing to see your due date come and go with no sign of labour. Although the majority of babies arrive after the due date, mostly within 10 days, waiting for the first sign of labour can seem like the longest part of your pregnancy. Do not be too despondent, and keep filling your diary with things to do in the days following the expected date of delivery to take your mind off things.

did you know?

Raspberry leaf tea is reputed to soften and 'ripen' the cervix which can help to trigger contractions.

There is an enzyme in fresh pineapple that is also reputed to be a natural inducer of labour.

Get your midwife to check the date when your baby is due, working from the last day of your period or from your scan. At the beginning of pregnancy, the odd day here or there does not seem very important, but when you have a date to be induced it can make all the difference!

effects on your baby

The placenta, which is your baby's source of nutrition, will eventually start to age and not work as well if your baby is very overdue. If the placenta does not function properly, your baby may not be getting all of the nourishment that she needs.

Nobody can say exactly when your labour is supposed to start because a 'normal' gestation is anywhere between 37 and 42 weeks of pregnancy. If you do not want to be induced, talk to your obstetrician or midwife. They should offer to monitor your baby's heartbeat at least twice a week with an electronic monitor, and to measure the fluid around your baby with ultrasound. You will also be advised to monitor your baby's movement as a guide to her wellbeing. Women are usually offered an induction of their labour 7–14 days after their due date.

getting labour started

If you are past your due date, there are things you can try to get labour going. None of these methods will trigger labour unless your baby is ready to be born but, if you have had problems during your pregnancy, such as bleeding or the threat of premature labour, check with your midwife or doctor first.

Nipple stimulation Use a shower attachment or a breast pump to stimulate your nipples. This may encourage your body to release the hormone oxytocin, which makes your uterus contract and sets off labour. You would probably need to do this for several hours, several times a day, but it is worth a try!

Sex After making love, lie down for as long as you can with your legs raised on a couple of pillows. This allows the semen to bathe the cervix, which can help to soften it and encourage labour to start.

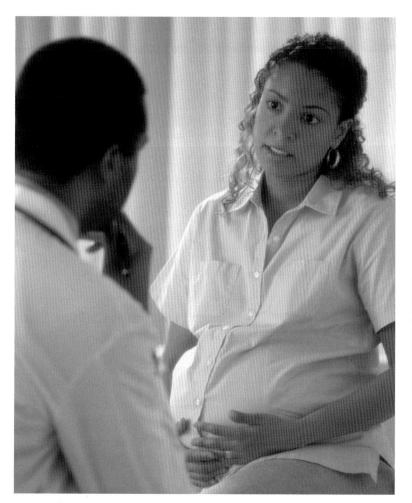

Counting the days after your baby's EDD can make you feel a bit frustrated, but be patient. Most labours will start naturally within a few days. Talk through the options with your midwife or doctor.

Semen is a natural source of the hormone prostaglandin, which is used in hospitals to induce labour.

Orgasm If neither you or your partner feel like sex, which is not uncommon towards the end of pregnancy, masturbation can help labour. When aroused, your body releases the hormone oxytocin, which can cause your uterus to contract, leading to labour.

Reflexology There is a pressure point on the foot that can stimulate contractions of the uterus, but you should consult a qualified reflexologist about this.

Walking Taking a long walk may encourage your baby in the right direction and also puts pressure on the cervix, which is good for getting labour going. Make sure that you are with someone and not in the middle of nowhere – walking around a shopping centre is just as effective as a walk in the country.

Spicy foods If spicy foods are part of your normal diet, they probably will not get you going. The idea is to eat something that will loosen your bowels, which can irritate the uterus and kick start labour. Eating the contents of a fruit bowl or a few slices of raw courgette can often have the same effect.

> ' I got thoroughly fed up with family and friends calling me and asking "Have you had it yet?" Did they really expect me to say "Yes, last week – but we forgot to tell you"? '
>
> Alison, mother of
> 8-week-old Thomas

shared experiences

> ' Every day that I went past my due date seemed like an extra week. The trouble was I had not bothered arranging to do or go anywhere as I assumed that I would have had the baby by then. Those 8 days seemed like the longest of my life! '
>
> Betty, mother of
> 10-week-old Charlotte

hospital birth

For many women, having a baby is their first experience of being in hospital. Suddenly finding yourself in an unfamiliar environment, surrounded by strange equipment, can be very unnerving. Ideally, part of your antenatal care should include a tour of the maternity unit where your baby will be born. You will have the opportunity to see the equipment and familiarize yourself with the environment.

what will be there

It is worth making an effort to learn what the various instruments are used for as this will help to reduce anxiety. If you do not see this equipment until you are in labour, you will probably be too preoccupied to ask questions about their functions.

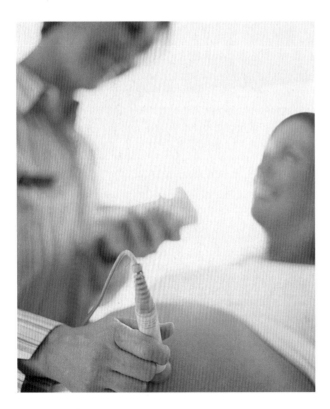

During labour your midwife will periodically monitor your baby's heart rate using a doppler to ensure that he is not in any distress.

the bed

Your hospital room will probably be dominated by the bed, which is usually in the centre so that people can move around it. The rooms are often not very big so, if the midwife is at one side of the bed, your partner will need to move to the other side to stay close to you.

The design of the bed will enable it to be raised or lowered, either manually or electronically, and it can have stirrups inserted in case you need to have a forceps or a ventouse delivery. Many beds can be converted into birthing chairs by removing the end and putting the head upright. Ask the midwife to show you the various options, because these will make you consider the possible positions in which you could give birth – if you choose to stay on the bed for the birth.

equipment

There will usually be several items of equipment in the room. These will include:

A cardiotocograph (CTG) to monitor your baby's heartbeat and your contractions (see page 239).

A Doppler, which is a hand-held device for listening to your baby's heartbeat (see page 159).

Gas and air (Entonox) which may be piped through a tube in the wall of the room or in a canister, and has either a mouthpiece or a facemask attached to it. You will have a canister of gas and air to use even if you are in a bath or on the floor rather than on the bed.

Emergency equipment should be available in all rooms and will include oxygen in case you need it. If there is a chance of your baby needing oxygen when he is born, a resuscitaire will probably be brought into the room. This is a trolley, with a space for the baby to be checked over, a lamp and a heater to keep him warm, and oxygen and suction should he need it.

A sphygmomanometer to measure your blood pressure. Your blood pressure will be checked at various times throughout labour.

other aids

There are a number of things that you could consider using during the birth, but you may have to ask about them because they may be stored elsewhere in the hospital, or you may need to provide them yourself.

Birthing aids such as a bean bag, birthing chair, birthing ball or rocking chair, can be very useful for encouraging a more active birth.

Birthing pools are increasingly used and many maternity units have more than one delivery room with a pool.

Extra comforts may be available, such as a cassette- or CD-player, so ask in advance. Music can be very useful during labour and you might like to choose a selection that you will find relaxing.

getting to know the staff

If the birth is completely straightforward, there will be no need for you to see anyone other than the midwives looking after you, as they are the experts at looking after healthy women in labour. However, there are occasions when you will meet other staff on the delivery ward, such as:

An obstetrician A doctor specializing in the care of women who have complications during pregnancy, labour or the postnatal period.

An anaesthetist A doctor specializing in anaesthetics, who would put an epidural in position. If you had to go to an operating theatre, an anaesthetist would be there, not only to provide an epidural or general anaesthetic but also to help out if excessive bleeding occurs.

A pediatrician A doctor specializing in babies and child health who will check your baby after the birth. A paediatrician would be present at instrumental deliveries or if any problem was anticipated with your baby, for example, premature labour.

Students Looking after women in labour is obviously an essential part of a student's training, but your permission should always be asked first.

Other staff There will also be a number of other people on the labour ward, for example, healthcare assistants, porters and theatre staff.

‘When I was in labour my waters went and they were slightly green. The midwife explained that my baby had opened her bowels (passed meconium), which we knew could be a sign that the baby was distressed. The resuscitaire was pushed into the room but my partner and I both knew what it was because we had had the chance to see it on our tour of the unit and we did not feel at all frightened.’

Louisa, mother of
3-month-old Katie

shared experiences

‘Although we would have liked a home birth, it just wasn't possible. But, with some music and home comforts we brought in, we managed to make the hospital environment seem much more relaxing, which definitely made giving birth seem less daunting!’

Matthew, father of
2-week-old Louis

water birth

Women are often attracted to water during labour in the same way that they take a bath if they have menstrual pain or backache or feel stressed. If you would like a water birth consider hiring a birthing pool, either to use at home or to take to the maternity unit if it does not have one already. Remember that hospital birthing facilities are subject to availability, that is, on a first come, first served basis.

'The water felt so fantastic. I stayed on my knees and leaned on the side of the pool, as this was the most comfortable position. At 5.50 am I pushed out my baby in the water and steered him to the surface myself. It was just incredible. Barry cut the umbilical cord and held him.'

Jayne, mother of
9-month- old Gabriel

shared experiences

'I had a water birth and the minute I got into the pool the difference was amazing. I'd been feeling the contractions across my lower back but the warm water relieved this and I was able to switch off completely and relax.'

Paulette, mother of
2-week-old Grace

advantages

The use of water during labour can have many benefits. Studies have shown that it helps you to relax, which in turn reduces pain and the need for analgesia. Being in a room with a pool is often more relaxed and less clinical, and you may find that you get one-to-one care with the midwife, which also helps you to cope. If necessary, you can still use gas and air in a pool, although you cannot use any other form of pain relief.

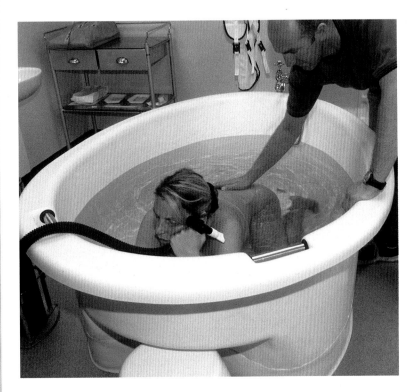

If you are keen on a water birth, many hospitals can now offer a birthing pool. Alternatively, you can hire one to use at home.

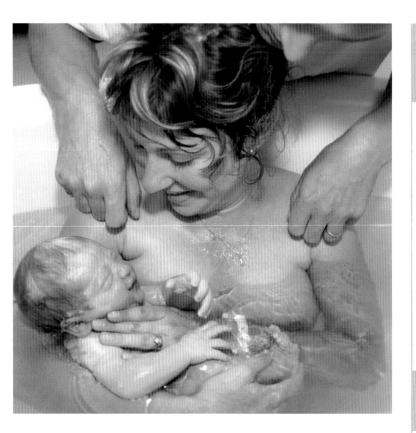

Your baby will take her first breaths when she is lifted to the surface of the water. Once this has occurred, her body can stay in the water, against yours, to keep her warm while her head stays above the water.

Not all women would be encouraged to use a birthing pool but, if you are considered low risk and have good midwifery care, it carries no more risks than a conventional birth. Even if you do not fancy the idea of giving birth while in the water, it is worth trying the pool just for labour and then getting out for the delivery – if you feel up to moving by then.

things to consider

There are certain considerations when giving birth in a birthing pool.

- It is important to be in established labour when you get into the pool and, ideally, your cervix should be at least 5 cm dilated. Getting into the pool too early in labour can actually slow down your contractions.
- Drink plenty of water while you are in the pool. It is important not to become dehydrated or overheated while you are in there.
- If your labour slows down, get out and move around. You can always get in again later.
- Even in a pool, you may still need encouragement to change position. You could try getting on all fours, leaning over the side of the pool or squatting.

Q **Is there any danger that my baby will breathe under the water?**

A Your baby will breathe when given the right stimulation. When she is exposed to air, the change in temperature and the hands on her body trigger her breathing, so the water in the pool must be kept at 37°C while your baby is born and the birth must be 'hands off'. The midwife will allow your baby to emerge into the water and then one of you can gently guide her to the surface, where she will take her first breath.

Q **Do I have to be naked in the pool?**

A Some women are happy to strip off completely in the pool, while others prefer to keep something on. A top that does not 'balloon' in the water is most practical. Women never really know how they are going to react until their labour, but midwives are happy to go along with whatever you find comfortable.

Q **What about the placenta?**

A If you decide to deliver the placenta naturally then there is no reason why you should not stay in the pool. However, if you want to have an injection of an oxytocic drug, the injection should not be given under the water.

home birth

Research shows that if your pregnancy has been straightforward and you are not considered high risk it is just as safe to have your baby at home as in hospital. With a hospital birth you are more likely to end up with interventions, and you have a greater risk of infection. Even if taken to hospital during labour, you are still less likely to end up with a caesarean section than someone booked for a hospital birth.

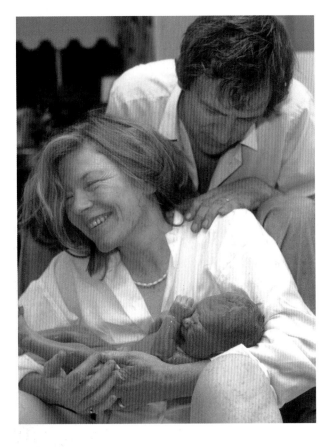

Having a baby at home has a special significance for the many couples who opt for this type of delivery.

advantages

The biggest advantage of having your baby at home is being in a familiar, comfortable environment with none of the elements of uncertainty and fear that can inhibit labour in a hospital. You have the freedom to move around as you wish, and to have as many people with you as you choose – or you may just prefer the privacy, knowing that members of staff are not going to walk through the door. Women who have a home birth are more likely to feel in control and relaxed than those who give birth in hospital.

preparing for a home birth

If you choose to have your baby at home, your midwife will generally bring the delivery equipment to your house at around 37 weeks and leave it there. There is little preparation involved in a home birth but there are a few things that you can do to make things easier.

things you can do

Have a list of contact numbers to hand for when labour starts, for example, your midwife's mobile number or the telephone number of the community midwife's office (the local labour ward should be able to contact the community midwife if you cannot get through). There are also a number of other sensible preparations you can make before you go into labour:

- Walk around your house to see how you can use the furniture during labour. Ideally you want to remain upright and walking around. Try putting a cushion on a table and leaning over it, or leaning on the kitchen worktop. Is it the right height? Can you adapt and use what is around you?

- An adjustable reading lamp will be useful when the midwife checks your perineum afterwards to see whether you need any stitches. You could also have a torch handy for the same purpose.
- If you have other children, it is useful to have someone to take care of them, just in case you have to be transferred into hospital, rather than having to wake them up and take them to stay elsewhere once your contractions have started. You need to know that they are being looked after in order to stay relaxed.
- Find some plastic sheeting, (for example, a ground sheet or an old shower curtain) to protect your mattress or carpet. Old sheets or towels can also be useful.
- Pack a bag for the hospital 'just in case'.

options for pain relief

Choosing to have a home birth makes a huge difference to women's ability to cope with the contractions. Because of this, and the one-to-one care that they get from the midwife, many women find that they do not need pain relief when they have a home birth. Most women use what is around them – they walk around, listen to music, eat and drink, and generally stay relaxed, which is the secret of staying in control of your labour.

Many women, whether at home or in hospital, find a soak in a warm but not hot bath to be a great source of pain relief but some drugs can be used at home.

- You can use gas and air (Entonox) to take the edge off the pain. Your midwife will bring some canisters to your home and you can breathe it through a mouthpiece or a facemask.
- Some doctors will prescribe meptazinol or pethidine, for the midwife to give you. However, some midwives are reluctant to use this at home because it makes the baby drowsy.
- Alternatively, you could hire a TENS (transcutaneous electrical nerve stimulation) machine, which works by blocking the pain impulses and encouraging your body to produce natural pain relievers. Check with your midwife whether she will be able to bring one with her or whether you should hire one.

dealing with problems

Midwives are trained and equipped to deal with emergencies should they occur. However if there are signs that all is not well during labour, your midwife may decide to transfer you to hospital.

You should discuss any reasons that she might have for doing this beforehand. They would include:

- Your baby showing signs of distress during labour, including opening his bowels
- Very slow progress of the labour
- Any bleeding during labour
- High blood pressure
- Signs of infection.

'Our baby was born at 3 am. Afterwards Rob and I sat on the bed with the midwives, drinking champagne. At 8 am our two-year-old daughter, Ruby walked into the room. It seemed like the most natural thing in the world. I said "Do you remember that I had a baby in my tummy? He has come out now, and he is called George." Then we all went downstairs and had some breakfast.'

Annie, mother of 2-year-old Ruby and 8-week old George

shared experiences

'When Peter and I heard the nurses at our antenatal group discussing home birth, we thought they were mad. But as the classes progressed, we gradually came to see the birth as a natural, rather than medical, process. I was keen to avoid any intervention and learned that staying relaxed was the best way to avoid potential problems – and staying at home was the key to being relaxed.'

Louise, mother of 3-week-old Noah

labour:
an overview

The uterus is made of muscle, which tenses and relaxes during a contraction. At the bottom is the cervix, which also forms the top of the vagina. As part of the birth process, changes must occur in the cervix in order for the baby to pass through and into the birth canal. The cervix will gradually get softer and thinner, and then it will start to dilate (open) in preparation for the birth.

contractions

Women describe the pain associated with contractions in various ways, for example as severe menstrual cramp, persistent backache or a wave of discomfort that peaks and then subsides. In the short term, the contractions vary in intensity, rather than getting progressively longer and stronger. However, overall, they become more frequent and last for longer as the birth approaches.

- **Latent phase** mild irregular tightenings, gradually lasting longer and becoming more frequent.
- **Stage 1** more rhythmical and intense, lasting for 30–60 seconds and occurring at 5–10-minute intervals.
- **Stage 2** sensation of contractions change. Usually feel expulsive with an overwhelming urge to bear down and push. Usually last around a minute, at least every five minutes.
- **Stage 3** relatively painless contractions of the uterus to expel the placenta.

what is labour?

Women often feel angry when, after a 20-hour marathon, the midwife records their labour as 8 hours. This is because the definition of labour is the onset of regular contractions with dilatation of the cervix. If you are getting contractions but your cervix has not started to open (dilate), this is still regarded as early labour (latent phase), which is different from established labour, that is, the point of no return.

Established labour is divided into three stages:
Stage 1 from the start of regular contractions and the opening of the cervix until the cervix has fully dilated (10 cm). With a first baby this takes an average of 10–12 hours.
Stage 2 from full dilatation of the cervix to the birth of the baby. When the cervix is fully open you will be able to push the baby down the birth canal. With a first baby, this takes an hour on average. The second stage is often shorter in subsequent pregnancies.
Stage 3 from the birth of your baby to the delivery of the placenta and membranes (the bag of fluid that surrounded your baby). This can last between 10 minutes and an hour.

the onset of labour

If you develop any signs of labour before 37 weeks of pregnancy, you should contact the labour ward immediately. However, your baby may arrive at any time between 37 and 42 weeks of pregnancy and, in practice, only 5 per cent of babies arrive on their due date. You may have mild, irregular contractions for days before labour starts in earnest, so do not rush to the hospital unless you have any obvious complications, for example, if your baby is in the breech position (bottom down) or if you have been booked for a caesarean section.

Enjoy the excitement of knowing that things are probably starting to happen, but try to pace yourself. There is no reason why you should not take a gentle walk with your birth partner, but you should also conserve your energy as much as possible by eating, drinking and resting in the comfort of your home. It is probably not wise to tell too

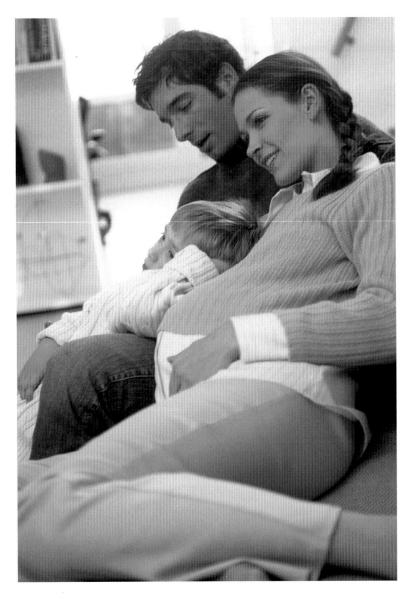

Spending time together as a family is particularly precious near the end of your pregnancy, as it might be some time before 'normal' family life resumes after the new baby's arrival.

' When I woke up that morning I knew I was going to go into labour, although I had no contractions. I just felt different, almost premenstrual. By lunchtime I had diarrhoea, and by teatime my contractions were 5 minutes part. Molly was born at 6 o'clock the following morning. '

Helen, mother of
14-week-old Molly

shared experiences

' When I had a show we just looked at each other, unsure what to do. We had been to antenatal classes, read every pregnancy book and magazine, and there we were, frozen to the spot with a mixture of fear and excitement. It is a good job we did not rush off to the hospital because it was still a week before the contractions started, and then 10 hours after that Jacob was born! '

Paula, mother of
4-month-old Jacob

many people what is happening or you might be indundated with phone calls from well-meaning friends and relatives wanting regular updates on your progress.

Keeping relaxed is the key to coping with labour. The longer you stay at home the better. A new environment is bound to make you tense, and a labour ward is no exception. It is natural to be excited about going into hospital but being there does not mean that your baby will arrive any quicker. In fact, many women find that the contractions stop once they get to hospital because anxiety inhibits their labour. Therefore, unless your waters break, or the contractions are strong and 5 minutes apart, it is too early to turn up at the maternity unit.

Your community midwife may be able to visit if you are unsure whether or not you have gone into labour. However, as a general rule, if you have any doubts, your labour has probably not started.

positions for labour and birth

Although women in the West have traditionally given birth lying on their backs, this is not the most effective position for either labour or delivery. Women who remain mobile and adopt a more upright position during labour, and who stand, sit or squat to deliver, generally have an easier time. Labour tends to be shorter, less painful and requires less intervention.

> 'Keeping mobile during labour was fantastic. I could pace my own labour. When I stood up the contractions were strong and regular and when I sat down they slowed down. I felt totally in control.'
>
> Nessy, mother of
> 9-week-old Gemma

shared experience

In the last weeks of your pregnancy, practise the positions on these pages a couple of times to see how they feel. You will not find which are the most effective and comfortable for you until you are in labour. However, do not stick to just one position but move between them as your body dictates, with your birth partner's help if you need it.

pre-labour

In the early stages, before you go into established labour, try to stay as relaxed as possible. Do not sit around waiting for the onset of labour, but take your mind off it by finding something to do. This is a good time to practise your breathing techniques (see page 233). During the day alternate between periods of rest and periods of keeping mobile. However, if you go into early labour during the night, there is no need to leap out of bed and start pacing around. This will just tire you out.

stage 1

During this stage of labour, while your cervix is dilating and your uterus is rising and tipping forwards, it makes sense to adopt positions that help these processes and assist in stretching the ligaments that join the bones of your pelvis.

Being upright, whether walking around or resting across a chair, ensures that your baby's head is pressing on your cervix, which will encourage contractions, speed up dilation of the cervix and move your baby's head down and deeper into the pelvis. Imagine carrying a dining table through a doorway. It would need to be tilted from side to side, in the same way that your baby needs encouragement to descend through the pelvis. Changing positions and walking around can help him to move further down.

When you are having contractions during this stage, adopt positions where you are leaning forwards so that your contractions work with gravity rather than against it, pushing your uterus forwards.

Positions where your thighs are flexed and wide apart help to open your pelvis, so there is more room for your baby to manoeuvre.

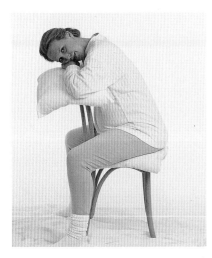

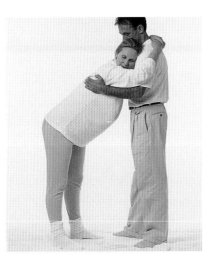

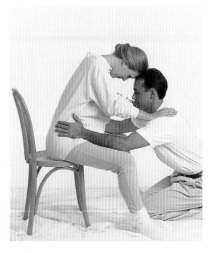

When you feel like resting rather than moving around, it is better to opt for a chair than a bed or an armchair. Pad the seat with a pillow and sit back to front, with your legs either side of the chair back. Relax onto another pillow placed under your chin.

When a contraction comes while you are walking around, stand with your hands around your birth partner's neck, lean forwards and let him support some of your weight in a reassuring hug until the pain subsides. You can also support yourself by leaning against a wall, worktop or a piece of heavy furniture.

Sit halfway back on a chair, with your knees apart and leaning onto your birth partner for support and reassurance.

keeping mobile

In stage 1 of labour, it is important to walk about as much as you can between contractions. This affects the speed of the contractions, your ability to cope with them and also the progress of the labour. On the whole, women who keep mobile during stage 1 have shorter labours and need less pain relief.

However, if your contractions start in the middle of the night, do not leap out of bed and start pacing around because it is also important that you go into labour rested and with sufficient energy to see you through the next few hours.

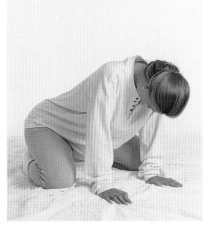

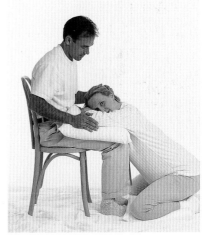

Kneel on something soft like a large flat cushion or a folded blanket, spreading your knees to make space for your bump and leaning forwards onto your hands. This position is good for stretching your pelvic ligaments. Rocking yourself gently in this position can help to turn your baby if he is facing forwards.

Kneel on something soft and lean into your birth partner's lap with your thighs either side of his feet. You could also adopt this position leaning onto an armchair or your bed.

stage 2

As with labour, many women deliver lying on their back because no one has suggested an alternative. In fact, this is not an ideal position because you are again working against the effects of gravity. It also places extra stress on the perineum, meaning that you are more likely to tear or need an episiotomy (see page 252).

Upright positions make pushing easier during this stage because you are then working with gravity, not against it. In addition, your baby has more room to move because your coccyx is swung back out of the way. Try the following positions with your birth partner before you go into labour.

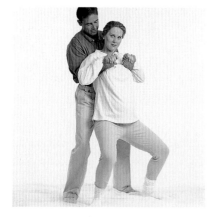

Your birth partner stands behind you, with his hands under your arms for support. He could lean on a wall to support his back, bending his knees as you bend yours and push on the floor or he could support you from in front.

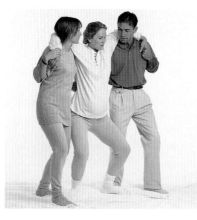

Stand or semi-squat, being supported on either side. As you push and bend your knees, your helpers should bend their knees too, taking your weight so that your feet remain on the floor, giving you something to push against.

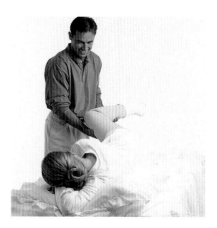

Lie on your left side with your knees bent. Your birth partner supports your upper leg as you push into the contractions. This can be a good position for getting rid of the last lip (the anterior lip) of the cervix.

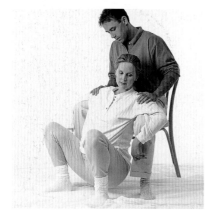

If you are getting too tired to stand, try this alternative. Squat between your birth partner's legs and lean into his lap with your feet flat on the floor and your arms over his knees. This position can be adapted for sitting on a bed, if you are securely propped up with pillows.

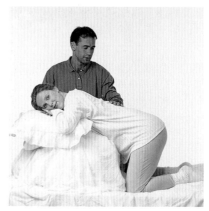

Kneel on the floor or bed, leaning onto pillows or a beanbag. This position may help you to feel secure with something to push against. The midwife can deliver your baby from behind. You could also be on all fours, with your middle supported on the pillows or a beanbag.

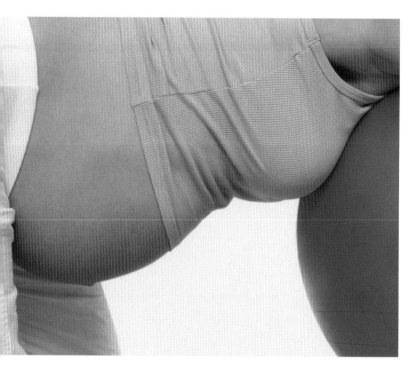

Leaning on a large, inflatable birthing ball if you need to rest between contractions, works in the same way as kneeling on all fours but with the added advantage that you don't have to support your own weight.

breathing

You already unconsciously change your breathing pattern according to what you are doing, for example, when drifting off to sleep, exercising, or sinking into an armchair at the end of a day. Nobody had to teach you to do this, it is automatic. Likewise, any kind of stress automatically affects your breathing. It will become faster and shallower, from the upper part of the lungs, and will cause tension in your shoulders.

During labour, the majority of women find that the stress of being in an unfamiliar environment and coping with contractions makes them tense. Therefore you need to find a breathing technique that will keep you relaxed and tension free. When you feel Braxton Hicks tightenings (see page 95), practise taking slow, deep breaths, just as you will when in labour.

breathing techniques

- Sit or stand comfortably, with loose shoulders, hands and face.
- Breathe in deeply through the nose and out through the mouth.
- Relax your body as you breathe out.
- As you breathe, find something on which to focus. During labour you could look into your partner's eyes or picture an image in your mind.
- During labour, if you get the urge to push before your cervix is fully dilated, panting through the contraction, or using gas and air, will help you to stop pushing, and reduce the pressure on the cervix. The best position to relieve pressure on the cervix is on all fours, with your head and chest down and your bottom in the air. Alternatively lie on your left side. Practise taking two short in and out breaths, followed by a longer one. Pant, pant, blow.

breathing and relaxing

- Hold a piece of ice in your hand while you practise your breathing. When the ice starts to feel uncomfortable, concentrate on your breathing and try to 'remove yourself' from the sensation.
- During labour your partner should remind you to keep your face relaxed. If your face is relaxed it is very difficult to tense other parts of your body.
- Do not worry if you forget what to do when you are in labour. A midwife will be there to give you reminders.

stage 1 of
labour

Stage 1 of labour is the longest, lasting from the start of regular contractions and the opening of the cervix until the cervix is dilated to 10 cm (fully dilated). It is then that the baby's head is able to pass through it. Though long, this stage is not relentless as, in between contractions, you will have the opportunity to move around and chat to your partner if you wish.

dilation of the cervix

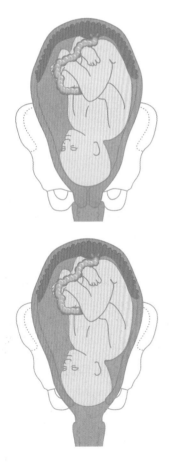

During stage 1 of labour the regular contractions move the cervix forwards in your pelvis, soften it and make it thin out and open so that your baby can pass through the birth canal during stage 2.

Before labour begins, the cervix is like a small, thick tube with a dimple in it, which nestles at the top and to the back of your vagina. The cervix moves forward, softens and thins and then gradually start to open.

Putting a finger into a cervix that is 1 cm dilated feels a bit like putting a finger in a nostril! As the cervix gets thinner and more stretchy, it feels more like a hole in a lump of bubble gum. Because of the amount of stretching and softening that needs to take place, the longest part of labour can often be the dilation of the cervix to 4–5 cm.

signs of labour

There are a number of signs, but experiencing any of them does not necessarily mean that you will go into labour immediately.

a 'show'

A show is the jelly-like; blood-streaked 'plug' of mucus that has been preventing infection from getting into your uterus. It often comes away from the cervix at the beginning of labour, although it can still be a few weeks before labour begins. There is no need to tell anyone about this. It is your own sign that there is a good chance of labour starting within the next few days – but it is not a guarantee!

contractions

In early labour, these tightenings of your uterus feel similar to period pains. You may also get backache. Although these niggling aches and pains can go on for days before labour becomes established, it does not mean that they are without effect. As well as having to move forward, your cervix also has to soften, become thinner and dilate, which often happens in the days before labour starts in earnest.

Once you are having regular contractions that are lasting for longer than 30 seconds and are spaced only 5 minutes apart (10 minutes apart if this is not your first baby), or you are struggling to cope with the pains, contact your midwife or labour ward. If you are capable of talking through a contraction, it is too early to go to the labour ward.

waters breaking

The breaking of your waters (amniotic fluid) usually happens during labour with the force of a contraction, but it can also happen before labour begins. If it does, contact your midwife or labour ward, who can confirm whether labour has started if you are unsure. A midwife will also listen to your baby's heartbeat and probably take a swab from your vagina to check for infection in case you do not go into labour soon afterwards.

Once their waters have broken, most women find that their contractions start within 24 hours. If you do not go into labour, the midwife will tell you how to check for signs and symptoms of infection, for example, by looking for changes in the colour and the smell of the amniotic fluid.

diarrhoea

This can occur shortly before labour begins and can be regarded as nature 'clearing you out' before the birth. Again, there is no need to rush to the labour ward. It may be some time before the contractions really start.

establishing labour

Once you are getting strong, regular contractions, your midwife can do a vaginal examination to establish just how far into labour you are. Most women lie in a semi-upright position on the bed, while the midwife gently examines them using two gloved fingers. She can feel how far your cervix is dilated and also confirm the exact position of your baby.

The midwife will check and record on your notes things such as your blood pressure, pulse and temperature, and ask you questions about the time you felt labour begin.

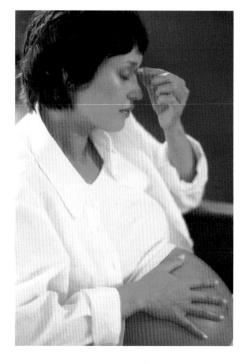

During the first stage of labour, if you can cope with the contractions, you are better off staying in your own home.

waters

Most women's waters break during labour because of the force of the contractions. However, even if your waters do break before labour starts, it will probably be with a trickle rather than a gush. Many women are not even sure that their waters have broken because it feels more like a dribble of urine. In this case, it is advisable to wear a sanitary towel and see whether it continues. If your waters do break, tell your midwife so that she can check you and your baby before labour begins. If you are worried that your waters might break while you are out and about, wearing a sanitary towel when you go out may give you more confidence.

It is now considered best to leave the membranes (bag of waters) to break by themselves. Once the waters break, the baby's head, which was being cushioned by the amniotic fluid, drops further down into the cervix, which can cause stronger contractions. If your membranes are left alone, you may find that both you and your baby can cope better without such direct pressure on your cervix.

However, there are times when it might be advisable to break the waters, for example, if labour is induced or needs speeding up, or if monitoring indicates the baby is becoming distressed.

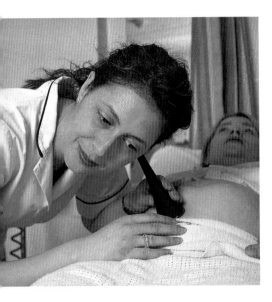

During labour your midwife or doctor will want to listen to the baby's heartbeat every 15 minutes or so, using a trumpet like pinnard or a hand-held Doppler probe.

monitoring the baby

Some babies show signs of distress during labour and for this reason your baby's heartbeat should be monitored. There are various ways of doing this.

dopplers and pinnards

During pregnancy your midwife will have listened to your baby's heartbeat using a hand-held instrument, such as a Doppler or a pinnard (see page 159). A pinnard is a type of ear trumpet that she places on your abdomen and through which she can hear your baby's heartbeat. Many women prefer the Doppler because the sound is amplified so that they can hear the heartbeat as well. If your pregnancy has been straightforward and no problems are anticipated during the birth, research suggests that this is the best way of monitoring the baby's heartbeat during labour.

If your baby opens her bowels inside you (passes meconium), which can be a sign of distress, or if you are given certain medications, for example, an epidural or oxytocic drugs, it is safer to have continual monitoring of the baby's heartbeat.

cardiotocograph (ctg)

This instrument consists of two transducers which are held in place on your abdomen by elastic belts and connected to a monitor. The monitor provides a print-out of the baby's heartbeat and also the

---

Q If I labour in water, how can my baby's heartbeat be monitored?

A If you labour in a birthing pool your baby's heartbeat can easily be monitored using a hand-held Doppler. Some Dopplers are designed to work under the water but, if one of these is not available, all you have to do is lift your bump above the surface of the water so that the midwife can listen in. Even while you are in the water the midwife can lean over and do a vaginal examination, check your blood pressure, or whatever else may need to be done to monitor your and your baby's wellbeing.

Q I hate internal examinations. Do I really need to have more?

A Nothing would ever be done without your consent but internal examinations during labour give valuable information about the progress of labour and you will be keen to know what progress you are making. If you are nervous, share your fears with your midwife, or mention them in your birth plan. Internal examinations are sometimes uncomfortable but it helps to empty your bladder first and to relax your muscles, either using the breathing exercises learned at your antenatal classes, or breathing some gas and air. Once you are in established labour, you will be given an internal examination approximately every 4 hours. Knowing what stage of labour you have reached can help you to make decisions about pain relief.

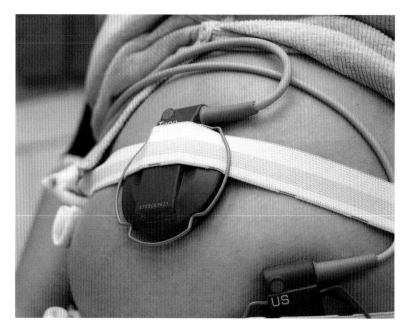

A cardiotocograph machine gives a continuous readout of your baby's heartbeat so that the midwives and doctors can see how your baby is coping with the stress of labour.

uterine contractions. The monitor can be moved about so, unless you have an epidural, which restricts your movement, you can still stay upright or get out of bed. If everything is going smoothly, there is no need for continual monitoring. However, there are many instances where continuous monitoring is necessary, for example, premature labour, use of oxytocin or an epidural, or signs of distress in the baby.

fetal scalp electrode (FSE)

Sometimes there are problems picking up an accurate and continuous reading of the heartbeat with the abdominal transducers, often because of the baby's position. In this case it may be necessary to use an FSE. The midwife or obstetrician will carry out a vaginal examination to determine the position of your baby and then attach a small metal clip to your baby's scalp. This is linked by a lead to the CTG (see above).

transition

Many women experience a period of transition between stages 1 and 2 of labour. This can present itself in different ways. For some women it is a period of rest: the contractions ease off, while nature prepares you for the exertion of birthing your baby in stage 2. Other women start to lose heart, feel unable to cope and stop thinking positively.

Midwives often recognize this transition period and know that, with encouragement, it will pass. Some women vomit during this stage, which is another positive sign that they are approaching stage 2 of labour. Other women begin to get an urge to 'bear down', although the cervix may not yet be fully dilated. It is hard to fight the urge to push but you should be encouraged to 'breathe through it', and to turn onto your knees with your bottom in the air, which will help to take the pressure off the cervix.

The trouble with labour is that you can get totally overwhelmed by the pain and all your good intentions for a natural birth go out of the window. I always tell pregnant friends and colleagues to just focus on keeping upright and active. Having done it twice I can guarantee it helps with the pain and speeds things up.

Wendy, mother of 3-week-old Erin

shared experiences

I had to be monitored because of the epidural. But the CTG was like having a TV on in the room. We all just stared at it.

Ceri, mother of 8-week-old Sophia

stage 2 of
labour

This stage lasts from full dilation until the birth. The contractions are described as expulsive and feel very different from those during stage 1, and many women find it easier to cope with them. The contractions cause an overwhelming urge to bear down and push out your baby, which is why women become more vocal at this stage, making involuntary noises with the effort of bearing down.

signs

The onset of stage 2 can be confirmed by a vaginal examination, although many midwives find this unnecessary because there are often other signs that the cervix is fully dilated.

These other signs include:
- Involuntary grunting with the effort of the contraction
- A heavy, blood-stained show (different to the show in early labour)
- Bulging of the back passage
- A slight dip of the baby's heartbeat with the contraction.

the baby's head crowns

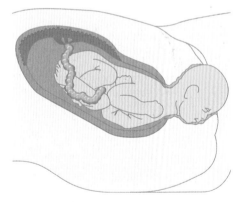

When the baby's head does not slip back between contractions, it is said to have crowned.

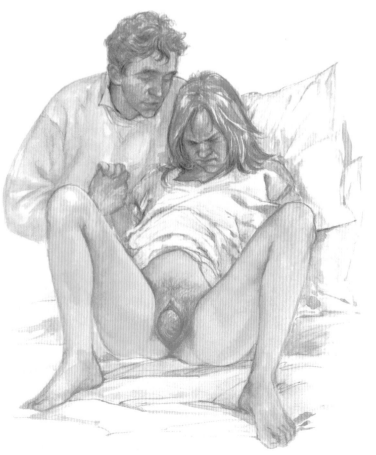

birth

There are always exceptions to the rule, but most women in the second stage of labour will feel an overwhelming, involuntary urge to bear down and push. It builds up like a wave and is impossible to fight, and some women even describe the feeling as sexual. Some women initially find the feeling scary as it is so powerful, not painful, but it becomes far less scary if you stop fighting it and just go with the feeling. Most women find it a relief to do so and push as their body tells them to. The best thing for you and your baby is simply to listen to your body and push spontaneously. If you do this, you will naturally give three or four short pushes, lasting about 5 seconds each, with every contraction. Research suggests that if you push spontaneously, it is better for you and the baby.

If you have an epidural and, because of this, cannot feel the contractions for yourself, the midwife can feel them by placing her hand on your abdomen and will tell you when to push. An upright position is best during stage 2, so that gravity can help your baby come down the birth canal. However, you may need encouragement to keep changing positions to help the the progress of the birth.

With each contraction, your baby will start to move down the birth canal until a small part of his head is visible. With a first baby, the head will slip back between contractions but, eventually, the head stays in position and more of it can be seen. This is called crowning and some women experience a burning sensation at this point.

Q Will I open my bowels during this stage of labour?

A   Many women have diarrhoea as a first sign of labour, and this is nature's way of clearing out the bowel before labour starts. A lot of women still open their bowels during labour and, if this is going to happen, there is nothing that you can do to stop it. 'Holding back' will make you more uncomfortable. If your bowels do not open when you push, it will feel as if they are, so you probably will not know for certain. During stage 2 of labour the baby's head puts pressure on the rectum, which is why you feel the need to open your bowels. This is a sign that the birth is imminent.

the baby's head emerges

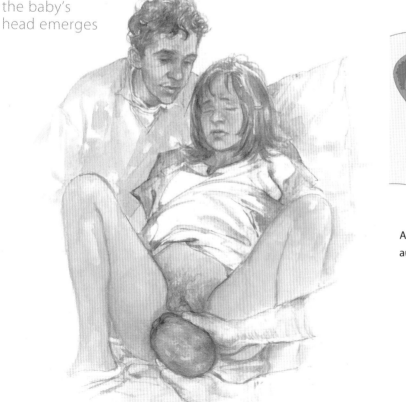

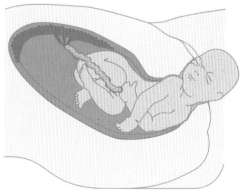

As soon as the head emerges, your baby will automatically turn it to one side.

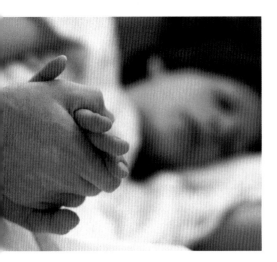

The midwife may ask you to pant rather than push at this point, in order to control the delivery of your baby's head and reduce the risk of tearing. Once a small part of your baby's head appears, reach down and touch it. Many women find this helps them to focus on where they are pushing, as well as giving them the encouragement of knowing that they are making progress and that the birth is not far off. Once his head is out, you will probably feel a sense of relief. Your baby will turn his head to come in line with his shoulders. which are turned to one side. The midwife will gently feel around his neck for the cord, which she can slip over his head.

The rest of your baby will be born with the next contraction. The first shoulder will emerge from under your pubic bone. Your midwife will gently lift this shoulder and your baby's head up to give the second shoulder (the one nearer the spine) more room. The rest of his body will then slip out easily accompanied by a further rush of amniotic fluid.

Your baby can then be placed directly onto your abdomen, either naked or, if you prefer, wrapped up. The cord can then be clamped and cut, either by the midwife or by your birth partner.

Even though you are probably feeling exhausted by now, you can take comfort from the knowledge that your new baby will be with you in just a matter of minutes.

the baby is born

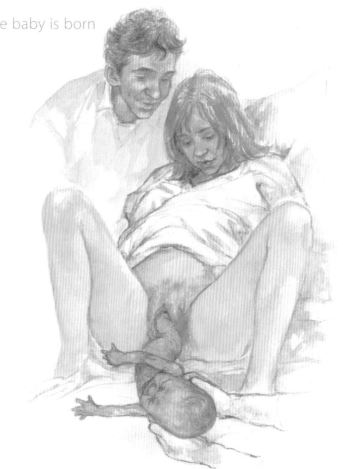

Q **I'm expecting twins. Will labour and birth be twice as painful for me as for mothers having just one baby?**

A Having twins does not automatically mean that labour and birth will be any longer or harder than for one baby. In fact, because twins are delivered earlier and are usually smaller than average, delivery may be even quicker and easier.

When your baby's head has emerged, he will turn it to one side and your next contraction will push out the rest of his body. Once his shoulders are delivered the rest of his body will slither out. Your new baby has finally arrived.

special deliveries

breech birth If your baby is in a breech position (see page 218), you will probably be advised to have a caesarean section, particularly for a first baby, if your baby is not in a 'frank breech' position, or is thought to be quite large. If your baby is found to be in a breech position when you are already in labour you may also be advised to have an emergency caesarean, unless it is too late and the birth is imminent. Ultimately the decision is yours so make sure that you are confident that you have had lots of information from your midwife or doctor.

twin and multiple births The majority of twins are delivered in hospital and you will probably be advised to have an epidural in case you need an emergency caesarean or an assisted delivery for the second twin. Both babies are usually continuously monitored during labour.

In some hospitals, it is policy to deliver twins in an operating theatre (even for vaginal deliveries) or in a larger delivery room, for safety and to accommodate a midwife and a paediatrician for each baby, as well as the obstetrician.

Although around 60 per cent of twin deliveries are by caesarean section, it is possible to have a normal delivery if the presenting twin is in a head-down position. If the first twin is in the breech position, your obstetrician will usually advise a caesarean section. During labour, an emergency caesarean may be required, either because labour is not progressing well or because there is evidence of fetal distress.

After the birth of the first twin, the second twin may be lying across the uterus, in which case it may be possible to turn him into either a breech or a head-down position so that he can be delivered vaginally.

You may be advised to have an epidural because of the higher risk of a caesarean section. After your first twin has been born, the obstetrician will confirm the position of the second twin and break the waters if necessary. Usually, you will be given a hormone drip to make sure that your contractions continue. The second twin is usually born within 20 minutes of the first.

Occasionally, he will show signs of distress, in which case you will be given an assisted delivery or a caesarean section. You will also be given a hormone drip after the birth. This encourages the uterus to contract to lessen the risk of bleeding because of the large area covered by the placenta.

Triplets or more are usually delivered by caesarean section. Much depends upon the position of your babies when you go into labour.

'It was a shock in labour when the midwife did a vaginal examination and said she could feel the baby's bottom, not his head. All along, everyone had thought he'd been head down.'

Paula, mother of
2-year-old John

shared experience

meconium

Your baby's first bowel movement is called meconium. It is a dark green-black tar-like substance, which can be passed during labour, particularly if your baby becomes distressed. Meconium is made up of different waste products, including bile pigment, mucus, amniotic fluid, lanugo and cells from the wall of the bowel.

stage 3 of
labour

The third stage of labour is the delivery of the placenta, which is expelled by contractions of the uterus. There are two ways of managing this stage: naturally (physiologically) or with an injection (actively). You should be given the opportunity to discuss the options beforehand, or put it in your birth plan, but how it is managed will depend partly on the nature of the birth.

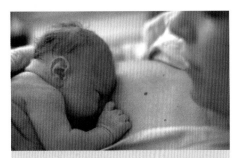

did you know?
Putting your baby to the breast will stimulate your body to release oxytocin. This makes the uterus contract, helping with the delivery of the placenta.

natural management

Women who have given birth naturally, with no intervention, often want to complete the process naturally, without drugs. Once the baby is born, the cord is left attached until it has stopped pulsating, when it is clamped and cut. The uterus will contract naturally, but it can take longer to expel the placenta. Blood loss tends to be heavier but this is seldom a problem as long as the mother is healthy and not anaemic.

It is perfectly normal to get the shakes after the delivery of the placenta. Your legs may feel wobbly as a result of change in body temperature and loss of fluid, as well as the sheer effort of childbirth. All being well, you will now be given a chance to spend some special time with your baby, so that you can get to know each other, before she is checked over.

active management

Immediately after the birth, the midwife will inject an oxytocic drug (ergometrine plus oxytocin) into your thigh. This is a synthetic hormone that causes the uterus to contract and the placenta to detach from the wall of the uterus. You will feel a contraction and the midwife will place one hand on your stomach while she gently pulls on the cord with the other hand. The blood loss tends to be lighter using this method, although the drug can make some women vomit.

The ergometrine can cause a rise in blood pressure, so, if you have high blood pressure, you will be given an alternative drug, oxytocin, intravenously. If you had an intervention during labour, for example, an induction, epidural, or an instrumental delivery, and are at higher risk of bleeding, it is advisable for the third stage to be actively managed.

complications?

The midwife will check the placenta to make sure that it is complete. Occasionally the placenta fails to separate from the wall of the uterus, or does so only partially, and a small amount of placenta left in the uterus can result in heavy bleeding and infection.

If various efforts to expel the placenta, for example, putting the baby to the breast and encouraging the mother to empty her bladder, have failed it will have to be removed manually in an operating theatre. This procedure is undertaken under spinal anaesthetic and the mother would be given a course of antibiotics afterwards in order to reduce the risk of infection.

stitches

After the delivery of the placenta, the midwife will check your vagina and perineum for any tears or grazes. A small tear that is not bleeding will heal naturally if kept clean and dry. A cut or a larger tear that involves muscle as well as skin will need stitching soon after the birth. You will be given a local anaesthetic in the area before the stitches are put in. The stitches do not need to be removed because they will dissolve. If you have had an assisted delivery, the doctor will stitch the cut as soon as the placenta is out and while your legs are still raised.

stitching procedure

In hospital, your legs will be placed in stirrups with your feet higher than your hips. You will be injected with a local anaesthetic a few minutes before the stitching begins. The muscle is aligned and stitched first and then the skin. You may be able to use gas and air while you are being stitched, although the local anaesthetic should provide enough pain relief. If the stitching is still painful, ask the midwife or doctor to stop until you are comfortable with the pain relief. The procedure usually takes about 20 minutes. At a home birth, the midwife will probably ask you to sit on the edge of the sofa or bed while she inserts the stitches.

Q **If I need stitches after the birth, could they burst open when I first open my bowels?**

A Opening your bowels will not make your stitches burst, but straining can make them feel uncomfortable – so make sure that you try to open your bowels in the first 2 or 3 days after the birth.

To avoid constipation, drink plenty of water, eat fresh fruits and vegetables, and start your pelvic floor exercises. Using a hospital toilet can be inhibiting and this does not help when you are trying to pass a stool for the first time after the birth. It can help psychologically to hold a sanitary towel against your stitches, to give the area some support. The midwife can give you a syrup to soften the stool and make it easier. Worrying about it will only delay things further.

'During my pregnancy I used to worry about having stitches after the birth. When I tore, I was not even aware it was happening. The midwife put the stitches in as I was cuddling Annabel, and to be honest I did not give it a second thought.'

Sue, mother of
6-week-old Annabel

shared experiences

'After I had given birth I felt the "loss" of my pregnancy. I actually missed my bump and all the allowances I had to make for it!'

Kai, mother of
10-week-old Robyn

unusual labours

There are times when everything does not go quite according to plan with a birth. Some babies appear before time and rapidly, while others take a lot longer than average. One thing is certain: everyone's experience of labour and childbirth will inevitably be slightly different and therefore your labour is unlikely to match your expectations in every respect.

sudden and fast birth

Many couples worry that the labour will progress so quickly that their baby is unexpectedly born at home or on the way to the hospital. This is called precipitate labour. It is unusual for this to happen, particularly with a first baby, and is more common in women who have already had a child. There are rarely any problems if a baby is born quickly. Problems are far more likely to occur in a labour where there is very slow progress. If you feel that your labour is progressing very quickly, you can always call your midwife to attend you at home or telephone for an ambulance rather than risk a car journey to the hospital. Women who have had a previous precipitate labour may prefer to go into hospital and be induced in a subsequent pregnancy, or have a planned home birth, rather than risk a journey in labour.

Premature babies can be born very quickly as the cervix does not have to be 10 cm dilated. If you show any signs of labour before 37 weeks of pregnancy it is very important to go straight to the maternity hospital, using an ambulance if the contractions are strong.

what to do in an emergency

Your partner will probably be reassured if he knows what to do in the event of a sudden birth – even if it never happens:

- If you feel the urge to push, get down on all fours, with your bottom in the air, and try to 'pant' through the contractions. This can help to delay the delivery.
- Have some clean towels ready to dry and wrap your baby and to put underneath you.
- If there is time, your partner should wash his hands.
- If your baby's head is visible, your partner should encourage you to pant and 'breathe' your baby out rather than push.
- Putting his hand on your baby's head will help to 'control' the speed of the birth.
- When your baby's head is out, stay calm and do not try to pull out the rest of her body. The body will be born with the next contraction.

'I know now why it is called labour. It is the hardest work I have ever done over 24 hours. It did not help that I was not allowed to eat and drink. How can you do the work without any energy? By the time the doctor told me I would need a caesarean I was absolutely exhausted, I just wanted the contractions to stop.'

Marlene, mother of 15-week-old Ian

shared experience

Your partner should carefully run a finger around your baby's neck and, if he can feel a cord, try to gently loop it over the baby's head.

- Support your baby's head as her body is born to prevent her falling onto the floor.
- Dry your baby with a towel to stimulate her if she initially appears to be a bit floppy.
- Wrap her up and cuddle her, keeping the cord attached.
- Do not try to cut or pull on the cord.
- Put your baby to the breast to feed as soon as you wish. This will help the uterus to contract.
- If you feel the urge to push out the placenta after a contraction, do so, but otherwise leave it alone. If the placenta is expelled, still do not attempt to cut the cord.
- Your partner should keep both of you warm. Hopefully, help should soon be at hand.

prolonged labour

Although an average first labour lasts about 10–12 hours, some labours are obviously much shorter while others are much longer. If you have had no problems during your pregnancy, the best thing you can do to keep your labour progressing is to stay at home for as long as possible. Many women find their labour slows down when they get to hospital.

There are a number of possible reasons for a prolonged labour and it is more common for first-time mothers than for women who have had a baby before.

tension

There is a cycle of events that midwives recognize all too readily, which is why you need encouragement during your labour to keep moving around for as long as possible.

- Your muscles tense whenever you feel anxious. The uterus is a muscle so tension can affect the contractions and slow them down.
- Rather than staying upright and moving about when you get to hospital, you may lie down on the bed. This can also slow down the progress of labour.
- If you are tense, you might find it difficult to deal with the contractions and ask for pain relief at an early stage of your labour. If you are given an injection of pethidine or an epidural this will confine you to the bed, in which case the contractions can slow down.

position of your baby's head

Your baby's position also determines the progress of your labour. In order for your baby's head to fit through your pelvis, she needs to have her chin tucked onto her chest. In some cases, the baby's chin is higher than this so that she has what is referred to as a 'deflexed head'. If the contractions are effective, your baby will tuck her chin down, but waiting for this can prolong labour.

'I woke up at 2 am with a grumbling stomach. I assumed it was something that I had eaten so I did not even bother to wake Will. I went to the bathroom and suddenly got the strongest urge to open my bowels. I shouted to Will as, all of a sudden, I realized that the baby was coming. It was the strangest feeling. I did not panic as I knew there was nothing I could do to stop it from happening. Jenny arrived at 2.20 am on the bathroom floor, where we both stayed until the ambulance arrived 5 minutes later. A midwife arrived soon after and checked us both over. I did not need stitches and there was no point in going to hospital. Although it was not planned it was still incredibly special, but next time we are planning a home birth. I have told the midwife that she will have to move in with me from 37 weeks of pregnancy!'

Sky, mother of
10-day-old Jenny

shared experience

what you can do to speed up the contractions

- Stimulate your nipples or clitoris. This will release the natural hormone oxytocin, which can get the uterus contracting.
- Have something to eat or drink – your body may be getting tired and running out of energy.
- Walk around, and go up and down some steps if possible.
- Pressure on a reflexology point near your ankle can stimulate the uterus to contract. Your partner can locate this point by putting his thumb on the inside of your ankle with his forefinger on the heel. The dip between these two points is linked to the uterus.

size of your baby's head

Labour will also be prolonged if your baby's head is large in proportion to your pelvis (see cephalopelvic disproportion, page 250). This is very rare. In this case, you may show signs such as a rise in temperature and pulse rate. A vaginal examination may show swelling on your baby's head. If these signs accompany slow progress, it may indicate that the head might not fit through the pelvis.

your baby's position

If your baby is in an occiput posterior position (see page 218), this can cause a prolonged labour. This is quite common. With regular contractions, most of these babies eventually turn round, but labour can be long and, at times, there may seem to be very little progress.

Because of the baby's position, you will probably feel much of the pain in your back, which can be distressing if there is a strong urge to push before the cervix is fully dilated. This is because the back of the baby's head is pressing on your back passage. A good position to adopt for this type of labour is on all fours, which takes the pressure off your back and allows your birth partner to massage you or put hot towels on the base of your back.

slow dilation

If progress is slow, the doctor may suggest an oxytocin drip to produce stronger and more regular contractions. It is also important to consider an effective form of pain relief, such as an epidural, as you may already be distressed and tired from a long labour.

If the cervix still does not dilate, despite the drip, a caesarean section will be necessary to deliver the baby. This may be a relief if you have genuinely had a prolonged labour or failure to dilate, even if this is not how you originally planned to give birth.

Some women have a rare condition called cervical dystocia, which affects the structure of the cervix. Some women are born with this, while others develop it as a result of scarring from infection and surgery. Despite strong uterine contractions, the cervix remains firm and does not dilate.

induced labour

Despite the best of intentions and well-scripted birth plans, some women need help getting into or speeding up labour and it is best to be aware of this, just in case it happens to you. Throughout your pregnancy, a lot of emphasis is placed on your due date, so you may be surprised to see that date come and go with no sign of labour.

Women should be offered an induction 7–14 days over their due date, as the placenta can start to deteriorate. Initially, this usually takes the form of a 'stretch and sweep', where the midwife gently inserts her gloved finger into your cervix and sweeps it around the bag of membranes. This can be done in your home or at the clinic. It can be a little uncomfortable, but it works in many cases.

reasons for inducing labour

There are various reasons for inducing labour, the most important being concerns about the welfare of the baby or mother. For example, labour may be induced if your blood pressure rises, or if you develop pre-eclampsia, although the initial approach is usually to try and lower your blood pressure by rest or medication.

However, there may be signs that high blood pressure is affecting the function of the placenta, which is your baby's source of food and oxygen and can affect his growth. Some babies are small for their age and the midwife might feel that their growth is tailing off, which again can be a sign of placental dysfunction. In both these cases, it may be necessary to induce labour. Some women, for example those with gestational diabetes (see page 81), have labour induced because their baby is getting very large.

Most women go into labour within 24 hours of their waters breaking. If this fails to happen within a day or two, there is a risk of the baby getting an infection, in which case the contractions may need a 'kick start'.

how labour is induced

The initial approach in inducing labour, particularly in the case of a first baby, is to insert a pessary or gel of prostaglandin (hormone) into your vagina. This softens the cervix and can start the contractions. However, this process usually needs to be repeated, and it may be a couple of days before the contractions begin. Once the cervix has started to dilate, the midwife can break your waters with an instrument that looks rather like a crochet hook. This will be a little uncomfortable but it should not hurt.

However, if you still show no signs of going into labour, then you may need an intravenous drip of oxytocin, a powerful hormone that makes the uterus contract. This requires close monitoring of both you and your baby because, in some cases, your body is not ready to go into labour and there is a danger of the uterus being overstimulated and your baby becoming distressed.

Being induced before your due date may increase the risk of a caesarean section, particularly with a first baby, so the decision should not be taken lightly.

speeding up labour with drugs

The majority of women go into labour spontaneously, but some women need help in speeding up their labour because the contractions can 'go off'. This happens particularly in cases where the mother has had an epidural, has been unable to stay upright, or if she has been in labour for a long time and the uterus is becoming tired. An intravenous drip of oxytocin should get the uterus contracting effectively, but both mother and baby need to be monitored closely (see above). The dosage of the drug is gradually increased until the contractions are approximately every 3–4 minutes.

'When I was induced I was worried that I would have to stay on the bed. The midwife still encouraged me to stand up, even with the drips and monitors attached.'

Jane, mother of 10-day-old Ned

shared experiences

'I would have preferred to go into labour naturally but it just was not happening. At the end of 18 hours, I got a live, healthy baby, which is what is important.'

Ruth, mother of 3-month-old Stephen

assisted deliveries

Forceps and ventouse are both types of assisted (or instrumental) delivery, in which instruments are used to assist with the birth of your baby. They can only be used during stage 2 of labour, so if your baby needs to be born quickly before this stage, she would be delivered by emergency caesarean section (see page 250). An obstetrician will perform both types of delivery.

'I never wanted a forceps delivery but when the midwife told me that my baby's heartbeat was slowing down as he was becoming distressed, I just wanted him to be born. I did not care how. My birth plan went out of the window but I was so relieved that David was alright that nothing else seemed important.'

Yvonne, mother of
3-week-old David

shared experience

reasons for assisted delivery

This type of delivery is commonly used if you have been pushing for a long time and your baby is making slow progress down the birth canal, particularly if she is showing signs of distress. This is more likely if progress has already been slowing during stage 1, perhaps indicating that you have a large baby or that the head is not in an occiput anterior (OA) position (see page 219).

ventouse/forceps trial

The obstetrician will carry out a vaginal examination in order to decide on the most appropriate instrument to help deliver your baby. This will depend upon the position of your baby and how far down the birth canal she is. If there is a significant chance that the instruments may still fail to deliver your baby then you will be advised to have the procedure attempted in the operating theatre. The obstetrician can then proceed to a caesarean section quite quickly. This is called a trial of ventouse/forceps. Your bladder will be emptied prior to the procedure, using a catheter, and your legs will be placed with your feet higher than your hips. Your midwife will stay with you throughout.

Q I noticed a mention of Vitamin K in an article about birth plans. What is this for and how is it given?

A Vitamin K helps blood clotting, and newborns do not have much of this vitamin. In rare cases, babies develop a problem known as haemorrhagic disease of the newborn (HDN), or Vitamin K deficiency bleeding, which can be fatal, so most babies are given Vitamin K either in the form of an injection after the birth, or as drops into the mouth (twice during the first week and, if breast-fed, again at 1 month old).

forceps delivery

forceps

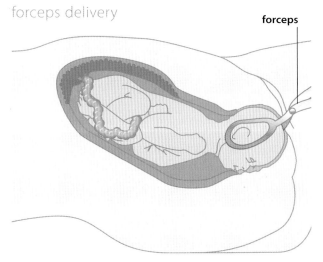

ventouse delivery

ventouse cup

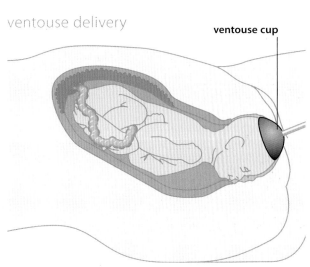

ventouse

A ventouse uses suction to help guide your baby out, and a metal or plastic cup is placed on your baby's head. The cup gets its suction either from a separate machine via a tube or from a hand-held device. While you push with each contraction, the obstetrician will gently pull the cup, guiding your baby out. It is not always necessary to have an episiotomy with this procedure.

forceps

Forceps are a pair of metal instruments that look rather like two large salad servers. They link together and are placed inside the vagina. The forceps cradle the baby's head and guide her out, although you still need to push with the contractions. Forceps known as Kielland's are used to help turn your baby if she is facing the wrong way. Neville Barnes' or Wrigley's forceps are used to guide and lift your baby out. As with ventouse, episiotomy is not always necessary, but is performed in many cases to help the baby's delivery.

effects on your baby

The delivery can cause distress or trauma to your baby, so it is usual to have a paediatrician in the room, with a resuscitaire (see page 222). In any case, you may have had an assisted delivery because your baby was already showing signs of stress, so it is a wise precaution to have a paediatrician and equipment to hand.

Babies who have had a ventouse delivery commonly have a bump on the back of their heads. This is usually reddish purple in colour and can be quite prominent. Forceps can sometimes leave two red marks on the side of your baby's head, but any bruises or bumps should go down within the first week.

Because of the bruising, these babies are more likely to develop jaundice. Occasionally, a baby appears irritable after an instrumental delivery, so it may be best not to let too many different people handle her for the time being.

With a forceps delivery, the mother will usually have a local anaesthetic or an epidural (see pages 256–257). Sometimes, particularly with a 'lift-out' ventouse, no anaesthetic is needed.

caesarean section

A caesarean section is a major operation involving an incision through the skin and muscles of your abdomen, and into the uterus, in order to deliver your baby. Unless there are medical grounds that make it the safest form of delivery for your baby, electing to have a caesarian section is not a decision you should take lightly. In the majority of cases the recovery time is much longer after a caesarian section.

'I wanted to be involved, so I asked if they'd take the screen down at the crucial moment so I could see James being born. It was amazing. First his head appeared, and then the rest of his body emerged. Although the delivery happened very quickly, it took a while for them to stitch me. To be honest, I wasn't bothered about that because by then I had my beautiful baby to cuddle!'

Cheryl, mother of
3-week-old James

shared experience

types of caesarean section

There are three types of caesarean section, depending on when the decision to perform the operation is made (the surgical procedure itself is the same):

Elective where the decision that a caesarean section is necessary is made before labour. There are many reasons for this decision, for example: a breech position of the baby, a previous caesarean, active herpes in the mother or her pelvis is deemed too small for the baby's head (cephalopelvic disproportion, or CPD).

Emergency where the caesarean is unplanned. In this case, the baby may have started to show signs of distress in early labour, or there has been very little progress. One of the causes for a decision to be made at this stage is when CPD (see above) is discovered once labour has already commenced.

Crash which is a true emergency. If the mother does not already have an epidural in place, she would need a general anaesthetic because the baby needs immediate delivery. Reasons for this include placental abruption, a prolapsed cord or severe signs of distress with the baby's heartbeat.

the operation

A caesaraean is no different from any other operation and you should remove any jewellery or nail polish. The top of your pubic hair will be shaved and the midwife will insert a catheter into your bladder just prior to the operation. A needle (a venflon or canulla) will be put into your hand through which fluid will drip in case your blood pressure falls. It takes about 10 minutes from the first incision until the delivery of your baby, and about another 40 minutes for the stitches to be put in the layers of muscle, fat and skin.

The procedure will not hurt but you will be aware of the pushing and pulling inside of you. Some women describe it as 'someone washing the dishes inside of their stomach'. The scar is just below the bikini line and will fade in time.

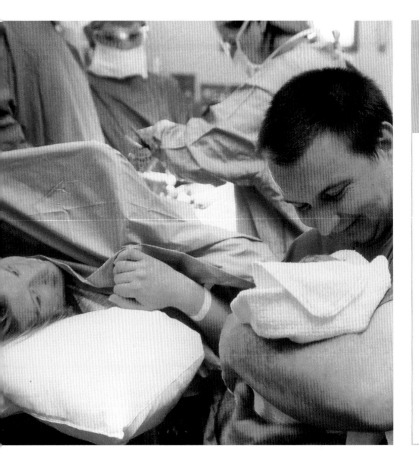

Your partner will probably be only too happy to cuddle his new baby while you are being stitched up.

anaesthesia

You will usually be given a spinal block or epidural so that you can stay awake during the operation and hold your baby soon afterwards. A general anaesthetic may be advisable if any complications are anticipated, for example, if there is a risk of heavy bleeding, as with placenta praevia (see page 114).

what happens afterwards?

A caesarean involves major surgery and problems can occur if your do not have enough rest and support afterwards. Being unable to do such a simple task as lifting or holding your baby can be frustrating. However, your midwife can show you different positions that can help, for example, placing a pillow on your lap, lying down or holding your baby under your arm to feed her. It is important to continue your pelvic floor exercises because the muscles may have lost tone during your pregnancy. However, you should avoid other forms of exercise (including driving, lifting and housework) for at least the first 6 weeks. Make the most of any help that is offered as you will need time to recover from the operation as well as having a new baby to look after.

Q I am going to have a caesarean section, as my baby is breech. My midwife has said that I can have a 'spinal'. Is this different from an epidural?

A A spinal block is similar to an epidural but involves injecting the anaesthetic into your back and then removing the needle. With an epidural, a fine plastic catheter is inserted into your back and left so that the drug can be topped up during labour. A spinal is quicker to insert and provides a short but very effective dose of anaesthetic. Because of this, spinals tend to be used for caesarean sections and, if necessary, towards the end of labour or sometimes for a ventouse or forceps delivery.

Q How much will my partner actually see?

A If your partner goes into the operating theatre with you, he will see very little of what is going on. Once everything has been set up and the anaesthetist has put your spinal block in position, a screen will be placed across you so that nothing can be seen from the top of your chest downwards. Your partner will sit next to you, close to your head, so he can only see your head and shoulders. As the baby is lifted out, he will be shown to you and then checked over by the midwife or paediatrician.

episiotomy
and tears

An episiotomy is a small cut made at the entrance to your vagina to give your baby more room during the birth. In the 1970s, it was a fairly routine procedure, particularly with a first baby. Nowadays, the main reasons for an episiotomy are the need for a quick delivery because the baby is showing signs of distress or forceps are needed for the birth.

Q Is it better to be cut or to tear?

A You may be fortunate enough not to have a tear or a cut, especially if you keep upright and moving as much as you can during your labour. Generally, it is better to tear than be cut, as tears may just involve the skin rather than going through the muscles, whereas a cut goes through both skin and muscle. Also tears appear to heal better and are more comfortable than a cut. If you tear, you may not even need stitches, as a small tear will heal by itself, as long as it is kept clean to reduce the risk of infection. However, in some circumstances, it is preferable to have an episiotomy.

Although it may sound daunting, once you are in labour it becomes much less of an issue. If you need an episiotomy, the midwife will get your consent first and then inject some local anaesthetic in the area where the cut is to be made. The area is very thin at the height of a contraction, and it is then that the incision is made – with one quick snip of a pair of sterile scissors. You are more likely to need an episiotomy if you need an instrumental delivery.

preventing tears

Some women do tear during childbirth and there is no guarantee that this will not happen. However, there are steps you can take to reduce the risk. Massage the area with wheat germ or sweet almond oil to make it more supple, and practise your pelvic floor exercises so that you become more aware of that area and can relax it when it comes to pushing out your baby.

As your baby's head is delivered the midwife will ask you to 'pant', not push, in order to control the speed at which the head is delivered and to reduce the chance of tearing. Even if you do tear, it does not necessarily mean that you will be stitched. Small tears have shown to heal just as well if they are kept clean.

position of tears

The most common tear goes from the entrance of the vagina towards your back passage. This area is called the perineum. A first-degree tear involves only the skin; a second degree tear involves skin and muscle; while a third-degree tear, which is less common, involves the lining or muscles of the back passage.

Sometimes tears are towards the labia or clitoris, and these can be extremely sore, particularly when passing urine. Drink plenty of fluids to dilute your urine and keep a jug by the toilet so that you can pour water over the urine as you empty your bladder, to make the discomfort more tolerable. Stitches do not have to be removed, as they will dissolve.

pain
relief

You can never judge in advance what pain relief, if any, you will want during labour, but it is important to be aware of the options and the effects they can have on your labour. Keep an open mind because many factors will influence your labour, including your baby's position, whether or not labour is induced, and even the shape of your pelvis.

There are many ways of dealing with contractions apart from using drugs. The main thing for you and your partner to accept is that you cannot cure the pain, only find ways of coping with it. Keeping active, by staying on your feet and moving around, will make a great difference to the labour and your ability to cope with the contractions.

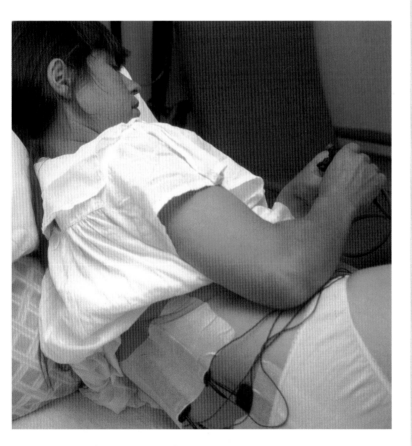

Views on how effective a TENS machine is are polarized. They can be a useful distraction from the pain, although you may not find they offer total pain relief.

'At first it seemed important to me to give birth naturally but I had assumed everything would be straightforward. I got to 7 cm dilated only using gas and air but stuck there for 4 hours because the baby was lying in an awkward position and the midwife advised me to have an epidural. I could not believe how different it felt, the pain relief was absolutely brilliant. I could not move my bottom half but I did not care. I thought I would be really disappointed not to have given birth naturally, but I gave it a go. It was the right decision as it was still another 6 hours until Ruth finally arrived.'

Vanessa, mother of
6-week-old Ruth

shared
experience

natural pain relief

PAIN RELIEF TYPE	WHAT TO DO	HOW IT WORKS
relaxation	Learn how to release the tension in your muscles, using breathing (see page 233). Relax your face, which will automatically relax your other muscles. Focus on some mental image or listen to a special piece of music, to distract you from the contractions and help you to relax through them.	Relaxing tense muscles encourages the body to produce endorphins, which are natural painkillers.
water	Relax in a warm bath. If you have backache, take a shower and aim the showerhead at the base of your spine. A hot-water bottle, or towels soaked in warm water, placed on your back may help, particularly if you have backache during labour.	The warmth relaxes the muscles, reducing tension and pain, and helping your body to produce natural endorphins.
massage and aromatherapy	You will be reliant on your partner for this (see pages 59 and 60). Research suggests that, just by visualizing your partner's hand massaging you, your body will release oxytocin, which helps the contractions to keep coming. Try putting a few drops of clary sage, jasmine or rose on a handkerchief to inhale during labour.	Massage is soothing and comforting, as well as relaxing tense muscles.
transcutaneous electrical nerve stimulation (TENS)	A TENS machine consists of a small portable handset and sticky electrode pads that you attach to your back.	With every contraction the machine releases small electrical impulses that block the pain and encourage the body to release endorphins.
hypnotherapy	Courses are available in different techniques such as hypnobirthing.	Uses self-hypnosis, deep relaxation, visualizations, anxiety management and breathing techniques to keep the mother feeling positive and in control.

ADVANTAGES	DISADVANTAGES	EFFECTIVENESS
Safe for mother and baby. You can keep active. Even if you are having a vaginal examination, or waiting for an epidural or pethidine to take effect, it helps to know how to relax.	None.	Relaxation will help you to cope with pain.
Safe for mother and baby. Suitable either at home and in hospital. Water supports the weight of your body and you can change positions easily.	None.	These measures will help you cope with pain by making you more relaxed, so the experience of pain is reduced.
Safe for mother and baby. Can work well in almost any position. Can be used with other methods of pain relief.	You may not feel like being touched when it comes to labour. Some essential oils should not be used during pregnancy – check with an aromatherapist.	Massage can be effective in helping you to cope – particularly with backache during labour.
Safe for mother and baby. Can be used at home and in hospital. Mother is in control of its use. Movement is not restricted. Easily removed if it does not work.	May need to be hired from a major drugstore or baby-care shop. (Not all maternity units have them, or they might be in use when you need them.) Cannot be used in a birthing pool.	Reports vary. Some women find TENS irritating or inadequate. Others say they could not have managed without it. It may be most helpful during early labour.
Safe for mother and baby. Can be used at home and in hospital. Mother is in control. Movement is encouraged. No equipment is necessary.	Courses are not universally available and may be expensive.	Mothers who have used the technique report less pain, shorter labour, less stress, fewer complications and medical or surgical intervention, quicker recovery times and better bonding with their babies.

medicated pain relief

PAIN RELIEF TYPE	WHAT HAPPENS	HOW IT WORKS
gas and air (entonox)	A mixture of nitrous oxide and oxygen that is inhaled through a mouthpiece or facemask.	Provides mild analgesia. Relieves tension.
pethidine or meptazinol	Narcotic drugs that are injected into the buttock or thigh by a midwife. They take 20 minutes to have an effect and last for up to 3 hours.	Mood-altering, producing relaxation and drowsiness. Relieves tension and anxiety, which can prolong labour.
epidural	A fine tube, inserted by an anaesthetist into the base of the spine, through which anaesthetic is introduced. This can either be topped up by the midwife, as required, or given continuously through an infusion pump.	Numbs the area from the waist down.
spinal block	An anaesthetist injects anaesthetic into the fluid around the spinal cord to provide short-lasting but very effective pain relief and then removes the needle.	Numbs the area from the waist down.

ADVANTAGES	DISADVANTAGES	EFFECTIVENESS
Safe for mother and baby. Mother controls its use. No restrictions on movement. Can be used in a birthing pool. Clears quickly from the system. Helps to establish a breathing pattern for each contraction. Can be used with other methods of pain relief.	May produce nausea.	Excellent for taking the edge off the pain – it will hurt, but you do not care so much!
Given by midwife, so readily available.	Crosses the placenta and can make your baby sleepy even after the birth – can be serious if given close to delivery. The baby needs to be closely monitored. May produce nausea, which can be counteracted by another drug. Mother may be confined to bed because of sleepiness.	Effective for women who are tense. Takes the edge off the pain. Some women find it hard as they can feel the contractions but are too sleepy to push.
Can lower blood pressure if it is very high. Will not affect the baby – unless blood pressure drops.	Anaesthetist needs to be available to administer an epidural. Mother must keep still while it is administered – difficult during contractions. Mother may need to be catheterized. A drip must be set up in case blood pressure falls. Risk of severe headache, if needle accidentally pierces the sheath around the spinal cord. Movement is severely or totally restricted. Can slow contractions – so a drip might be needed to speed things up. Mother cannot feel contractions so may need to be told when to push.	The most effective form of pain relief, which works in 90 per cent of cases. Unfortunately some women only feel the effects of an epidural down one side.
Can lower blood pressure if it is very high. Will not affect the baby – unless blood pressure drops.	Anaesthetist needs to be available and mother must keep still. Mother usually catheterized. Same risk of severe headache as epidural. Movement is restricted. Nausea is a common side-effect. Can take about 5 hours to wear off.	Very effective for fast pain relief for unplanned caesareans and some instrumental deliveries.

first few moments for you
and your baby

Nothing can prepare you for how you will feel when you first see your baby. Babies are often blue when they are born, but their colour changes as soon as they take their first breath. He may be covered in vernix, the white sticky lubricant which has kept him waterproof during his weeks in the amniotic fluid. If you want your baby to be placed onto your belly when he is born, let the midwife know.

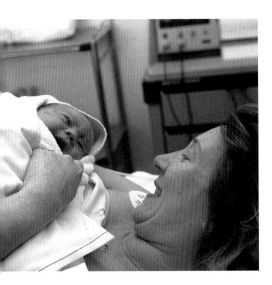

Eye-to-eye contact is a natural part of saying 'hello' to your new little bundle. At this age, he can focus his eyes for short distances.

contact

Whether you are breast-feeding or bottle-feeding, try to have some skin-to-skin contact with your baby immediately after the birth, to start the bonding process. Cuddle and stroke your baby, and give him an opportunity to smell and feel the warmth of your skin and listen to your voice talking to him.

Think about the surroundings into which he has been born. Ask if the lights can be dimmed and the noise kept to a minimum so that the birth is less of a shock for him.

feeding

If you have decided to breast-feed, you may want to put your baby to the breast soon after the birth. Babies have very strong sucking reflexes during the first hour and often latch on really well. Putting your baby to the breast also causes a reflex that helps your uterus contract, which reduces the amount of bleeding. However, your baby may be too exhausted and not particularly interested in feeding – after all, he has had a tiring, stressful few hours as well.

Some babies need an early feed to help boost their blood-sugar level, especially if they needed any medical attention when they were born and used up a lot of energy to get their heart and lungs working well.

If you need help with breast-feeding the midwife will be there to advise you. Once you feel confident, try putting your baby to the breast yourself and then asking the midwife to check that he is latched on properly. Some babies latch on immediately, but the majority need to learn what to do. To start with, your baby may only take a few sucks at a time, but this is quite normal. He is discovering what to do, getting to know your smell – and stimulating your breasts, which will help to produce more milk.

It can take a couple of weeks to get the hang of breastfeeding: just because your baby is not interested at first does not mean that you cannot do it.

Q **Will my partner be allowed to cut the cord?**

A Many partners love the thought of being the one to cut your baby's cord, and find it symbolic that they are making that separation between you and your baby. Occasionally the cord is around your baby's neck, in which case the midwife will slip it over his head or clamp and cut it. Otherwise there is no reason why your partner cannot do it. Even if he is not keen at the moment, it is worth asking him again because he may change his mind when the baby is born.

Q **What happens after the placenta is out?**

A Soon after you have given birth, the midwife will check over you and your baby. She will make sure that your baby is breathing regularly and that there are no obvious problems. She will put her hand on your tummy to feel that your uterus is well contracted so that the blood loss is not too heavy. If you have torn during the birth, or had an episiotomy, the midwife will stitch it as soon as she can. However, not every tear needs stitching – it depends on how deep it is, and whether or not it is bleeding. Your midwife will look at it and assess the damage.

time together

In the period after the birth, it is important that you, your partner and your baby spend some time together in order to get to know each other. Your baby does have to be weighed and measured, but there should be no rush to get this done immediately. After all, the measurements are not going to change drastically in a few hours. The midwife will make sure that you are comfortable and that the bedding is changed for you.

You will probably be desperate for a cup of tea and a light snack after all your exertions, and these will be brought to you in the room. This is a very special time, but you may still be shocked and exhausted after the delivery.

After coping with contractions every couple of minutes, and then the effort of pushing out your baby, it can seem really bizarre when it all suddenly stops. Your body is resting, the pain has gone, and you have this amazing baby in your arms – who, only minutes earlier, was your bump.

'Nothing prepared me for how I would feel when I saw her for the first time. It was just incredible that the bump that we had talked to for the last 9 months was now gazing up at us.'

Sheri, mother of 10-day-old Elizabeth

shared experiences

'I did not fancy the idea of my baby being put straight onto my stomach so the midwife wrapped him in a towel and then placed him in my arms.'

Amy, mother of 2-week-old Daniel

your baby's
appearance

Beautiful though she will seem to you, your baby may not quite match up to the newborn babies seen in glossy magazines. If you had an assisted delivery, she may still have some marks or bumps and her head may be rather elongated or even lop-sided. All this is normal and will resolve in time. She will be covered in creamy-white vernix and may be streaked with blood.

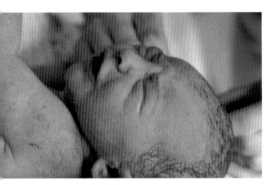

To make sure that everything is as it should be, your midwife or doctor will give your baby a thorough check in the few minutes after she is born.

On top of your baby's head, near the front, is a 'soft spot', or fontanelle, where the skull bones have not fused together. Do not worry about touching it because there is a tough layer of skin beneath it. There may be signs of swelling, which is quite normal if there has been pressure on the head during the delivery, and this will have been noted along with the results of other early tests.

Her eyes may also be puffy as a result of pressure during the birth but any severe discharge could be a sign of infection. Any birthmarks will be drawn to your attention, although it is quite usual for babies to have little pink marks, often called 'stork marks', which gradually fade. Her temperature will be checked because newborn babies can lose heat quite quickly – particularly if they are small or have a low Apgar score. Some babies have a blue area on their tummy or back, a bit like a bruise. The are called 'Mongolian spots' and are often found in babies of African, Asian, Mediterranean, Native American or Canadian origin.

the Apgar score

Parents often ask when their baby will be checked, unaware that their baby's first check took place at 1 minute of age. This Apgar test (after the doctor who devised it) is repeated again at 5 minutes. Five categories are assessed, which are each given a score of 0, 1 or 2, the total being out of 10. The categories include:

Colour Parents are often surprised that babies do not immediately come out pink but are tinged with blue. However they do pink up quickly after their arrival – especially after a good cry. In non-white babies, the inside of the mouth, the whites of the eyes, the soles of the feet and the palms are examined.

Heart rate Newborn babies should have a heart rate of over 100 beats per minute.

Breathing This should be strong and regular, as it will be if your baby is crying.

Muscle tone Your baby should be able to actively move her arms and legs.

Response/Reflex Your baby should respond to stimulation, such as being dried with a towel or handled. A healthy baby will have a score of 7 or higher, whereas a baby with a score lower than 7 may need time to recover from the birth. A baby with a very low score may need medical attention.

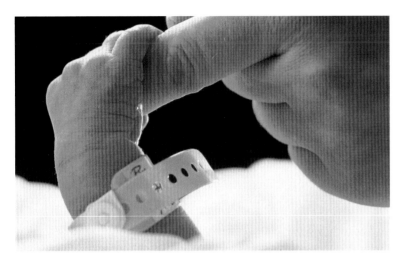

Tender touches and skin-to-skin contact can calm and soothe your baby. If she is born in hospital, she will get a name bracelet moments after she is born to make sure that everybody knows that she is yours.

early health checks

The paediatrician will carry out a thorough series of checks within the first few days, or this may be done by your doctor if he visits you.

Head and neck This involves checking the skull bones and fontanelle; the eyes, ears and nose; the roof of the mouth, to make sure that the palate has formed properly; and the neck for any signs of cysts.

Heart sounds and breathing 'Innocent' heart murmurs may be heard in the first few hours as her circulatory system adjusts. If the murmur continues, her heart may be scanned before you leave hospital.

Spine The doctor will hold your baby and run his thumb down the bones in her back (vertebrae) to check that the bones are in the right place and that there are no obvious abnormalities of the spinal cord.

Hips The doctor will bend your baby's legs up and turn them out to check for signs of a condition called congenital dislocation of the hips (CDH). This is when the ball at the top of the thigh bone (femur) does not fit properly into the socket of the pelvis or is dislocated. Many babies have 'clicky hips' where pregnancy hormones have made the ligaments loose. This is nothing to worry about and will improve with time.

Hands, feet, arms and legs The doctor will check the feet for signs of them turning turn in excessively (talipes). This is often related to the baby's position in the uterus and will correct itself. He will also look at the creases on your baby's palms – there are usually two. A single crease may indicate Down's syndrome, in which case further checks would be made. He will also check the tone and strength of the limbs.

Genitals and anus Babies commonly have swollen genitals after birth and a baby girl may have some vaginal discharge for a couple of days. The doctor will check that the genitals are formed properly and that a boy's testicles are in his scrotum (not undescended). The doctor will also check with you that your baby has opened her bowels (passed meconium, see page 241).

Reflexes The doctor will check the baby's reflexes, which are present at birth and indicate that the central nervous system is working correctly.

'I could not stop gazing at Alex when he was born. It was incredible to think that, for all those weeks he had been my "bump" and now, at last, here he was.'

Lindy, mother of
8-week-old Alex

shared experiences

'I was a bit shocked by how blotchy and spotty she was when she was born, but the midwife told me that nearly all babies have small, white facial spots – called milk spots – in the first few days. They disappeared within a few weeks and her skin is beautiful now.'

Caroline, mother of
8-week-old Freya

premature babies

All babies born before 37 weeks of pregnancy are deemed premature, although a baby born at 24 weeks is obviously going to need a lot more help than one born at 36 weeks because he is still very immature. In the United Kingdom, approximately 7 per cent of babies are born prematurely and in the United States about 11.5 per cent of babies are premature.

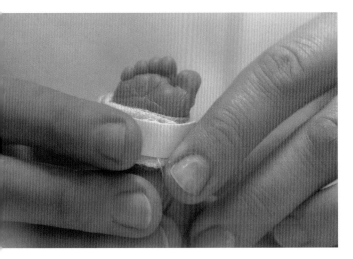

Drops of blood are often taken from a baby's foot if blood tests are needed when he is premature and in special care.

reasons for early birth

Sometimes labour just starts unexpectedly early. At other times, labour may need to be induced before 37 weeks because there are serious concerns about the wellbeing of the mother and baby, for example, if the mother has severe pre-eclampsia or if the placenta is not functioning properly. Women with a multiple pregnancy, for example, twins – or especially triplets – are more likely to go into early spontaneous labour.

Early labours tend to be quicker as the cervix does not have to dilate to the full 10 cm to allow a small baby to pass through (see page 244). However, an early labour can come as a great shock because you are seldom totally prepared.

care of premature babies

Many premature babies need help with their breathing because it is not until the final weeks of pregnancy that their lungs are fully mature. A mechanical ventilator may be used to push air in and out of your baby's lungs.

Also, small babies do not have much fat laid down and can lose heat very easily. If they get cold, they will not feed and their blood-sugar level will fall (hypoglycaemia). Many premature babies are therefore cared for in an incubator, where they can be kept warm.

Small babies are unable to suck at the breast at first, so it is important for you to express milk so that your baby can be given it through a tube. Expressing your milk ensures that you will have a good milk supply when he gets bigger and stronger and can be put to the breast.

Premature babies are also more prone to infection and, unfortunately, being premature is the single biggest cause of death in babies. Although the survival rate of premature babies has increased over the last few years – and many premature babies soon catch up with their full-term peers, the number of babies born prematurely has not reduced significantly. Also, there is an increased risk of disability amongst premature babies, particularly in those born extremely early.

coping with a premature baby

When you are not practically or emotionally prepared, the early arrival of your baby can be quite overwhelming. You may find that his condition varies from day to day, depending on how early he was born, and that there are times when it is a matter of two steps forward and one step back.

If you have other children, you may have difficulty dividing your time between everyone. It is also difficult to make any plans because it is usually impossible for anyone to predict exactly when you will be able to take your baby home.

Parents have a vital role to play, even when a premature baby is on the special-care baby unit. If you are unable to put your baby to the breast you will still be encouraged to express your breast milk so that it can be given to your baby via a tube. There should be facilities on the unit for doing this. Your baby will recognize your voice so talk or sing to him, even if you cannot hold him.

Most babies on a special-care unit will be in an incubator. This is a plastic cot with a lid, which has a thermostat to control the heat so that the baby does not get cold. There is a port hole through which you can touch and stroke your baby. Parents are encouraged to provide as much of the care as possible in this unit, and you will be expected and encouraged to help with feeding, washing your baby and changing his nappy.

risk factors for premature birth

It is difficult to identify which women are most at risk, but certain factors are known to increase the risk of having a premature baby.

- Smoking
- Use of recreational drugs
- Very high caffeine intake
- Previous premature birth
- Previous cervical surgery
- Certain pregnancy-related medical conditions, for example, cholestasis (see page 79).

Premature birth is also associated with infections so it is important to have your urine checked regularly at the antenatal clinic. Also tell your doctor or midwife if you have any unusual vaginal discharge. They can confirm any infection and advise appropriate treatment (see also page 99).

'I never dreamt that our baby would be born early. We had nothing prepared but the only thing that mattered was that she was alright. The members of staff on the special-care baby unit were amazing. We will never be able to thank them enough for the care that they gave Millie and I will never forget the day we were able to bring her home.'

Julie, mother of
5-month-old Millie

shared experience

special-care
baby units

The special-care baby unit (SCBU) is a separate ward run by specialist nurses and paediatricians. Although it deals mostly with premature babies, there are other babies who also need to spend some time here. Especially after a full-term pregnancy, it can be a huge shock to new parents to find that their baby has a problem that requires special care.

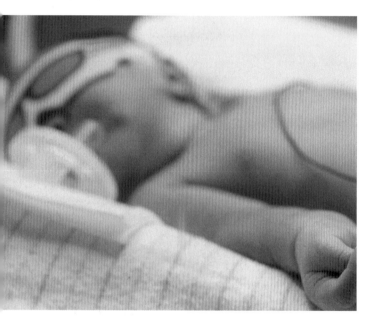

It can be incredibly upsetting to see your baby wired and tubed up in a special-care unit, but it is reassuring to know that she is being looked after by specialists and is receiving the best care available.

Parents can find an SCBU quite daunting, because it is full of beeping machines and alarms sounding on cots. Although the staff are used to this, parents tend to assume that every alarm is a sign of something seriously wrong, which is often not the case. Many babies have a fine cable attached to a pad on their foot or hand, monitoring their pulse rate and oxygen levels. If a baby moves or knocks against the pad, it may sound an alarm because it needs to be repositioned.

special-care babies

The majority of babies are born without problems but, if there is any concern, they are best being cared for by specialist staff. There is a high ratio of carers to babies in SCUBs. The care can range from a few hours of observation to intensive life support.

The specialist staff in the SCBU will encourage you to participate in the care of your baby and will explain what is going on so that you feel involved. Some babies develop breathing difficulties soon after birth, making a 'grunting' sound as they breathe. Initially they may just be observed and encouraged to have an early feed, but if the difficulties persist they may have an infection. The paediatrician will arrange for the baby to have some screening tests, including a chest X-ray, swabs, lumbar puncture, and urine and blood analysis, and may recommend a course of antibiotics. Other babies develop severe jaundice and need a course of light therapy (phototherapy); some have a very low blood-sugar level, a structural abnormality, or they may have inhaled meconium during the birth.

How long a baby stays in the SCBU depends on the problem and how well she responds to treatment. SCBUs often have different 'areas', depending on the level of specialist care that the baby needs. As a baby improves she will move areas, until she is ready to go home.

coping with the news

With so many screening tests available nowadays, parents assume that any significant problems or disabilities will be picked up during the pregnancy, but this is not always the case. Some medical conditions or disabilities, such as cerebral palsy, are not always identified before the birth.

Your initial reaction may be denial, thinking that the professionals have made a mistake. More commonly, the feeling is guilt. What did I do wrong? Did I eat or drink something to affect my baby? Although you will be reassured that you are not to blame, you will still feel guilty and blame yourself. It can help to get in touch with an organization where you can talk to other people with similar experiences. These groups can be a great source of comfort, advice and hope.

Sometimes, despite all the efforts of the medical team, a newborn baby dies. Dealing with this tragedy is one of the hardest things new parents will ever have to do. It is important that both parents are open about their feelings of loss so that they can learn to accept them and can support each other through the grieving process. If your baby dies, you will still be encouraged to spend time with him, having cuddles and building some memories. You will be offered counselling which can help and strengthen you in your bereavement.

Q **My friend's baby was jaundiced and had to stay in hospital for a few days. Is this unusual?**

A   Jaundice is very common in newborn babies and usually appears on the third day after the birth, disappearing by a week. The baby's skin develops a slight yellowish tinge due to the presence of bilirubin, a pigment produced by the breakdown of red blood cells. This is a normal process and, in most cases, does not need treatment. Your baby will excrete the bilirubin as she soils her nappies, so the more she feeds the sooner this will happen. Your midwife may ask if she can take a small amount of blood from your baby's heel to check the level of jaundice. However, if your baby is alert and feeding well, the midwife may not think this necessary.

A few jaundiced babies need to stay in hospital for a couple of days for a course of phototherapy, and this could be what happened to your friend's baby. For this treatment, the baby lies in a cot under a fluorescent light, which speeds up the process of clearing the jaundice. Some babies are more prone to jaundice, for example, premature babies or babies who have had an instrumental delivery. Occasionally, it can indicate an underlying disorder, but it usually clears up without treatment.

'The first time I saw him properly was in the special-care unit. I felt as if he did not belong to me as everyone else was talking about him and telling me about his progress. I kept myself together but I felt like picking him up and running out of there with him. He was my baby, not theirs!'

Ruth, mother of
12-week-old Stevie

shared experiences

'I had never intended to breast-feed but when Jack had a chest infection and went to the special-care unit, the nurses encouraged me to breast-feed. I was so glad that I did this as I felt that it was something that I could do for him that nobody else could.'

Esther, mother of
3-week-old Jack

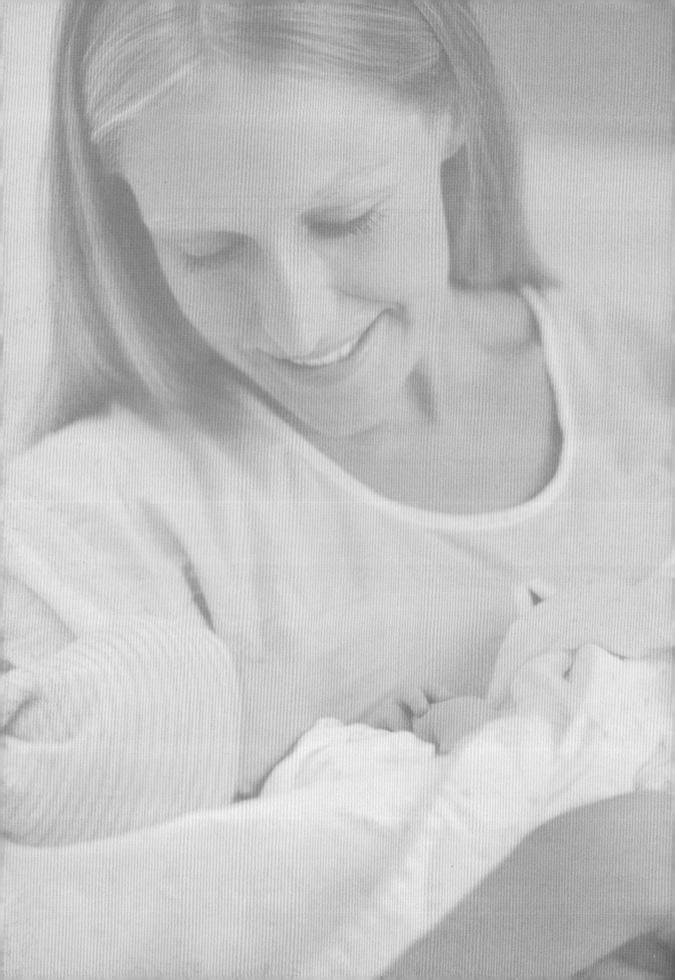

the first
few days

At last, you meet the tiny person who has been growing inside you. In the few days after he is born, you can feel like you never have a moment to rest – feeding, changing nappies and clothes, and getting him to sleep can seem to take up so much time. It's a good idea to have some help – from your partner, mother or sister, or friend – because, as all your time is taken up with your baby, someone needs to look after you.

hospital
routines

Every hospital has its own routines, which are there for your benefit as well as that of the staff. Being away from home with your new baby can be quite daunting, so be prepared and make sure that you know what to expect. Most hospitals have unrestricted visiting hours for partners but other visitors may only be allowed to visit during certain hours of the day.

' Being in hospital after the birth had its pros and cons: it was great to be brought regular meals without having to prepare them myself, but the noise was incredible. I was so hypersensitive to the sound of babies crying that I could hear the sound in my head for hours after I returned to the peace and quiet of my home. '

Phoebe, mother of
9-month-old Rachel

shared experiences

' I took in my own pillow case and it was lovely to have that familiarity when I lay down to sleep. '

Lizzie, mother of
10-day-old Hazel

preparation

Take some luxury toiletries with you to pamper yourself and a large fluffy towel for a shower or bath, as well as suitable clothes to change into (see page 217).

There is no need to sit around in your nightdress each day. When your partner visits you, let him spend time with your baby while you soak in a bath and get changed into clean clothes. You are in hospital because you have had a baby, not because you are ill, so there is no reason for you to stay in bed.

baby care

Nobody expects you to know what to do immediately. Many women have never even held a baby before and, not surprisingly, need help and support with caring for their baby. There are often nursery nurses or healthcare assistants working on the postnatal ward, as well as the midwives, and all of them will be pleased to show you and your partner how to top-and-tail your baby, change a nappy, wind your baby and so on.

visitors

Most maternity units are happy for two people to be in the labour ward with you during the birth. However, once your baby is born, they will probably prefer other visitors to wait until you have gone to the postnatal ward. This ensures that there are not too many people wandering around and that the dignity of other women who are still in labour is respected. An emergency situation can arise very quickly and it is best not to have a corridor full of visitors when staff members are trying to push a trolley into the operating theatre.

length of stay

If you have had a normal delivery, you can usually have a wash or a bath on the labour ward, change your clothes, have something to eat and drink, and then move to a postnatal ward. Some women choose to go home directly from the labour ward if there have been no complications – particularly if they have had midwife-led care and are confident about feeding their baby. However, women usually go to the postnatal ward after an hour or so and stay in overnight, especially if this is a first baby.

How long you stay in hospital depends on a number of factors:

Type of delivery If you have had a caesarean section you will probably stay in for 4–6 days.

Blood loss If you have lost a lot of blood, you may feel a bit wobbly and may even need a blood transfusion.

Pre-eclampsia If you have had high blood pressure during your pregnancy, it still needs to be monitored after the birth to make sure that it settles down.

Your baby's condition If your baby was premature and was taken to a special-care unit, you may want to stay in for a few days so that you can be close to her.

Feeding Some babies take a few days to learn how to feed, either from the breast or the bottle.

Infections If you or your baby show any signs of infection, you may need a course of intravenous antibiotics, which will take a few days to take effect.

checks

After the birth, the midwife will check both you and your baby each day to make sure that you are both well enough either to go home or, more commonly, to a postnatal ward. She will make sure that you are recovering well from the birth, that your blood loss is not too heavy and that any problems, such as a rise in blood pressure, are identified. She will also check that your baby is thriving, feeding well and that her cord is clean and dry.

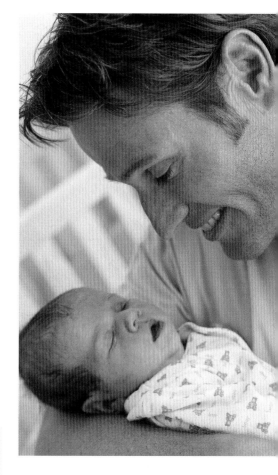

Those early days offer lots of chances for cuddles with your newborn. It is great, too, if your partner is around to let you have a rest or a chance to sleep in between feeds.

Q **If I am tired, will the midwives look after my baby overnight?**

A This does not tend to happen nowadays because it is much better if your baby stays with you. However, if you have been particularly poorly, a member of staff may offer to look after your baby for a while so that you can get some rest. Staying with your baby at night is part of the process of getting to know each other – learning each other's sounds and smells, and feeding her when necessary. Even if you feel tired, which is inevitable, you will probably be more relaxed having your baby with you, where you can see her, rather than wondering whether every cry you hear is your baby!

your body
after the birth

Many women look in the mirror when they get home and compare their body with a half-deflated balloon, so you are not alone! Do not expect to be able to squeeze yourself into your pre-pregnancy jeans yet. Not only have your muscles and skin been stretched, but you may also be retaining quite a lot of fluid (oedema). Your body also needs time to recover after the birth.

'I had an episiotomy with my daughter and tore with my son so both times I needed stitches. I was incredibly lucky in that they never bothered me – some of the other mothers in my parentcraft classes suffered horribly afterwards.'

Georgina, mother of 6-month-old Sam

shared experiences

'Your body may never be the same after the birth, but it is quite surprising how little you care. I had no trouble with weight, but my episiotomy scar gave me trouble for a full four months afterwards, and I won't even get started on my lost cup size!'

Victoria, mother of 7-month-old Jonas

swelling

Once you are home, you may find that your feet and legs become swollen, in which case raise your feet when resting, or sleep with a pillow under your feet. You will gradually lose the excess fluid as you pass urine.

stitches

Any stitches given after a vaginal delivery will dissolve, so they do not have to be removed. However, you need to keep the area clean and dry. A daily soak in the bath can make a big difference to how you feel. Adding four drops of lavender oil to the bathwater may help and you may prefer to sit on a rubber ring. If you have had a tear or a cut (an episiotomy), your midwife will check that the area is healing and that there are no signs of infection.

A caesarean section involves different types of stitches: some dissolve but others have to be removed by the midwife on about the fifth day after delivery. Most women do not find this painful because the area often still feels numb. If you are worried, you can always take a couple of painkillers beforehand.

bleeding

After the birth you will have a blood loss – called lochia – which is similar to a heavy period. This can last for up to 6 weeks, even after a caesarean. However, the flow should become a lot less after the first week and will become more of a brownish discharge, gradually becoming lighter. Use sanitary towels, not tampons because these can cause infection.

If you notice any clots on your sanitary towel, show them to your midwife. She can examine them to make sure that it is only blood. Very occasionally, the clots contain a piece of placenta, which means that not all of the placenta has been expelled. If the blood loss is heavy, or smells bad, tell your midwife because this could indicate an infection and you may need some antibiotics.

after pains

Once you have given birth, your uterus shrinks, taking about 6 weeks to return to pre-pregnancy size. As it contracts in the first few days, you may feel 'after pains', which are similar to period pains. These pains are stronger with a second or subsequent baby and are more noticeable when you are breast-feeding. Any pains should respond to mild painkillers, a soak in a warm bath or a hot-water bottle held against your stomach. Your midwife will check your uterus by gently pressing on your abdomen.

bladder and bowels

Your bladder should return to normal after the birth of your baby, but you may feel bruised from the delivery. Passing urine may sting, especially if you have had a tear. If this is a problem, try passing urine in a warm bath or pour a jug of lukewarm water between your legs while you are sitting on the toilet. Drink plenty of fluids and resist the temptation to hold the urine for as long as possible because this will make you more likely to get an infection.

It may be a few days before you open your bowels again. You may find being in hospital inhibiting and want to take your time in the toilet and you may also be worried about the stitches (see page 243). Drink plenty of water and eat fresh fruit, vegetables and other fibre-rich foods. Also, remember that any codeine-based painkillers can cause constipation. If you still have not opened your bowels a few days after returning home, your midwife can arrange for a mild laxative.

breasts

Around the third day your breasts will become large, hard and engorged with milk. This will happen even if you decide to bottle-feed, but nowadays you will rarely be given medication to prevent this happening. The milk will come in and the discomfort will go after a couple of days, so wear a good support bra in the meantime.

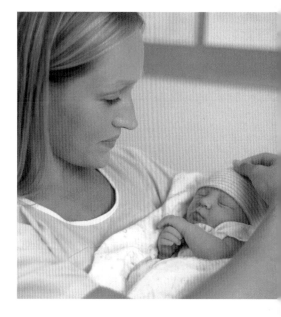

After the birth, focus on your baby and building a relationship with him and worry about getting into your jeans a bit later.

Q How long will it take to lose the weight I put on?

A Women vary in the amount of weight they gain in pregnancy and in the time it takes to return to their pre-pregnancy shape. You'll lose some weight almost straight away after the birth, and more weight is lost as the uterus contracts to its normal size. It is important not to do too much when you are a new mother, so rather than aiming to return to your pre-pregnancy weight as fast as possible, try to relax, feel good about yourself, and be assured that with all the exercise you get from looking after a new baby, you will soon lose the weight.

pelvic floor
exercises

The pelvic floor consists of a 'hammock' of muscles and ligaments, resembling a figure of eight, and stretches from your pubic bone (at the front) to the bottom of your backbone. This holds your bladder, bowel and uterus in place, as well as helping to close the outlets of the bladder and bowel. The muscles also play a role in love-making – their contractions increase the pleasure for both you and your partner.

pelvic floor muscles

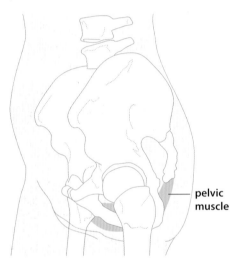

pelvic muscle

Regular exercise of the pelvic floor muscles will help to prevent such problems as stress incontinence as well as to make you more aware of them during the second stage of labour when you need to control them.

These muscles and ligaments come under strain during pregnancy and childbirth so it is important to maintain their strength by exercises. The weight of your baby during pregnancy places a strain on the muscles, but the hormone relaxin also softens and stretches them. If you have any strain or weakness in these muscles, you may leak urine – particularly when you cough, laugh, sneeze or exercise.

the importance of these exercises

Prolonged or repeated stretching of these muscles can result in permanent damage. If you ignore any weakness in your pelvic floor, you may develop conditions such as a prolapsed vagina, rectum, bladder or uterus. This is where the muscles fail to support the organs and start to 'drop', bulging into the vagina. This can result not only in urinary incontinence but also in lack of control over bowel movements. Surgery may be necessary to repair this.

when to start the exercises

There is no reason why you should not start doing these exercises as soon as you find out that you are pregnant. It is important to continue these exercises, not only during your pregnancy but also after the baby is born, in order to help yourself to regain the muscle tone. Do not leave it until after the birth because you will not be able to feel the muscles as well as you can now. All women should do these exercises throughout their lives to guard against stress incontinence (involuntary leakage of urine).

how to do these exercises

Sit comfortably, with your back straight and knees relaxed and held slightly apart.

• Imagine that you are trying to avoid breaking wind, or that you are 'holding on' to a desperate need to open your bowels. As you squeeze the muscles around your back passage you should feel the muscles move. Do not lift your buttocks or move your legs.

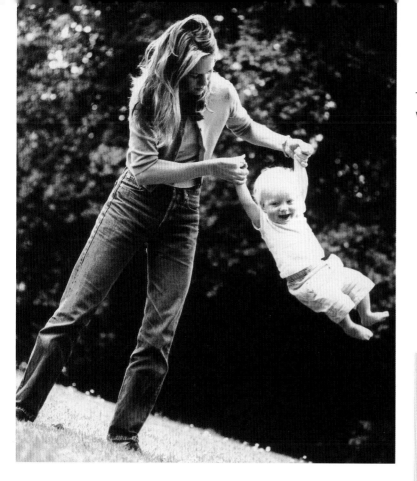

Taking time to do your pelvic floor exercises will pay off in later years.

- Imagine that you are sitting on the toilet to pass urine. Clench the muscles that you would use to stop the stream of urine and imagine drawing them up, like an elevator rising.
- Imagine that you are trying to grip a tampon in the vagina using your pelvic floor muscles.

In each case, relax the muscles quickly and then repeat the exercise. Try to combine the three exercises. Pull up the muscles quickly several times and then do the exercises again slowly. Think about the position of the different muscles and how they feel. Imagine the muscles as an elevator – rising three floors and stopping at each one. When they are on the top floor, lower them in stages, stopping at each floor! Repeat the exercises ten times, five times per day.

Check that you are doing the exercises properly by putting a finger into your vagina and feeling the muscles tighten as you clench. Develop an awareness of how your muscles feel when they are relaxed. This is important in the second stage of labour, when you are pushing out your baby. Tighten the muscles of your pelvic floor as you breathe in and then with each outward breath, slowly relax the muscles as much as possible.

Try to associate the exercise with another activity, for example when you have a drink or after you have passed water. It does not matter what position you are in – you could be standing, sitting, squatting or lying down. The great thing about these exercises is that you can do them anywhere and at anytime and no one else will be any the wiser about what you are doing!

> ' I have only just realized that my pelvic floor muscles have been weakened – almost 6 months after the birth – because I've gone back to work and promptly caught a cold … and every time I sneeze, I leak. '
>
> Cecilia, mother of 6-month-old Joshua

shared experience

your emotions
after the birth

In the first few days, you will probably experience a range of emotions, including relief, exhaustion, fear, anxiety and elation. Some women feel guilty because they assumed that they would fall head over heels in love with their new baby, but now find that it is something that grows gradually. Others are exhausted after giving birth, uncomfortable because of stitches and need time to get to know their baby.

'The love that I felt for Katie was overwhelming. I felt so frightened that something awful would happen to her if I left her alone for a minute. It was a relief to talk to my midwife and find out that I was not the first mother to feel like this.'

Helen, mother of
3-month-old Katie

shared
experience

Some women may feel regrets for not giving birth in the way that they had planned, disappointment that they are unable to breast-feed, or neglect because everyone else's attention is firmly focused on the newly arrived baby.

Often women feel that everything should get 'back to normal' as quickly as possible – expecting to fit into pre-pregnancy clothes, sleep through the night and have a tidy house. This is where many mothers feel disappointed – as if they have failed when this tiny baby dominates their lives day and night!

So many women talk about getting into 'a routine' but, in practice, there is no routine in the early days. Forget about the housework. Pick up your baby, cuddle him when he wants to be cuddled and feed him when he wants to be fed.

baby blues

Whether or not you decide to breast-feed, your milk will still 'come in' at about the third day. This coincides with a rush of hormones that can give you the 'baby blues'. It is completely normal to feel weepy, and your midwife will reassure you that, in the majority of cases, this passes in a short while. It can be useful to talk through the delivery with your midwife so that you can be sure of understanding everything that happened during the birth. However, nothing will prepare you for the changes in these first few days, not only in terms of your body but also the huge, and sometimes overwhelming, feeling of responsibility towards your baby.

postnatal depression

The 'baby blues' may continue, or they may not appear until a few weeks after the birth, which may mean you have postnatal depression. This affects approximately 12 per cent of women in different ways, for example, feelings of detachment, anxiety, inability to cope, weepiness and unhappiness. Some women regard this as a natural reaction to a life-changing event. For others there is a particular reason, for example,

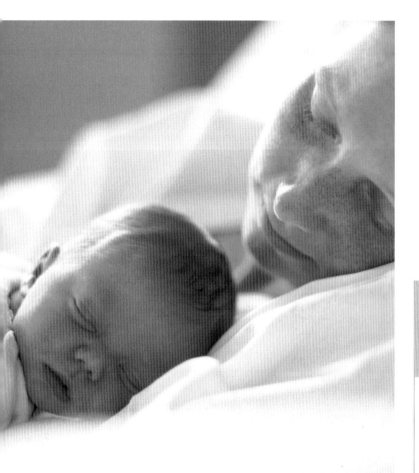

When your baby naps, grab the chance to close your eyes too. You can cuddle up together so long as you observe the rules for safe sleeping (see page 278).

their baby being on a special-care unit, a traumatic labour or insufficient support after the birth. Whatever the reason, you should tell you midwife, health visitor or doctor so that you can get help.

Often you can find support from groups of women who have had experience of postnatal depression. Nowadays, there is great social pressure for your life to return to how it was before you baby is born – your body, your home, routines and relationships – but the reality is that things have changed. Feeling low does not mean that you have failed as a mother – just that you need some support and help to get you through it.

The birth of a baby can have a great effect on your relationship with your partner and it is very easy to become competitive with your partner as to which of you is the most tired. Just acknowledge that you are both tired and both need to support each other. The chances are that you will both have times when you need some 'space' and 'time out' – even if it is just the luxury of an uninterrupted bath, half an hour watching television or a nap during the afternoon.

Q **After my baby was born I found life exhausting. How can I avoid it this time round without upsetting people?**

A It is only natural to want to show off your baby to the world, but some visitors can be hard work. You need to catch up on your sleep during the day, so it is a good idea to put a note on your door saying 'Mother and baby sleeping' or leave a message on your answering machine to say that 'Much as I would love to see people, the best time is between…' Most people would hate to intrude but, at the same time, they are genuinely excited about seeing your new baby. The most popular visitors are the ones that bring a cooked meal or take away a bag of ironing. Do not be shy of accepting help from friends and family if they offer. It will not only make them feel good but will also make a real difference, allowing you to spend time with your new baby and not worry about the other things.

feeding
your baby

Breast-feeding is undoubtedly better for your baby's health and development and 98 per cent of women are able to breast-feed. Nevertheless, it is not always possible either because of a medical condition or because the mother just does not feel comfortable with it. There is no reason to feel guilty: formula milk will meet your baby's dietary needs and there is no reason why she should not thrive on it.

breast-feeding

Breast milk is produced on a supply and demand basis. For the first two or three days, until your milk comes in, your breasts produce colostrum (a thick, creamy substance, packed with antibodies to protect your baby from infections and disease). The more your baby feeds at the breast, the more milk you will produce. The milk is made up of thirst-quenching foremilk, followed by a thicker hind milk.

Breast-feeding can be uncomfortable at first so you may need advice. Your midwife will advise you but you can prepare yourself by getting the telephone numbers of breast-feeding counsellors. Other women who have breast-fed can also give you support.

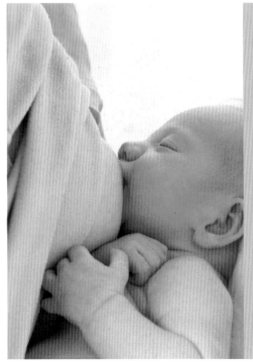

advantages of breast-feeding

There are many good reasons for breast-feeding if you are able to do so.
- Breast-feeding helps to protect your baby against serious infections of the ear and chest, as well as gastroenteritis (vomiting and diarrhoea).
- Breast-feeding helps to reduce the risk of eczema and asthma, particularly if you have a family history of these conditions.
- Some studies suggest that breast-feeding gives protection against ovarian cancer, breast cancer and hip fractures.
- Breast-feeding can help you to bond with your baby.
- Breast-feeding helps you to lose weight because it burns off any extra fat that you have accumulated during pregnancy.
- Breast milk is produced at the perfect temperature so there is no need for bottles and sterilizing units.
- Children who were breast-fed for 8 months or longer show a higher IQ score than those given formula milk.
- Breast-fed babies are less likely to be obese up to the age of 6 years.

In the first few days, while you are learning how to position your baby at the breast, your nipples may become sore. Then, on the third day, when your milk comes in, your breasts will feel large, hard and engorged. Do not worry – this is normal and does not last.

positioning

Nobody expects you to know how to position your baby at the breast but, if your baby does not latch on properly, your breasts will become very sore. You may need to experiment with different positions depending upon the type of birth and the size of your breasts.

- Make sure that you are comfortable.
- Hold your baby so that she is facing you so she does not have to turn her head towards you. Her head should be level with your nipple.

latching on

- Tease your baby with the nipple or let her smell your skin. As soon as she opens her mouth wide, bring her head to your breast.
- She should not only suck on the nipple but also have as much of the area around it (the areola) in her mouth as possible. If she only has the nipple in her mouth, break the seal with your finger, remove her from the breast and try again.
- When she is latched on properly her mouth should be wide open, with the nipple drawn deeply into her mouth. You will see the muscle in front of her ear working as she sucks.
- When she has finished suckling she will be content. This could take 5 minutes or 35 minutes. Place your little finger in your baby's mouth to release the seal; this will avoid painful pulling on your nipple.

bottle-feeding

When bottle-feeding, it is essential to follow the instructions about washing and sterilizing all equipment because babies can very easily pick up serious stomach infections.

- Wash bottles and teats thoroughly in warm soapy water, using a bottlebrush.
- Wash your hands thoroughly before making up feeds.
- Store prepared bottles of formula milk in a refrigerator for a maximum of 24 hours after they have reached room temperature.
- Do not keep the contents of a bottle for longer than half an hour after your baby has finished drinking.

Bottle-fed babies should still be fed on demand. Your baby will let you know when she is hungry and, unless she is jaundiced, very small or poorly, you should not wake her for a feed.

You may find that she will take more at some feeds than others and that she will feed more frequently at certain times of the day. It takes longer for babies to digest formula milk so they do tend to go longer between feeds. A newborn baby will probably take six or seven feeds in 24 hours and, in the first two or three days, will be taking approximately 60 ml at a feed.

did you know?
Research shows that your partner has the greatest influence on the way you feed your baby. Make sure that he is aware of the advantages of breast-feeding!

Applying Savoy cabbage leaves to the breasts can relieve engorgement. Keep the cabbage in the fridge until you need it.

Chamomile tea bags can help sore nipples to heal. After brewing the tea, store the bags in the fridge. Once they're cool, put them inside your bra against your nipples. Put a breast pad over them to protect your bra.

Breast-feeding helps your uterus contract and will also use up calories, which can help you lose some of the weight gained during your pregnancy.

about bottle-feeding

- If your baby seems hungry but does not take much milk at a feed, try using a larger teat, for example, a medium flow one. Some babies get tired quickly and give up feeding too early.
- Do not leave your baby to feed on her own, with the bottle propped up. She could easily choke.
- Do not increase the amount of powder in the feed just because your baby seems hungry. It can be very dangerous if the feed is not made up correctly.

your baby's
sleep

On average, your newborn baby will sleep for a total of 18 hours out of 24, but he will still keep you busy. He has developed his own sleeping pattern in the womb, so it is unrealistic to expect him to follow your sleeping pattern immediately now that he has been born. However, he will soon learn to distinguish between day and night and you will gradually be able to establish a routine.

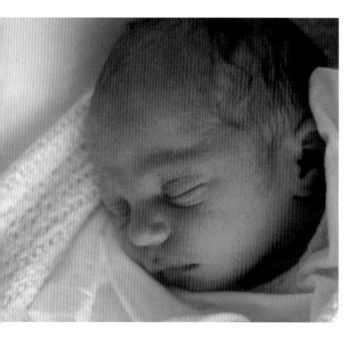

As a parent, you will never tire of gazing at your sleeping baby – in fact in the early months, your baby becomes the focus of every waking moment.

sleep patterns

As your baby grows and starts to feed less at night he will sleep for longer periods. By 4 months he will probably be sleeping twice as long at night as during the day. Make the most of his waking periods by talking to him and letting him kick on a mat on the floor. He is more likely to sleep soundly after some stimulation – it does not take much to tire a baby!

Being in a dark or quiet room will make no difference. Usually he will just like the security of being near you. After a few months, he will outgrow a carrycot or Moses basket, waking himself up by kicking or pushing against the sides.

Try to sleep while your baby is asleep during the day. This will help you to cope with sleepless nights. Understandably people will want to visit you, but try to limit visits to a certain time each day, so that there are periods when you know you will not be disturbed.

safe sleeping

Follow these guidelines to make sure that your baby sleeps safely:
- Place him on his back, with his feet at the bottom of the cot.
- Do not use a cot bumper or cover his head with a hat.
- Keep the room temperature at about 18 °C. At this temperature two blankets (not folded) should be sufficient.
- Blankets should come no higher than his shoulders, so that they cannot go over his head.
- Your baby's hands and feet often feel cool so feel his tummy or the back of his neck to judge his temperature.
- Never put your baby next to a radiator or heater, or give him a hot-water bottle.
- Do not let anyone smoke around your baby.

- Keep your baby in your room for the first 6 months, but only let him share your bed if you are breast-feeding.
- Never let your baby sleep in bed with you (even if you are breast-feeding) if you smoke, take drugs or have been drinking alcohol.
- If you have any doubts about the temperature of the room or how much bedding to use, ask your midwife or health visitor.
- Never sleep with your baby on a sofa.

calming your baby

Babies do cry and we cannot always tell why, which can be hugely frustrating. For much of the time they probably do not even know themselves. They are often more unsettled in the early evening, perhaps because they sense that you and your partner are tired. If you are feeling tense, take a deep breath and consciously relax your shoulders as you breathe out – babies easily sense any tension and will react to it by crying.

Ignore any advice telling you to leave your newborn baby to cry, unless you are totally at the end of your tether. In the longer term, your baby will feel more secure if he knows that you will respond to his crying and will be more relaxed. However it is worth allowing him to 'fuss' a little when you put him down, as he needs to learn to go to sleep on his own.

comforting a crying baby

Some of the methods used to comfort a crying baby may sound ludicrous but, when your baby is crying, you will try anything.
- Check whether his nappy needs changing.
- Offer him a feed – he may be having a growth spurt and want feeding more often.
- If you breast-feed and putting him to the breast comforts him, do not worry whether or not he is hungry or just sucking for comfort. Does it matter so long as he is content?
- Try winding him. Vary the positions: across your shoulder; seated on your lap while you support his head; or laid across your lap, having his back gently rubbed. If you think he still has tummy ache, try soothing him with a bath.
- Some babies like certain sounds, for example, the vacuum cleaner or running water. Record a tape of these noises and play it to your baby – you may find that he stops crying when he listens to the sounds.
- He may just want to be held, which is a perfect excuse for doing nothing except cuddle him.
- Whenever you feel unable to cope, put him in his buggy or take him out in the car – either of these can help to calm both of you!

twins

Some parents find that their babies settle better if they share the crib – after all, they are used to being in a small space where they can touch and see each other. If you let your babies sleep together, be sure to follow the rules for safe sleeping (see opposite). It is possible to buy a larger cot specifically designed for twins, although they will eventually need separate cots.

Inevitably, twins are exhausting. As well as caring for two babies you may be recovering from a caesarean section or a premature birth. Having good support when you leave hospital is essential. It can be worth contacting any local college that runs a nursery nursing course; they may be looking for somewhere to place a student, who can gain valuable experience while, at the same time, providing you with help.

caring for
your baby

Although in the early days, you may feel like you never have a spare moment, apart from feeding, newborns are actually fairly low maintenance. It can take time to work out what the different cries mean and what it is that your baby needs. As long as she is not hungry, has a clean nappy and is given plenty of cuddles, you will not go far wrong.

keeping your baby clean

Do not worry too much about bathing your baby in the first few days because she will not get very dirty. It is enough to 'top-and-tail' her with cotton wool and water, and to bathe her about twice a week.

top-and-tailing

You may find the following guidelines useful:

- Make sure that the room is warm and that everything you need is at hand. There is nothing so frustrating than starting to wash your baby and then realizing that you have left the towel in another room!
- Your baby might not like being uncovered so let her wear her nappy and vest and wrap her in a towel, holding her on your lap or on the changing mat.
- Begin by gently wiping her face with cotton wool and water – there is no need to use soap. Clean behind her ears, where milk tends to collect, but never try to clean inside them because the wax that you see inside the ear helps to protect her ear drum.
- Wipe any skin creases on her neck and make sure to dry them properly, patting them with a soft towel so that they do not become sore.
- Give her hands a wipe and dry them afterwards.
- You are now ready to change her nappy (see opposite). Clean your baby's bottom, wiping from front to back, that is, towards the back passage. Use a new piece of cotton wool each time to reduce the risk of spreading bacteria. It is not necessary to clean inside the vagina of a baby girl or to pull back the foreskin of a boy.
- Make sure that you dry her bottom thoroughly before putting on a clean nappy in order to reduce the risk of nappy rash.

- Your baby's skin is very sensitive so use warm water in the first few weeks. You may prefer to use wipes but, if your baby shows any sign of nappy rash, go back to water and cotton wool until it has cleared.

bathing

If you do not have a baby bath, a new washing-up bowl is perfectly adequate for bathing a newborn baby. She will have outgrown it by the time she is 3 months old. Some babies love a bath while others do not like the feeling of being exposed. Newborns need only a quick dip in the water while, at a few weeks old, she may prefer a few minutes soaking and splashing as part of her bedtime routine! Do not put too much water in the bath: about 6 cm deep will do. Test the temperature with your elbow or wrist to make sure that it is only just warm. Never leave your baby alone in the bath.

After her bath, you may like to massage her skin gently with a small drop of baby oil, but make sure the room is comfortably warm. If your baby develops cradle cap (a yellowish crust on the scalp) gently massage in some olive oil in the evening, washing it out the following morning with a gentle baby shampoo.

cord care

The cord will separate more quickly if it is open to the air and left dry, with the nappy folded over slightly. There is no need to bathe the cord unless it becomes sticky, in which case use cotton wool and water. Your midwife will check the cord daily, and it usually drops off by the tenth day, so you do not usually have to worry about it. If the area around it becomes inflamed or the cord begins to bleed, tell your midwife or doctor.

dressing your baby

In the first 2 or 3 weeks, you will be changing your baby's clothes frequently so you will need 6–8 stretch suits and the same number of vests or body suits. (Body suits are cosier in winter because there is no gap around the tummy.) For the first few months these can easily form the basis of your baby's wardrobe – just in progressively bigger sizes.

preparation

Do not buy too many clothes at first because you will probably get some as gifts. Also it is difficult to know what size clothing your baby will need until she arrives. Hand-knitted matinee jackets may be beautiful but they are often too ornate, with holes that can catch your baby's fingers or ribbons that can get into her mouth.

changing the nappy

Most people opt for disposable nappies, which are easy to use although not environmentally friendly. The main thing is to avoid getting nappy cream on the tabs, which makes them lose their stickiness. If this happens, just use some adhesive tape instead. Cloth nappies are cost effective, more comfortable to wear, and do not cause waste disposal problems. However they will need sterilizing, washing and folding after each use, although there are now many nappy-washing services who will do this for you.

swaddling

Babies often like the security of being swaddled but it is important that they are not overheated. Therefore you should only wrap your baby in lightweight material, as well as making sure that her head is not covered unless you are going outside. If your baby seems to settle better when swaddled, make sure that the swaddling is not too tight and is only of one layer, and that you place her on her back.

going outside

When you go outside, make sure that your baby wears a hat. In summer this will protect her from the sun. In winter it will keep her warm – try to get one that will cover her ears. If the weather is cold and your baby is in a pram, pull up the hood and cover her with a couple of blankets. If you carry her in a sling, a snowsuit might be useful, but she will not need a cardigan as well because your body heat will keep her warm.

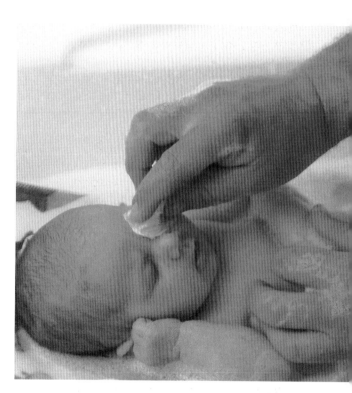

Bathtime may well become one of the times that you – and your partner – and the baby enjoy most together.

index

Executive Editor Jane McIntosh
Editorial Director Jane Birch

Executive Art Editor Geoff Fennell
Design 'OME Design
Illustrations Bounford.com, Patricia Ludlow (Linden Artists)

Picture Research Aruna Mather, Jennifer Veall
Production Controller Manjit Sihra
Index Indexing Specialists

acknowledgements

Alamy/Ace Stock Limited 273; /Nancy Brown 57 top right; /Jean-Michel Foujols/Stock Image 23 top centre left; /Sally and Richard Greenhill 226; /P. Gueritot/Stock Image 190; /imageshop-zefa visual media uk ltd 53; /Mark A. Johnson 210; /Butch Martin 266, 271; /Louise Mazzoni/Stock Image 201; /Medical-on-Line 236; /Janine Wiedel Photolibrary 217, 258; /S. Kirch/plainpicture 242; /John Powell Photographer 83 top right; /Shout 224, 225; /Stock Image 84 centre left, 158 bottom right, 168 centre right

Banana Stock 269, 276

Bubbles/Daniel Pangbourne 65 top centre; /Claire Paxton 208; /Loisjoy Thurstun 209; /Lucy Tizard 67 top left

Corbis UK Ltd/184 bottom centre left, 214-215, 229; /Annie Griffiths Belt 180 centre left; /Michael Keller 150 bottom right; /Laura Doss 193; /Ronnie Kaufman 200; /Layne Kennedy 240; /Rob Lewine 100 top left, 172 centre left; /Warren Morgan 15 top right; /Jose Luis Pelaez, Inc. 116, 130, 221; /RNT Productions 75 centre left; /Norbert Schaefer 8-9 ; /Allana Wesley 154, 182 centre right; /Larry Williams 134-135, 164 bottom right

Getty Images/Steve Allen 152 top right; /John Dowland 235; /Michael Salas 45 centre left top, 68 main; /Mark Scott 206; /UHB Trust 133 top left; /Caroline Wood 103 centre left

Octopus Publishing Group Limited/Frank Adam 42 picture 2; /Clive Bozzard-Hill 37; /Colin Gotts 50; /Jeremy Hopley 40 top left; /David Jordan 110; /Sandra Lane 42 picture 6, 96; /William Lingwood 42 picture 7, 42 picture 4, 42 picture 3; /David Loftus 40 bottom left; /Daniel Pangbourne 47 bottom right, 48 bottom left, 231 top left, 231 top centre, 231 top right, 231 bottom right, 231 bottom centre, 232 top centre, 232 top left, 232 top right, 232 bottom right, 232 bottom centre; /Lis Parsons 34; /Peter Pugh-Cook 36, 46 left, 46 right, 46 centre left, 46 centre right, 47 top right, 47 centre right, 48 top left, 48 top right, 48 bottom right, 49 left, 49 right, 90, 98; /William Reavell 42 picture 1, 59, 89; /Craig Robertson 35, 40 centre left bottom; /Russell Sadur 19 top right, 19 bottom right; /Gareth Sambidge 39, 60, 61; /Simon Smith 42 picture 5; /Karen Thomas 40 centre left top; /Ian Wallace 40 centre left

Angela Hampton/Family Life Picture Library 25 top right, 211, 253

Imagingbody.com 145 centre left, 153 bottom left

IPC Magazines 52 centre left, 54 centre left, 81 top right, 87 top left, 88 bottom left, 174 bottom left, 176 bottom centre left, 203

Oxford Scientific Films/Dr Derek Bromhall 163 top; /Neil Bromhall 171 top left; /Mantis Wildlife Films 163 bottom left

Photolibrary.com/Thomas del Amo 118 bottom centre; /Brand X Pictures 94 centre left; /James Braund 66 centre left; /Jeff Corwin 264; /Digital Vision 71 top right; /& Mayer Eisenhut 275; /Image 100 137 top left; /IT Stock 56 centre left; /Amy Neunsinger 102 top left; /Leanne Temme 194; /workbookstock 132 bottom left

Photodisc 4-5, 7 bottom right, 44 centre left, 63 top centre, 86 top left, 185 bottom right, 188

Photonica/Doug Plummer 64 centre left

Science Photo Library 169 centre right; /Steve Allen 145 bottom left; /Samuel Ashfield 111 top left; /Bernard Benoit/Kretz Technik 187 bottom left; /Christopher Briscoe 3 bottom centre, 261; /CNRI 138 centre right, 144 centre right; /Christian Darkin 21 centre right; /Tracy Dominey 251, 281; /Du Cane Medical Imaging Ltd 26 centre left; /Edelmann 113 top right, 170 centre right top, 171 bottom centre left; /Mauro Fermariello 31 top left, 262; /GE Medical Systems 125 top right; /Steve Gschmeissner 27 top right; /BSIP, LA/Filin.Herrera 126 centre left; /Ian Hooton 32, 58 bottom left, 76 bottom centre left, 78 top right, 123 top left, 192, 222; /BSIP, Laurent 124 bottom centre, 198, 237; /Dr Najeeb Layyous 125 bottom right, 153 centre left, 179 centre left top, 187 top left; /BSIP, MAY 146 centre right; /Matt Meadows 205 top, 205 bottom; /Hank Morgan 162 top right; /Prof.P.Motta/Dept.of Anatomy/University, "La Sapienza", Rome 13 top left; /Steve Percival 260; /A. J. Photo 127 centre right; /PH. SAADA/Eurelios 197 top; /James Stevenson 278; /Alexander Tsiaras 149 bottom left; /Paul Whitehill 233; /Zephyr 197 bottom

SuperStock/Pohlmann/Mauritius 167; /Juan Manuel Silva/Age Fotostock 195